297
Current Topics in Microbiology and Immunology

Editors

R.W. Compans, Atlanta/Georgia
M.D. Cooper, Birmingham/Alabama
T. Honjo, Kyoto · H. Koprowski, Philadelphia/Pennsylvania
F. Melchers, Basel · M.B.A. Oldstone, La Jolla/California
S. Olsnes, Oslo · M. Potter, Bethesda/Maryland
P.K. Vogt, La Jolla/California · H. Wagner, Munich

J. Langhorne (Ed.)

Immunology and Immunopathogenesis of Malaria

With 8 Figures and 6 Tables

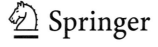 Springer

Jean Langhorne, PhD
Division of Parasitology
National Institute for Medical Research
The Ridgeway, Mill Hill
London, NW7 1AA
UK

e-mail: jlangho@nimr.mrc.ac.uk

Cover illustration: Interaction of Host Phagocytic Cells with Malaria Parasites. Lower right: a splenic dendritic cell phagocytosing a Plasmodium chabaudi schizont-infected erythrocyte (CD11c$^+$ MHC Class II+ DC (green), and PKH26-labelled schizont-infected erythrocyte (red), reproduced with permission of Cecile Voisine, Division of Parasitology, NIMR, UK. Upper left: P. berghei infection in the liver of C57Bl/6 mice ex vivo, sporozoities (green) localize temporarily in Kupffer cells. Reproduced with permission of Dr U. Frevert, NYU and Dr N. Steers, WRAIR, USA.

Library of Congress Catalog Number 72-152360

ISSN 0070-217X
ISBN-10 3-540-25718-7 Springer Berlin Heidelberg New York
ISBN-13 978-3-540-25718-9 Springer Berlin Heidelberg New York

Springer is a part of Springer Science+Business Media
springeronline.com
© Springer-Verlag Berlin Heidelberg 2005
Printed in Germany

The use of general descriptive names, registered names, trademarks, etc. in this publication does not imply, even in the absence of a specific statement, that such names are exempt from the relevant protective laws and regulations and therefore free for general use.
Product liability: The publisher cannot guarantee the accuracy of any information about dosage and application contained in this book. In every individual case the user must check such information by consulting the relevant literature.

Editor: Simon Rallison, Heidelberg
Desk editor: Anne Clauss, Heidelberg
Production editor: Nadja Kroke, Leipzig
Cover design: design & production GmbH, Heidelberg
Typesetting: LE-TEX Jelonek, Schmidt & Vöckler GbR, Leipzig
Printed on acid-free paper   SPIN 11362449   21/3150/YL – 5 4 3 2 1 0

Preface

Malaria is still a major global health problem, killing more than one million people every year. Almost all of these deaths are caused by Plasmodium falciparum, one of the four species of malaria parasites infecting humans. This high burden of mortality falls heavily on sub-Saharan Africa, where over 90% of these deaths are thought to occur, and 5% of children die before the age of 5 years. The death toll from malaria is still growing, with malaria-specific mortality in young African children estimated to have doubled during the last 20 years. This increase has been associated with drug resistance of the parasite, spread of insecticide-resistant mosquitoes, poverty, social and political upheaval, and lack of effective vaccines.

Failure of the host to control a malaria infection is in part related to the complexity of the parasite and the interaction with the immune system of the host. Although there is now considerably more investment in malaria research, and there are encouraging signs in vaccine development, we are a long way from understanding the nature and control of protective immunity or the pathological consequences of the host's response to Plasmodium. With the major advances in knowledge in basic immunology, inflammation, and the genomic information on the host, vector and parasite, we are now in a position to elucidate the key unknowns in the immune response to malaria. What initiates the immune response? How is it regulated? What are the mechanisms of immune evasion employed by the parasite? What are the key molecules of the parasite that induce protective immune responses?

The early interaction of the parasite with the host is important in determining the nature of the subsequent acquired response and the pathology associated with the severe complications of malaria such as cerebral malaria, severe anemia, and hypoglycemia. Thus the manner in which the malaria parasite activates the innate immune system and the cytokines and chemokines induced will all influence the magnitude of the inflammatory response and the types of T and B cell responses elicited. An understanding of these processes might enable us to determine the level at which host responses contribute to malarial disease, or might allow us to dissect out protective from pathological processes, and thus lead to some immunologically based intervention strategies.

Immunity to malaria develops slowly and protection against the parasite occurs later than protection against disease symptoms. Because of the different location of the parasite and the different antigens expressed at the liver and blood stages, the relevant immune responses and their specificity and regulation will not be same for the liver and blood stages of infection. A thorough understanding of the mechanisms and antigens recognized at both these stages, and the differentiation of immunity to disease and infection, will be important for the construction of an effective vaccine. For each stage of the infection there are several potential targets of the protective immune response; molecules on the surface of sporozoites, infected liver cells, blood-stage merozoites, and infected red blood cells have been identified. Genomic research will identify many more.

In addition to consideration of specificity of the protective response, particular parasite antigens may be specifically expressed in individuals under certain conditions. For example, despite acquisition of immunity through exposure to malaria, women in endemic areas have a high risk of severe malaria during the first and second pregnancy. A key feature of this is the accumulation of parasites in the placenta, which may be binding to placental endothelium via specific molecules that are not expressed on parasites in the circulation. Obviously if this is the case then understanding of the nature of these molecules, and how they relate to pregnancy-associated malaria, will be important.

The host response to malaria can clearly result in pathology. Glycosylphosphatidylinositols (GPIs) of the parasite, which anchor a range of Plasmodium molecules to cell surfaces, are considered likely candidates to induce host inflammatory responses, fever, and other pathology. Antibodies to these GPIs may ameliorate the severity of disease and thus could potentially be used therapeutically. One of the most severe complications of Plasmodium falciparum malaria is cerebral malaria (CM). The pathogenesis of CM is complex and not easy to dissect in the human host. Although not perfect replicas of the human disease, Plasmodium infections in rodents have given us significant insights into the role of inflammatory and regulatory responses in CM and therefore may be able to provide us with useful information for intervention and treatment.

Malaria infections are chronic, and immunity can wane rapidly despite the presence of some long-lived responses. Several questions arise from these observations. Are these manifestations of defects in the immune response specific to malaria infections or are they similar to responses to other infectious diseases? Why are some responses short-lived, and is chronic infection necessary to maintain immunity?

This collection of reviews addresses many of these important issues of malarial immunity and immunopathology. They are of interest not only to malariologists, but hopefully also to the broader immunological community. Strong interactions with and feedback from immunologists working in other infectious diseases and in basic immunology will help us to move the field of malaria immunology and therapeutic intervention forward more quickly.

London, February 2005   Jean Langhorne

List of Contents

List of Contributors

(Addresses stated at the beginning of respective chapters)

Achtman, A. H.   71
Anstey, N. M.   145

Beeson, J. G.   187
Belnoue, E.   103
Boutlis, C. S.   145
Bull, P. C.   71

de Souza, J. B.   145
Duffy, P. E.   187

Engwerda, C.   103

Grüner, A. C.   103

Ing, R.   25

Krzych, U.   1

Langhorne, J.   71

Rénia, L.   103
Riley, E. M.   145

Schwenk, R. J.   1
Stephens, R.   71
Stevenson, M. M.   25

Urban, B. C.   25

CTMI (2005) 297:1–24
© Springer-Verlag Berlin Heidelberg 2005

The Dissection of CD8 T Cells During Liver-Stage Infection

U. Krzych (✉) · R. J. Schwenk

Department of Immunology, Division of Communicable Diseases and Immunology,
Walter Reed Army Institute of Research, Bldg 503 Forest Glen Annex,
Silver Spring, MD 20910, USA
Urszula.Krzych@na.AMEDD.army.mil

Abstract   Multiple injections of γ-radiation-attenuated *Plasmodium* sporozoites (γ-spz) can induce long-lived, sterile immunity against pre-erythrocytic stages of malaria. Malaria antigen (Ag)-specific CD8 T cells that produce IFN-γ are key effector cells in this model of protection. Although there have been numerous reports dealing with γ-spz-induced CD8 T cells in the spleen, CD8 T cells most likely confer protection by targeting infected hepatocytes. Consequently, in this chapter we discuss observations and hypotheses concerning CD8 T cell responses that occur in the liver after an encounter with the *Plasmodium* parasite. Protracted protection against pre-erythrocytic stages requires memory CD8 T cells and we discuss evidence that γ-spz-induced immunity is indeed accompanied by the presence of intrahepatic CD44^{hi} CD45RB^{lo} CD62l^{lo} CD122^{lo} effector memory (EM) CD8 T cells and CD44^{hi} CD45RB^{hi} CD62l^{hi} CD122^{hi} central memory (CM) CD8 T cells. In addition, the EM CD8 T cells rapidly release IFN-γ in response to spz challenge. The possible role of Kupffer cells in the processing of spz Ags and the production of cytokines is also considered. Finally, we discuss evidence that is consistent with a model whereby intrahepatic CM CD8 T cells are maintained by IL-15 mediated-homeostatic proliferation while the EM CD8 T cells are conscripted from the CM pool in response to a persisting depot of liver-stage Ag.

1
Introduction

The participation of major histocompatibility complex (MHC) class I-restricted CD8 T cells as key effectors in protective immunity against pre-erythrocytic-stage malaria infection has been firmly established. Evidence supporting the effector function of CD8 T cells is based on studies in human [37,68] and animal [6, 93, 106] models of protection induced by radiation-attenuated (γ) plasmodia sporozoites (γ-spz) as well as from observations in malaria-endemic areas [34]. The effector function is associated mainly with the production of inflammatory cytokines such as interferon (IFN)-γ or tumor necrosis factor (TNF)-α that mediate elimination of the parasite within the hepatocytes by the nitric oxide (NO) pathway [72, 97]. CD8 T cells have also been shown to exhibit cytolytic activity against targets that express antigens belonging to the pre-erythrocytic-stage parasites [68]. Most important, liver memory CD8 T cells capable of rapidly producing IFN-γ accompany protracted protective immunity induced by γ-spz [6].

The overwhelming evidence for CD8 T cells as the key effectors mediating protection against pre-erythrocytic-stage parasites forms the basis for the development of the various platforms of pre-erythrocytic-stage malaria vaccines such as RTS,S, which has been shown to confer short-lived protection in both malaria-naïve [101] and malaria-exposed persons [80].

Despite the wealth of observations, complete understanding of protective CD8 T cells requires the resolution of critical questions concerning their induction, formation, and maintenance of immunologic memory, exquisite antigen specificity, and target antigens. These mechanisms are inextricably linked to the mode of processing and presentation of exo-erythrocytic antigens, processes that remain unexplored in the Plasmodia system. Consequently, most of our current understanding of the involvement of CD8 T cells during liver-stage malaria infection is still in the realm of hypotheses and ideas based on observations whose resolution continues to be hampered by the modus vivendi of this enigmatic parasite.

Extensive reviews of the literature on immune responses considered to play a role in anti-malarial protective immunity have previously been published in other books and journals [15, 36, 40, 41, 74]; however, responses that occur specifically in the liver during the liver-stage infection are less well understood. In this chapter we will concentrate on observations and offer hypotheses concerning CD8 T cell-mediated responses that are induced and/or occur in the liver during the encounter with the *Plasmodium* parasite.

2
Plasmodia Parasites in the Vertebrate Host

Malaria infection is initiated when sporozoites are inoculated into a vertebrate host from the salivary glands of an *Anopheles* mosquito. The sporozoites are transported via the blood to the liver where they invade hepatocytes, an obligatory venue for schizogony. The mechanism by which Plasmodia sporozoites enter and localize within hepatocytes has been partially delineated [10, 24, 25]. Maturation of liver-stage parasites is characterized by amplification and molecular changes marked by the acquisition of new protein antigens. The fully differentiated schizonts rupture and release thousands of merozoites that invade erythrocytes to initiate the erythrocytic phase of infection, hence the commencement of clinical malaria.

In the vertebrate host, the parasite exhibits three phases of development—sporozoite-, liver-, and blood-stage—which are morphologically distinct and express to some extent unique protein profiles. Some proteins, under certain conditions, are potent antigens for the induction of cellular or antibody responses that provide protective immunity against the infection or the disease. The circumsporozoite surface (CS) protein, for example, is a major sporozoite-stage antigen [76], and T and B cell responses specific for epitopes on the CS protein correlate with protection in humans [21] and mice [93]. Sporozoite surface protein 2 (SSP2) [88] or thrombospondin-related adhesion protein (TRAP) [86] and CS protein also facilitate sporozoite invasion of hepatocytes [25, 85]. As parasites develop and replicate within the parasitophorous vacuole in hepatocytes, they manifest liver-stage-specific antigens [31] that appear to be the major inducers of the powerful cellular immune responses against the pre-erythrocytic-stage parasite. Proteins that characterize the erythrocytic stage are thought to play a role in the invasion of red blood cells [40].

The liver, therefore, plays a key role in the life cycle of the protozoan *Plasmodium* parasite as the liver-stage is considered not only pivotal for the survival of the parasite, but also as a significant period for the induction, effector phase, and possibly the maintenance of anti-Plasmodia immune responses. Understanding immune events that occur in the liver during natural infection and in model systems of protective immunity will expand our knowledge of organ-specific immune responses to plasmodia antigens and thus facilitate exploitation of these responses to expedite progress in vaccine development against this serious infectious disease.

3
Importance of Liver-Stage Antigens in Protection During Natural Exposure to Plasmodia

Naturally acquired immunity is primarily directed against the blood-stage antigens and mediated by protective antibodies [15]. Liver-stage antigen 1 (LSA-1) [113] is considered the only Plasmodia antigen that is specifically expressed in the liver-stages, and LSA-1-specific T and B cell responses have also been observed among residents of malaria-endemic areas. Naturally acquired responses to LSA-1 peptides were first implicated in human protection in Gambia [34] with LSA-1 peptide Is6-(a.a.1786–1794) specific CTL responses in persons expressing the HLA-B-53 allele [35]. These and other observations showing an association between a mild form of malaria and the expression of HLA B-53 suggested that B53-restricted LSA-1-specific CTL responses confer protection against a severe form of malaria [35]. Studies conducted in other malaria-endemic regions also concluded that protective immunity in naturally exposed populations is directly linked to LSA-1-specific responses [8, 13, 43, 59, 66, 67, 71]. In some instances, protective responses that lasted over 6 months were associated with LSA-1 peptide-specific CD8 T cells producing INF-γ [13]. An examination of immune responses elicited with either the LSA-J peptide (a.a.1613–1636) or the B53-restricted ls6 epitope showed that INF-γ responses were associated with a prolonged time to reinfection as well as a reduced risk of developing malaria-related anemia in Gabonese children [67, 71]. Although LSA-1-specific responses characterized by other cytokines, such as IL-10 [60], or other lymphocytes, such as CD4 T cells or B cells [44], have also been linked to protection in *P. falciparum* endemic areas, the association between CD8 T cells that produce INF-γ or mediate cytolytic events is clearly evident during natural transmission.

CD8 CTL cells recognizing peptides of other exo-erythrocytic antigens, including LSA-3 [2], SALSA [7], and STARP [79], have been observed both in persons residing in areas of malaria endemicity as well as chimpanzees exposed to γ-spz. These responses are also considered to be associated with protective immunity.

In endemic areas, protective immunity to malaria develops gradually after multiple exposures over many years and, although associated with a decline in clinical manifestations of the disease, it decays rapidly once exposure to the parasite ceases. It is not clear why long-term protection does not persist. We hypothesize that the tolerant milieu of the liver, sequestration of the liver-stage antigens within hepatocytes, and relatively short duration of the liver-phase infection are in part responsible for the lack of memory CD8 T cells. Others postulate that a phenomenon known as altered peptide ligand resulting from polymorphisms at regions recognized by CD8 T cells induces antagonistic effects that interfere with the priming and the survival of memory T cells [81]. Furthermore, poor immunogenicity may also stem from inadequate immunizing doses or infrequent exposure, such as occurs in hypoendemic areas.

4
A Model of Protective Immunity Induced by Radiation-Attenuated Plasmodia Sporozoites

Exposure of humans [12, 84] and laboratory rodents [75] to multiple doses of γ-spz leads to sterile and lasting protection against the development of erythrocytic-stage infection after sporozoite challenge. γ-spz carrying the sporozoite-associated CS protein and SSP2 invade the liver where they undergo aborted development [112]. In hepatocytes, the parasite no longer produces CS protein de novo but begins to express liver- and blood-stage antigens [41]. Nonetheless, γ-spz fail to establish an erythrocytic-stage infection. It is believed that radiation partially retards the maturation of the parasite and that under-developed liver schizonts remain in the liver forming an antigen depot, a step that is considered critical for induction of local antigen-specific protective immunity [56]. Findings by Scheller and Azad [92] that protection is abrogated by primaquine, a drug that disrupts liver schizogony [5], support the notion that accumulation and persistence of liver-stage antigens are required for the induction and maintenance of protracted protection.

4.1
γ-spz Cause a Switch from Tolerance to Inflammation in the Liver: Role of IL-12 and IL-10

The liver is an immunotolerant organ. If the prevailing state of tolerance in the liver attracts infectious sporozoites and allows them to expand and continue their life cycle, then some event(s) induced by γ-spz must account for the reversal of tolerance to inflammation that is needed for the induction as well as persistence of adaptive immune responses [54]. The mode of the initial γ-spz interaction with toll-like receptor (TLR) molecules on cells of the innate immune system in the liver, including Kupffer cells (KC), could trigger a response that differs from that induced by infectious sporozoites. Before the invasion of hepatocytes, *P. berghei* sporozoites enter KC [82]. Naïve KC produce low levels of IL-10 but do not produce IL-12; however, within 6 h after a priming dose of γ-spz, they become high IL-12 responders. The inflammatory cytokine is balanced by equally prompt upregulation of IL-10. The levels of both cytokines abate after boost immunizations with γ-spz. In contrast, infectious sporozoites do not activate naïve KC to produce IL-12 and actually down-regulate IL-10 [100]. The importance of enhanced IL-12 levels before sporozoite challenge was demonstrated previously in a protection study based on administration of IL-12 in vivo [94]. Others have shown that IL-12 is a critical cytokine for the development of CD8 T cell responses to pre-erythrocytic-stage malaria [17]. We propose that a cascade of pro-inflammatory cytokines released during the phase of innate immunity induced by γ-spz leads to temporary local inflammation, which is perceived as a "danger signal" needed to trigger proper responses from the adaptive immune system [70].

4.2
Mode of Sporozoite Entry into Liver Antigen Presenting Cells

The molecular form of the sporozoites might also influence the mode of sporozoite entry into KC, which, in turn, might dictate intracellular localization of sporozoites, as has been recently shown for dendritic cells (DC) interacting with other parasites [11]. On the basis of studies conducted in vito [26, 82], the entry of infectious sporozoites is mediated by membrane:membrane fusion and parasites localize in a vacuole that does not co-localize with lysosomes so that the sporozoites avoid metabolic degradation before safely reaching hepatocytes. Frozen/thawed *P. berghei* sporozoites are phagocytized by KC [82], as are infectious sporozoites in the presence of *P. berghei*-immune serum [96]. However, neither the frozen/thawed nor infectious sporozoites induce protective immunity.

Conceivably, γ-spz could also be internalized by phagocytosis and channeled to phagosomes for metabolic degradation and export by MHC class II and I molecules. A significant upregulation of MHC class I is evident on KC after sporozoite challenge of γ-spz-immune mice. In sharp contrast, MHC class I molecules are downregulated on KC during infection of naïve mice [100]. Inflammatory cytokines are known to increase the expression of MHC class I:peptide complexes on antigen-presenting cells (APC) by inducing immune proteasomes for more efficient generation of antigenic peptides for entry into the ER and loading onto empty MHC class I molecules [49]. Accordingly, KC from γ-spz-immune/challenged mice present peptides and protein antigens to specific T cells, but the APC function of KC from mice infected with sporozoites is severely reduced [100]. Thus, the interaction between KC and γ-spz might ignite the inflammatory process that is presumed to reverse the tolerant state in localized areas of the liver, which favors the induction of liver-stage antigen-specific effector T cells.

5
CD8 T Cells Mediate Protective Immunity

Pioneering work by Weiss [106], based on in vivo depletion of CD8 T cells, unequivocally established CD8 T cells as key effectors in a rodent model of protection against malaria. By demonstrating a failure to protect β_2-microglobulin knockout (KO) mice, we confirmed [110] the critical involvement of CD8 T cells in protective immunity induced with γ-spz. More important, we established that effector CD8 T cells are MHC class I-restricted/dependent because protection is not transferred by γ-spz-immune (wild-type) wt cells to the β_2-microglobulin KO recipients since CD8 T cells must recognize peptides from *Plasmodium* antigens presented by MHC class I on APC in the liver. Target LSA peptides that are recognized by the effector CD8 T cells have not yet been defined, although we and others [18] are using the combination of genomics and bioinformatics approaches to reach this goal.

The need for proximity between effector lymphocytes and target hepatocytes has been revealed during both plasmodial [87] and viral infections [3]. For example, an adoptively transferred protective CD8 T cell clone specific for the CS protein homes to the liver and localizes in direct apposition to infected hepatocytes [87]. Earlier immunohistologic studies revealed that challenge of γ-spz-immune mice induces lymphocyte-rich infiltrates and granuloma formation around hepatocytes harboring the parasite [50]. By contrast, in naïve rats the cellular response occurs at the time of release of merozoites [51]. These observations led us to studies aimed at characterizing intrahepatic T cells and determining the conditions that contribute to the maintenance of these cells.

5.1
Are the Effector CD8 T Cells Induced in the Lymph Node or the Liver?

The initial site of induction of liver resident CD8 T cells remains unclear. It is possible that these cells arise in the liver after interaction with liver APC such as KC or DC that present either the sporozoite-stage antigens including CS protein or liver-stage antigens. Alternatively, these cells might be induced in a draining lymph node and during sporozoite challenge migrate to the liver, where they might undergo further expansion. Although lack of evidence supporting either scenario favors the prevailing view that T cell activation occurs as a result of interaction with DC in the lymph node, the possibility of a local or a site-specific activation of CD8 T cells remains very attractive and should be explored. There is some evidence that effector CD8 T cells migrate to sites of inflammation, such as the liver, after sporozoite challenge. For example, transferred TCR transgenic CD8 T cells specific for the *P. yoelii* CS protein peptide SYVPSAEQI are found in the liver, where they function as effector cells [91].

5.2
CD8 CD45RB^{lo} T Cells Persist in Livers of Mice Protected Against Malaria

P. berghei γ-spz-immune intrahepatic mononuclear cells (IHMC) contain CD4 and CD8 T cells with inducible CD44^{hi} CD25^{hi} and CD45RB^{lo} phenotypic markers [30]. Expression of CD45RB, an activation/memory marker that changes from CD45RB^{hi} to CD45RB^{lo} with increased antigen exposure and the state of cellular maturation [63, 95], differs between CD4 and CD8 T cells. CD4 CD45RB^{lo} T cells appear transiently and most revert to the RB^{hi} phenotype by 5 days after each immunization; a similar result is seen after challenge with infectious sporozoites [30]. CD8 CD45RB^{lo} T cells are present in naïve liver, but multiple immunizations with γ-spz stabilize and then increase the RB^{lo} phenotype. Enhanced frequencies of CD8 CD45RB^{lo} T cells coincide with the induction of sterile protection [30], which in C57Bl/6 mice requires three immunizations with *P. berghei* γ-spz [65].

These observations are in agreement with the transient expansion of T cells [1, 4] and the respective roles of CD8 T cells as effector [106] cells and CD4 T cells as inducer/helper cells [108]. It is possible that activation of CD4 T cells precedes that of CD8 T cells to create a favorable milieu in the liver for the induction, as well as for the prevention of attrition of Plasmodia antigen-specific CD8 T cells. This is particularly attractive because the liver is a site where activated CD8 T cells usually die by apoptosis [14].

5.3
Are Both IL-4 and IFN-γ Needed for Protection Induced by *P. berghei* γ-spz?

Liver lymphocytes from mice protected by *P. berghei* γ-spz rapidly produce enhanced IFN-γ with a peak response around 7 days after the challenge [6]. The release of IFN-γ, which coincides with the activation of CD8 T cells, is preceded by elevated production of IL-4, which declines when IFN-γ reaches its peak [56]. The reciprocal regulation between these two cytokines reflects the precise orchestration of functional activities among T cell subsets induced by γ-spz. It is likely that IL-4 in the liver is produced by NK T cells, whereas IFN-γ is primarily produced by CD8 T cells [6].

If NK T cells produce IL-4, their decline in the liver after immunization with γ-spz and/or challenge would favor development of a local inflammatory milieu for the induction of protective immunity. We observed that a challenge of *P. berghei* γ-spz-immune mice leads to a transient reduction of hepatic NK T cells [56]. A similar phenomenon was observed during infection with *Listeria*, where IL-4-producing CD4 NK TCRαβ^{int} liver lymphocytes decline early during infection, presumably to promote the development of Th1-type cells, which are essential for protection against *Listeria* [48]. Once immunity has been established, IL-4 might once again increase to promote the generation and/or maintenance of a memory pool that would include the long-lived CD8 T cells.

This notion is supported by several observations. For example, it has also been shown that an initial infection with *P. chabaudi chabaudi* induces Th1-type cells and, after clearance of the acute phase, there is a switch to a Th2-type response [61]. The survival of *P. yoelii* CS protein-specific CD8 T cells depends on IL-4 secreted from CD4 T cells [9]. In a preliminary study we also demonstrated that the most mature form of memory CD8 T cells (CD44^{hi}CD45Rb^{lo}CD27$^-$) is absent from CD4 KO mice owing in part to a reduced level of IL-4. Similarly, protective immunity induced in humans by *P. falciparum* γ-spz coincides with production of IL-4 by memory CD4 T cells [78]. This view is in agreement with the observation that the effector CD8 T cells decline after inflammation has subsided [4], whereas memory CD8 T cells persist in a state of stasis if they are supported by lymphokine-secreting memory CD4 T cells.

6
Function of CD8 T Cells: CTL Versus IFN-γ

Earlier studies identified CS protein- and SSP2-specific CD8 CTL to be the pre-erythrocytic-stage effectors in γ-spz-immune mice [52, 58, 89, 107] and in humans [19, 111]. Because CS protein is no longer synthesized once the parasite enters the hepatocytes, a mechanism must account for the recognition of CS protein determinants within the context of cell-surface MHC class I molecules expressed on the infected hepatocytes. Curiously, protective immunity is not interrupted in perforin and Fas KO mice, suggesting that the effects of CD8 T cells may not involve lytic activity [83]. Hence CD8 T cells that produce IFN-γ followed by the induction of nitric oxide synthetase (NOS) [53] might be physiologically more relevant to the process of elimination of liver-stage parasites.

IFN-γ was one of the first cytokines shown to inhibit the hepatic stages of rodent and human malaria both in vitro and in vivo. IFN-γ has both parasito-static and lytic effects on the developing liver-stage parasite [72]. Injection of IFN-γ protects mice against sporozoite challenge [23]. Moreover, immunization with γ-spz fails to generate protective immunity in IFN-γ receptor KO mice [102].

In *P. berghei*-immune mice the major source of IFN-γ is thought to be the CD8 T cell in the liver [6]. Secretion of IFN-γ by these cells would preclude the need for direct lysis of hepatocytes and also could account for suppression of parasite growth in surrounding hepatocytes by the few CD8 T cells that encounter infected hepatocytes. IFN-γ could also contribute to protection indirectly by upregulating MHC class I and class II molecules and B7–1 and B7–2 co-stimulatory molecules on both KC and hepatocytes. This, in turn, would further promote activation of effector T cells.

In the *P. yoelii* system, transgenic CD8 T cells specific for SYVPSAEQI have been shown to eliminate the parasite by a mechanism that depends on rapid INF-γ production [91]. Although the anti-parasitic activity is quite impressive, the long-term protective effectiveness of these cells has not yet been determined. The authors also propose that protection against *P. yoelii* sporozoite challenge could be achieved by a single T cell specificity, provided that this clone has previously undergone adequate expansion to increase its precursor frequency so that it would be effective against the load of infectious parasites [32].

In our view, long-term sustained protection requires various CD8 T cell specificities, particularly those belonging to proteins expressed during pre-erythrocytic liver-stage development. It could be envisaged that CS protein-specific CD8 T cells initiate the effector stage of protection because they are the first cells to produce INF-γ as soon as they encounter infectious sporozoites. Such a protective response, however, would be effective only for a short period after the infection. This interpretation might provide at least a partial explanation for the restricted expansion of the CS protein-specific T cells [32, 33]. Complete protection might require the subsequent activation of a second wave of CD8 T cells specific for epitopes other than the CS protein, as they would have to target hepatocytes by recognizing liver-stage antigens. Such concerted and functionally integrated effector function provided by CD8 T cells with multiple specificities might be necessary to provide protection that is not just short-lived but one that can be sustained.

7
Memory CD8 T Cells

7.1
Memory CD8 T Cell Subsets

The formation of optimally effective memory T cells, either from naïve populations or from antigen-expanded effector cells, is one of the cardinal features of antigen-specific immune responses elicited by infections or vaccinations and it is inextricably linked to long-lasting protective immunity [1]. On the basis of the cell surface markers indicative of activation (CD44, CD45RB, CD122), migration (CD62L), and functional response (IFN-γ), intrahepatic memory CD8 T cells generated by immunization with *P. berghei* γ-spz segregate into at least two distinct subsets: (a) the dominant, IFN-γ-producing $CD44^{hi}CD45RB^{lo}CD122^{lo}CD62L^{lo}$ phenotype, hence effector memory (EM); and (b) the indolent IFN-γ-producing $CD44^{hi}CD45RB^{hi}CD122^{hi}CD62L^{lo/hi}$ phenotype, hence central memory (CM). We propose that these functionally and phenotypically unique subsets of liver memory CD8 T cells form an interactive network involving different phases of cell activation and differentiation [6]. The co-presence of distinct subsets within the intrahepatic memory CD8 T cell pool in mice protected against malaria is consistent with an earlier view that virally induced memory CD8 T cells are organized into subsets on the basis of distinct functional activities and their maturation/activation status [22, 46, 90, 103, 109].

7.2
Effector Memory CD8 T Cells

Similar to the rapid responses mediated by influenza- and Sendai-specific effector memory CD8 T cells [39], intrahepatic γ-spz-immune EM CD8 T cells produce a copious amount of IFN-γ within 1–6 h after spz infection. Although the pool of EM T cells eventually contracts and the IFN-γ response diminishes, the IFN-γ-producing memory T cells persist at levels nearly threefold above those found in naïve mice. IFN-γ-producing EM CD8 T cells are still found in the livers of long-term (10 months) γ-spz-immune mice that maintain protracted protection against a re-challenge. Although EM phenotype liver CD8 T cells also accumulate with age in naïve mice, these cells produce comparatively low levels of IFN-γ. Liver CD8 T cells from mice infected with sporozoites also produce IFN-γ, yet these mice fail to be protected because the IFN-γ response is markedly delayed and the early absence of inflammation allows the onset of parasitemia [6].

7.3
Central Memory CD8 T Cells

The IFN-γ reactivity of the CM CD8 T cells exhibits a lag period and the responses are low and relatively short-lived. Therefore, these cells do not appear to be directly involved in the elimination of the parasite. Instead, by acquiring the $CD122^{hi}$ phenotype, the CM CD8 T cells most likely engage in homeostatic proliferation, which qualifies them to function as a reservoir to maintain the size of memory CD8 T cell pools [69]. CD8 $CD44^{hi}CD122^{hi}$ T cells have been shown to be highly dependent on IL-15 for proliferation and survival [45]. Studies of Sendai virus-specific memory CD8 T cells present in the lung airways demonstrate the co-presence of two memory CD8 T cell subsets, one of which is maintained in the lung by homeostatic proliferation [38]. The maintenance of memory pools is one of the prerequisites of a memory T cell response because attrition, particularly of the effector CD8 T cells, is inevitable during any infection [4].

8
Mechanisms for Maintenance of Protection Induced by Radiation-Attenuated Sporozoites

8.1
Are Memory T Cells Needed for Long-Term Protection?

One of the key questions is whether memory T cells are required for maintenance of protection induced by γ-spz. Evidence from our laboratory indicates that the persistence of memory CD8 T cells ($CD44^{hi}CD45RB^{lo}$) correlates with the maintenance of protective immunity, which in C57Bl/6 mice lasts for nearly 1 year after the last immunization with *P. berghei* γ-spz [6]. Interestingly, the persistence of memory phenotype CD8 T cells was restricted to liver lymphocytes, because splenic T cells from the same group of γ-spz-immune mice showed no phenotypic differences from splenic T cells from naïve mice [30].

The persistence of memory CD8 T cells in the liver can be accounted for by at least two mechanisms. First, some of the memory T cells detected after immunization may be long-lived memory cells derived from the effector T cells. Second, the $CD44^{hi}CD45RB^{lo}$ CD8 T cells in the livers of long-term immune mice may be derived from cells that constantly ingress to the liver in response to the liver repository of Plasmodia antigens. Although it appears unlikely that they traffic to the liver from the spleen, because $CD44^{hi}$ CD8 T cells were not present in the spleens of animals with long-term immunity, it is possible that they traffic from the draining celiac lymph nodes, although this also remains unknown. Irrespective of whether maintenance of protection relies on long-lived intrahepatic memory T cells or T cells that constantly ingress to the liver, both require a repository of Plasmodia antigens [6].

8.2
The Liver Is a Depot for Attenuated Exo-erythrocytic Forms

One of the cardinal requirements for induction of protection is the accumulation of threshold amounts of Plasmodia antigens in the liver. However, there is ample contradictory evidence with respect to the antigen requirement for the persistence of memory T cells [29, 73, 77]. On the basis of results from our laboratory, the persistence of accumulated antigens in the liver is critical for the maintenance of protective immunity [6]. Administration of primaquine at the time of immunization with γ-spz results in a loss of protective immunity [6, 92], which correlates with a decrease of EM but not CM phenotype CD8 T cells in the liver [6]. In another system [32] primaquine did not appear to affect the functional activity of CD8 T cells that are responsive to an epitope on the CS protein of *P. yoelii*. These results are indeed expected, as the primary action of primaquine is against liver-stage development, without affecting the sporozoite-stage.

The disruption of the intrahepatic-stage parasite development prevented the formation of a local antigen depot, which impeded the conscription of CM into EM CD8 T cells. Although most of the results particularly from viral systems argue convincingly against the need for antigen to maintain long-lived memory CD8 T cells [62, 73], we suggest that antigen requirements might be quite different in instances where a parasite exhibits tropism to an immune-privileged organ, such as the liver in Plasmodia infection. The liver antigen repository may be sufficient to play a unique role in distinguishing the "locally" activated liver memory T cells from those found in the spleen or lymph nodes.

The hypothesis regarding the need for a depot of liver-stage antigen also explains in part the need of intermittent boost immunizations with γ-spz to maintain protective immunity induced in humans by immunization with *P. falciparum* γ-spz [78]. There is evidence in other systems that T cell memory is maintained only if a protracted restimulation of effector T cells is maintained, either by some form of persisting antigen or by cross-reacting environmental antigens [114]. Therefore, the need for an accumulation of antigen may not only signify that a threshold concentration is necessary to generate a T cell response, but it may also indicate that a certain level of antigens is required to maintain memory T cell response, and hence protection.

The precise cellular location of the malaria antigen depot in the liver has not been established. In principle, hepatocytes can function as APC. Although there is no evidence that hepatocytes present Plasmodia antigen to T cells, because so few hepatocytes become infected by the invading spz, they also might be inefficient as APC. Even if the numbers of infected hepatocytes did not limit the APC activity, it is presumed that their intracellular function must be altered to benefit the parasite, and hence the capacity for antigen processing and presentation might be diminished. Evidence from Leishmania infection suggests the parasitophorous vacuole is resistant to the formation of acidified phagolysosomes for a proper intracellular degradation of parasitic protein antigens. Instead, MHC class II molecules enter this vacuole where they undergo degradation [16].

It is interesting that infectious and denatured *P. berghei* sporozoites localize within distinct intracellular vacuoles of KC and only denatured parasites localize within phagolysosomes. It is likely that γ-spz taken up by KC also localize within phagolysosomes, because we have observed that γ-spz are rapidly degraded within these cells (U. Krzych, N. Steers, U. Frevert, unpublished observations). Although evidence is still lacking, it is nonetheless possible that KC process the ingested γ-spz and present spz antigens to CD8 T cells. This most likely occurs by a cross-presentation mechanism whereby antigens from phagosomes gain entry into the MHC class I pathway. It has recently been shown that exogenous particulate antigens can enter the MHC class I pathway as a result of phagosome–ER fusion [27]. After phagocytosis and phagolysosomal degradation, protein antigens are retrotranslocated to the cytoplasm to gain access to the proteosomal complex for further processing and TAP-dependent translocation either to the ER or the phagosome for loading onto MHC class I molecules [42]. In addition to γ-spz antigens, KC or DC that phagocytize necrotic, infected hepatocytes could also engage in cross-presentation of liver-stage antigens. Of note, however, we are unable to stimulate liver memory CD8 T cells with *P. berghei* CS protein peptides ([55] and D. Berenzon, unpublished data). Investigation of the cross-presentation of Plasmodia antigens derived from the partly developed liver-stages parasites would most significantly expand our understanding of the nature of antigens and the type of APC that are involved in the induction and maintenance of liver memory CD8 T cells.

8.3
Maintenance of Central Memory CD8 T Cells by IL-15

It has been established that IL-15 promotes the survival of long-term memory CD8 T cells by maintaining their homeostatic proliferation, whereas IL-2 stimulates both the initial expansion and subsequent contraction of T lymphocytes [57, 64, 98, 99, 105]. In a preliminary experiment, we have observed that immunization with γ-spz caused upregulation of IL-15 mRNA in KC, but not in cells isolated from spleens of γ-spz-immune mice. Is IL-15 in the liver involved in the maintenance of local CD8 T cells? We have already demonstrated [6] that CM CD8 T cells express a high density of CD122. Moreover, although this T cell subset proportionately represented a much smaller fraction of the liver CD8 T cells, twice as many CM T cells (80%) were CD122^{hi} than EM T cells (39%), which expressed primarily CD122^{lo}. This ratio of CD8 CD44^{hi}CD45RB^{hi}CD122^{hi} to CD8 CD44^{hi}CD45RB^{lo} CD122^{lo} T cells was maintained for 14 days after spz challenge of γ-spz-immune mice. Moreover, we have also shown that only the CM CD8 T cells proliferate in vitro in the presence of IL-15 and that these cells are severely reduced in IL-15 KO mice (D. Berenzon, manuscript in preparation). The enhanced sensitivity of the CM CD8 T cells to reduced levels of IL-15 suggests that this subset preferentially expands upon exposure to elevated levels of IL-15 in the liver. It also implies that an optimal protective response requires the compartmentalization of CD8 T cells, with each subset performing not only a unique role, but also relying on distinct regulatory mechanisms.

Il-15 is produced by a variety of cell types (although not by T cells) in response to signaling via the TLR or exposure to type I IFN. IL-15 acts in an autocrine fashion and induces IL-12. There is evidence [20] that APC retain IL-15 bound to the IL-15Rα chain to transactivate CD8 T cells expressing the IL-15Rβγc complex. Both IL-7 and IL-15 promote the survival of CD8 effector T cells during the contraction phase of an acute response, but IL-7 seems to be critical for the differentiation of CD8 effector T cells into CD8 memory T cells [47]. The role of IL-7 in the maintenance of Plasmodia-specific CD8 memory T cells remains to be investigated.

9
Presence of Both CD8 Effector and Central Memory T Cells Is Needed for Effective Memory Responses

What is the relationship between the CM and the EM CD8 T cells? We explored this issue using IL-15 KO mice (D. Berenzon, manuscript in preparation).The results from protection studies were surprising. Like wt mice, IL-15 KO mice were protected against a challenge that occurred within 7 days after the last boost immunization with *P. berghei* γ-spz. Protection was short-lived, however, as at re-challenge 2 months later, the IL-15 KO mice became parasitemic. Analysis of the CD8 T cell subsets shortly after the challenge, when the IL-15 KO mice were protected, showed an accumulation of EM CD8 T cells and a very small pool of CM CD8 T cells. It appears, therefore, that in the absence of IL-15, EM CD8 T cells develop perhaps directly from naïve CD8 T cells. Without the provision of IL-15, and hence the reservoir of memory CD8 T cells, however, the EM cells cannot be sustained during re-challenge, at which time we observed an absence of CM CD8 T cells and a drastic reduction in the EM CD8 T cells. These preliminary observations strongly support our hypothesis that EM T cells are conscripted from the CM CD8 T cells in a continuous, albeit slow process that occurs in the liver as a result of an increased antigen load after repeated immunizations with γ-spz (Fig. 1). The process could also occur during infection, when large numbers of EM CD8 T cells would be most needed to combat the parasite. In either case, the cells in the CM CD8 T cell pool are maintained under the influence of IL-15 that is upregulated by γ-spz in KC. Upon encounter with specific antigen from the liver repository, the CM CD8 T cells would be driven to differentiate into the $CD44^{hi}CD45RB^{lo}CD122^{lo}$ phenotype that is easily triggered by infectious sporozoites to produce IFN-γ [6]. The EM T cells might also proliferate to antigens, a notion that is consistent with the recent findings showing antigen-specific proliferation of terminally differentiated memory $CD8CD45RA^{+}CD27^{-}$ T cells [104].

10
Apoptosis of Intrahepatic CD8 T Cells Is Decreased During Protection

If during malaria infection memory CD8 T cells are either induced in or travel to the liver, these cells will encounter formidable challenges. According to the Responder Trap hypothesis [14], activated CD8 T cells that traffic to the liver to kill infected hepatocytes will themselves be eliminated. One of the mechanisms of activation-induced cell death may involve Fas/FasL-mediated apoptosis [28]. In our preliminary experiments, we have observed that CD8

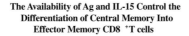

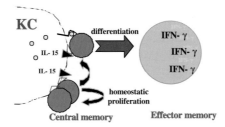

Fig. 1 CD8 T_{EM} cells are primarily sensitive to the availability of liver-stage antigen (Ag) but the maintenance of CD8 T_{CM} cells depends on the provision of IL-15/IL-7. In the liver, the conscription of CD8 T_{CM} cells into the CD8 T_{EM} cell pool could be a continuous, albeit slow process resulting from an increased Ag load after repeated immunizations with γ-spz. The process could also occur during infection, when large numbers of CD8 T_{EM} cells are most needed to combat infection. In either case, the T_{CM} cell pool would expand under the influence of upregulated IL-15 in the KC during exposure to γ-spz. Upon encounter with specific Ags from the liver repository, CD8 T_{CM} cells would be driven to differentiate into the T_{EM} cells that are easily triggered to produce IFN-γ

CD45RB^{lo} T cells isolated from livers of mice protected against malaria are spared from apoptosis. In contrast, CD8 T cells isolated from livers of mice infected with *P. berghei* are rapidly eliminated. It appears that CD8 T cells induced by Plasmodia antigens persist as a memory T cell pool in the livers of long-term protected mice. The requirements for memory T cell activation and maintenance in the liver are currently being investigated.

11
Summary

In summary, MHC class I-restricted CD8 T cells have been shown to function as key effectors in protective immunity against pre-erythrocytic-stage malaria infection in residents of malaria-endemic areas and human and animal models of protection induced by radiation-attenuated Plasmodia sporozoites. The effector function is associated mainly with the production of inflammatory cytokines such as IFN-γ or TNF-α that mediate elimination of the parasite within the hepatocytes by the nitric oxide pathway. The success of protection induced by γ-spz depends on the long-lived intrahepatic memory CD8 T cells, which reside in distinct sub-populations as CD8 CM and CD8 EM T cells.

While the CD8 EM T cells are maintained by the antigen-driven conscription of the CD8 CM T cells, the latter representing a very broad spectrum of antigen-specific T cells are maintained by IL-15 (Fig. 1). This arrangement assures a steady availability of antigen-specific T cells should they be required to combat an infection. The dependence on specific antigen essentially controls the balance between the two phenotypes and the differential expression of IL-15R prevents the EM CD8 T cells from becoming activated in the event of sporadic co-infections. However, it is the activated status of the intrahepatic memory CD8 T cells [6] that really distinguishes them from the memory CD8 T cells in the spleen and lymph node as it represents the sentinel of a local, organ-specific infection.

Acknowledgements The authors would like to express their thanks to Drs. Dmitri Berenzon, Nick Steers and Clara Brando, Ms Lisa Letellier and Mr. Isaac Chalom, whose work and dedication during the past several years made this chapter possible. The authors also acknowledge help and support of Dr. D. Gray Heppner. This research was supported in part by a grant from the National Institutes of Health (UK) and the US Army Materiel Command. The views of the authors do not purport to reflect the position of the Department of the Army or the Department of Defense.

References

1. Ahmed R, Gray D (1996) Immunological memory and protective immunity: understanding their relation. Science 272:54–60
2. Aidoo, M, Lalvani A, Gilbert SC, et al. (2000) Cytotoxic T-lymphocyte epitopes for HLA-B53 and other HLA types in the malaria vaccine candidate liver-stage antigen 3. Infect Immun 68:227–232
3. Ando K, Guidotti LG, Wirth S, et al. (1994) Class I-restricted cytotoxic T lymphocytes are directly cytopathic for their target cells in vivo. J Immunol 152:3245–3253
4. Badovinac VP, Porter BB, Harty JT (2002) Programmed contraction of CD8(+) T cells after infection. Nat Immunol 3:619–626
5. Bates MD, Meshnick SR, Sigler CI, et al. (1990) In vitro effects of primaquine and primaquine metabolites on exoerythrocytic stages of *Plasmodium berghei*. Am J Trop Med Hyg 42:532–537
6. Berenzon D, Schwenk RJ, Letellier L, et al. (2003) Protracted protection to *Plasmodium berghei* malaria is linked to functionally and phenotypically heterogeneous liver memory CD8+ T cells. J Immunol 171:2024–2034
7. Bottius E, BenMohamed L, Brahimi K, et al. (1996) A novel *Plasmodium falciparum* sporozoite and liver stage antigen (SALSA) defines major B, T helper, and CTL epitopes. J Immunol 156:2874–2884
8. Bucci K, Kastens W, Hollingdale MR, et al. (2000) Influence of age and HLA type on interferon-gamma (IFN-gamma) responses to a naturally occurring polymorphic epitope of *Plasmodium falciparum* liver stage antigen-1 (LSA-1). Clin Exp Immunol 122:94–100

9. Carvalho LH, Sano G, Hafalla JC, et al. (2002) IL-4-secreting CD4+ T cells are crucial to the development of CD8+ T-cell responses against malaria liver stages. Nat Med 8:166–170

10. Cerami C, Kwakye-Berko F, Nussenzweig V (1992) Binding of malarial circumsporozoite protein to sulfatides [Gal(3-SO4)beta 1-Cer] and cholesterol-3-sulfate and its dependence on disulfide bond formation between cysteines in region II. Mol Biochem Parasitol 54:1–12

11. Cervi L, MacDonald AS, Kane C, et al. (2004) Cutting edge: dendritic cells copulsed with microbial and helminth antigens undergo modified maturation, segregate the antigens to distinct intracellular compartments, and concurrently induce microbe-specific Th1 and helminth-specific Th2 responses. J Immunol 172:2016–2020

12. Clyde DF, Most H, McCarthy VC, et al. (1973) Immunization of man against sporozite-induced falciparum malaria. Am J Med Sci 266:169–177

13. Connelly M, King CL, Bucci K, et al. (1997) T-cell immunity to peptide epitopes of liver-stage antigen 1 in an area of Papua New Guinea in which malaria is holoendemic. Infect Immun 65:5082–5087

14. Crispe IN, Mehal WZ (1996) Strange brew: T cells in the liver. Immunol Today 17:522–525

15. Day KP, Marsh K (1991) Naturally acquired immunity to *Plasmodium falciparum*. Parasitol Today 7:68–71

16. De Souza Leao S, Lang T, Prina E, et al. (1995) Intracellular *Leishmania amazonensis* amastigotes internalize and degrade MHC class II molecules of their host cells. J Cell Sci 108 (Pt 10):3219–3231

17. Doolan DL, Hoffman SL (1999) IL-12 and NK cells are required for antigen-specific adaptive immunity against malaria initiated by CD8+ T cells in the *Plasmodium yoelii* model. J Immunol 163:884–892

18. Doolan DL, Southwood S, Freilich DA, et al. (2003) Identification of *Plasmodium falciparum* antigens by antigenic analysis of genomic and proteomic data. Proc Natl Acad Sci U S A 100:9952–9957

19. Doolan DL, Wizel B, Hoffman SL (1996) Class I HLA-restricted cytotoxic T lymphocyte responses against malaria—elucidation on the basis of HLA peptide binding motifs. Immunol Res 15:280–305

20. Dubois S, Mariner J, Waldmann TA, et al. (2002) IL-15Ralpha recycles and presents IL-15 In trans to neighboring cells. Immunity 17:537–547

21. Egan JE, Hoffman SL, Haynes JD, et al. (1993) Humoral immune responses in volunteers immunized with irradiated *Plasmodium falciparum* sporozoites. Am J Trop Med Hyg 49:166–173

22. Ehl S, Klenerman P, Aichele P, et al. (1997) A functional and kinetic comparison of antiviral effector and memory cytotoxic T lymphocyte populations in vivo and in vitro. Eur J Immunol 27:3404–3413

23. Ferreira A, Schofield L, Enea V, et al. (1986) Inhibition of development of exoerythrocytic forms of malaria parasites by gamma-interferon. Science 232:881–884

24. Frevert U (1994) Malaria sporozoite-hepatocyte interactions. Exp Parasitol 79:206–210

25. Frevert U, Galinski MR, Hugel FU, et al. (1998) Malaria circumsporozoite protein inhibits protein synthesis in mammalian cells. Embo J 17:3816–3826

26. Frevert U, Sinnis P, Cerami C, et al. (1993) Malaria circumsporozoite protein binds to heparan sulfate proteoglycans associated with the surface membrane of hepatocytes. J Exp Med 177:1287–1298

27. Gagnon E, Duclos S, Rondeau C, et al. (2002) Endoplasmic reticulum-mediated phagocytosis is a mechanism of entry into macrophages. Cell 110:119–131

28. Galle PR, Hofmann WJ, Walczak H, et al. (1995) Involvement of the CD95 (APO-1/Fas) receptor and ligand in liver damage. J Exp Med 182:1223–1230

29. Gray D, Matzinger P (1991) T cell memory is short-lived in the absence of antigen. J Exp Med 174:969–974

30. Guebre-Xabier M, Schwenk R, Krzych U (1999) Memory phenotype CD8(+) T cells persist in livers of mice protected against malaria by immunization with attenuated *Plasmodium berghei* sporozoites. Eur J Immunol 29:3978–3986

31. Guerin-Marchand C, Druilhe P, Galey B, et al. (1987) A liver-stage-specific antigen of *Plasmodium falciparum* characterized by gene cloning. Nature 329:164–167

32. Hafalla JC, Morrot A, Sano G, et al. (2003) Early self-regulatory mechanisms control the magnitude of CD8+ T cell responses against liver stages of murine malaria. J Immunol 171:964–970

33. Hafalla JC, Sano G, Carvalho LH, et al. (2002) Short-term antigen presentation and single clonal burst limit the magnitude of the CD8(+) T cell responses to malaria liver stages. Proc Natl Acad Sci U S A 99:11819–11824

34. Hill AV, Allsopp CE, Kwiatkowski D, et al. (1991) Common west African HLA antigens are associated with protection from severe malaria. Nature 352:595–600

35. Hill AV, Elvin J, Willis AC, et al. (1992) Molecular analysis of the association of HLA-B53 and resistance to severe malaria. Nature 360:434–439

36. Hoffman SL, Franke E, Hollingdale MR, et al. (1996) Attacking the infected hepatocyte. ASM Press, Washington DC

37. Hoffman SL, Franke ED (1994) Inducing protective immune responses against the sporozoite and liver stages of *Plasmodium*. Immunol Lett 41:89–94

38. Hogan RJ, Cauley LS, Ely KH, et al. (2002) Long-term maintenance of virus-specific effector memory CD8+ T cells in the lung airways depends on proliferation. J Immunol 169:4976–4981

39. Hogan RJ, Usherwood EJ, Zhong W, et al. (2001) Activated antigen-specific CD8+ T cells persist in the lungs following recovery from respiratory virus infections. J Immunol 166:1813–1822

40. Holder AA (1996) Preventing merozoite invasion of erythrocytes. ASM Press, Washington DC

41. Hollingdale M, Krzych U (2000) Immune responses to liver-stage parasites, vol. 80. Karger, Basel

42. Houde M, Bertholet S, Gagnon E, et al. (2003) Phagosomes are competent organelles for antigen cross-presentation. Nature 425:402–406

43. John CC, Sumba PO, Ouma JH, et al. (2000) Cytokine responses to *Plasmodium falciparum* liver-stage antigen 1 vary in rainy and dry seasons in highland Kenya. Infect Immun 68:5198–5204

44. Joshi SK, Bharadwaj A, Chatterjee S, et al. (2000) Analysis of immune responses against T- and B-cell epitopes from *Plasmodium falciparum* liver-stage antigen 1 in rodent malaria models and malaria-exposed human subjects in India. Infect Immun 68:141–150

45. Judge AD, Zhang X, Fujii H, et al. (2002) Interleukin 15 controls both proliferation and survival of a subset of memory-phenotype CD8(+) T cells. J Exp Med 196:935–946

46. Kaech SM, Tan JT, Wherry EJ, et al. (2003) Selective expression of the interleukin 7 receptor identifies effector CD8 T cells that give rise to long-lived memory cells. Nat Immunol 4:1191–1198

47. Kaech SM, Wherry EJ, Ahmed R (2002) Effector and memory T-cell differentiation: implications for vaccine development. Nat Rev Immunol 2:251–262

48. Kaufmann SH (1993) Immunity to intracellular bacteria. Annu Rev Immunol 11:129–163

49. Khan S, van den Broek M, Schwarz K, et al. (2001) Immunoproteasomes largely replace constitutive proteasomes during an antiviral and antibacterial immune response in the liver. J Immunol 167:6859–6868

50. Khan ZM, Vanderberg JP (1992) Specific inflammatory cell infiltration of hepatic schizonts in BALB/c mice immunized with attenuated *Plasmodium yoelii* sporozoites. Int Immunol 4:711–718

51. Khan ZM, and Vanderberg JP (1991) Eosinophil-rich, granulomatous inflammatory response to *Plasmodium berghei* hepatic schizonts in nonimmunized rats is age-related. Am J Trop Med Hyg 45:190–201

52. Khusmith S, Charoenvit Y, Kumar S, et al. (1991) Protection against malaria by vaccination with sporozoite surface protein 2 plus CS protein. Science 252:715–718

53. Klotz FW, Scheller LF, Seguin MC, et al. (1995) Co-localization of inducible-nitric oxide synthase and *Plasmodium berghei* in hepatocytes from rats immunized with irradiated sporozoites. J Immunol 154:3391–3395

54. Krzych U, Guebre-Zabier M, Schwenk R (1999) Malaria and the liver: tolerance and immunity to attenuated *Plasmodia sporozoites*. Wiley-Liss

55. Krzych U, Jareed T, Link HT, et al. (1992) Distinct T cell specificities are induced with the authentic versus recombinant *Plasmodium berghei* circumsporozoite protein. J Immunol 148:2530–2538

56. Krzych U, Schwenk R, Guebre-Xabier M, et al. (2000) The role of intrahepatic lymphocytes in mediating protective immunity induced by attenuated *Plasmodium berghei* sporozoites. Immunol Rev 174:123–134

57. Ku CC, Murakami M, Sakamoto A, et al. (2000) Control of homeostasis of CD8+ memory T cells by opposing cytokines. Science 288:675–678

58. Kumar S, Miller LH, Quakyi IA, et al. (1988) Cytotoxic T cells specific for the circumsporozoite protein of *Plasmodium falciparum*. Nature 334:258–260

59. Kurtis JD, Hollingdale MR, Luty AJ, et al. (2001) Pre-erythrocytic immunity to *Plasmodium falciparum*: the case for an LSA-1 vaccine. Trends Parasitol 17:219–223

60. Kurtis JD, Lanar DE, Opollo M, et al. (1999) Interleukin-10 responses to liver-stage antigen 1 predict human resistance to *Plasmodium falciparum*. Infect Immun 67:3424–3429

61. Langhorne J, Gillard S, Simon B, et al. (1989) Frequencies of CD4+ T cells reactive with *Plasmodium chabaudi chabaudi*: distinct response kinetics for cells with Th1 and Th2 characteristics during infection. Int Immunol 1:416–424

62. Lau LL, Jamieson BD, Somasundaram T, et al. (1994) Cytotoxic T-cell memory without antigen. Nature 369:648–652

63. Lee WT, Yin XM, Vitetta ES (1990) Functional and ontogenetic analysis of murine CD45Rhi and CD45Rlo CD4+ T cells. J Immunol 144:3288–3295

64. Li XC, Demirci G, Ferrari-Lacraz S, et al. (2001) IL-15 and IL-2: a matter of life and death for T cells in vivo. Nat Med 7:114–118

65. Link HT, White K, Krzych U (1993) *Plasmodium berghei*-specific T cells respond to non-processed sporozoites presented by B cells. Eur J Immunol 23:2263–2269

66. Luty AJ, Lell B, Schmidt-Ott R, et al. (1999) Interferon-gamma responses are associated with resistance to reinfection with *Plasmodium falciparum* in young African children. J Infect Dis 179:980–988

67. Luty AJ, Lell B, Schmidt-Ott R, et al. (1998) Parasite antigen-specific interleukin-10 and antibody responses predict accelerated parasite clearance in *Plasmodium falciparum* malaria. Eur Cytokine Netw 9:639–646

68. Malik A, Egan JE, Houghten RA, et al. (1991) Human cytotoxic T lymphocytes against the *Plasmodium falciparum* circumsporozoite protein. Proc Natl Acad Sci U S A 88:3300–3304

69. Masopust D, Vezys V, Marzo AL, et al. (2001) Preferential localization of effector memory cells in nonlymphoid tissue. Science 291:2413–2417

70. Matzinger P (1994) Tolerance, danger, and the extended family. Annu Rev Immunol 12:991–1045

71. May J, Lell B Luty AJ, et al. (2001) HLA-DQB1*0501-restricted Th1 type immune responses to *Plasmodium falciparum* liver stage antigen 1 protect against malaria anemia and reinfections. J Infect Dis 183:168–172

72. Mellouk S, Maheshwari RK, Rhodes-Feuillette A, et al. (1987) Inhibitory activity of interferons and interleukin 1 on the development of *Plasmodium falciparum* in human hepatocyte cultures. J Immunol 139:4192–4195

73. Murali-Krishna K, Lau LL, Sambhara S, et al. (1999) Persistence of memory CD8 T cells in MHC class I-deficient mice. Science 286:1377–1381

74. Nardin EH, Nussenzweig RS (1993) T cell responses to pre-erythrocytic stages of malaria: role in protection and vaccine development against pre-erythrocytic stages. Annu Rev Immunol 11:687–727

75. Nussenzweig RS, Vanderberg J, Most H, et al. (1967) Protective immunity produced by the injection of x-irradiated sporozoites of *Plasmodium berghei*. Nature 216:160–162

76. Nussenzweig V, Nussenzweig RS (1989) Rationale for the development of an engineered sporozoite malaria vaccine. Adv Immunol 45:283–334

77. Oehen S, Waldner H, Kundig TM, et al. (1992) Antivirally protective cytotoxic T cell memory to lymphocytic choriomeningitis virus is governed by persisting antigen. J Exp Med 176:1273–1281

78. Palmer DR, Krzych U (2002) Cellular and molecular requirements for the recall of IL-4-producing memory CD4(+)CD45RO(+)CD27(-) T cells during protection induced by attenuated *Plasmodium falciparum* sporozoites. Eur J Immunol 32:652–661

79. Pasquetto V, Fidock DA, Gras H, et al. (1997) *Plasmodium falciparum* sporozoite invasion is inhibited by naturally acquired or experimentally induced polyclonal antibodies to the STARP antigen. Eur J Immunol 27:2502–2513

80. Pinder M, Reece WH, Plebanski M, et al. (2004) Cellular immunity induced by the recombinant *Plasmodium falciparum* malaria vaccine, RTS,S/AS02, in semi-immune adults in The Gambia. Clin Exp Immunol 135:286–293

81. Plebanski M, Lee EA, Hannan CM, et al. (1999) Altered peptide ligands narrow the repertoire of cellular immune responses by interfering with T-cell priming. Nat Med 5:565–571

82. Pradel G, Frevert U (2001) Malaria sporozoites actively enter and pass through rat Kupffer cells prior to hepatocyte invasion. Hepatology 33:1154–1165

83. Renggli J, Hahne M, Matile H, et al. (1997) Elimination of *P. berghei* liver stages is independent of Fas (CD95/Apo-I) or perforin-mediated cytotoxicity. Parasite Immunol 19:145–148

84. Rickman KH, Beaudoin RL, Cassels JS, et al. (1979) Use of attenuated sporozoites in the immunization of human volunteers against falciparum malaria. Bull WHO 57:261–265

85. Robson KJ, Frevert U, Reckmann I, et al. (1995) Thrombospondin-related adhesive protein (TRAP) of *Plasmodium falciparum*: expression during sporozoite ontogeny and binding to human hepatocytes. Embo J 14:3883–3894

86. Robson KJ, Hall JR, Jennings MW, et al. (1988) A highly conserved amino-acid sequence in thrombospondin, properdin and in proteins from sporozoites and blood stages of a human malaria parasite. Nature 335:79–82

87. Rodrigues M, Nussenzweig RS, Romero P, et al. (1992) The in vivo cytotoxic activity of CD8+ T cell clones correlates with their levels of expression of adhesion molecules. J Exp Med 175:895–905

88. Rogers WO, Malik A, Mellouk S, et al. (1992) Characterization of *Plasmodium falciparum* sporozoite surface protein 2. Proc Natl Acad Sci U S A 89:9176–9180

89. Romero P, Maryanski JL, Corradin G, et al. (1989) Cloned cytotoxic T cells recognize an epitope in the circumsporozoite protein and protect against malaria. Nature 341:323–326

90. Sallusto F, Lenig D, Forster R, et al. (1999) Two subsets of memory T lymphocytes with distinct homing potentials and effector functions. Nature 401:708–712

91. Sano G, Hafalla JC, Morrot A, et al. (2001) Swift development of protective effector functions in naive CD8(+) T cells against malaria liver stages. J Exp Med 194:173–180

92. Scheller LF, Azad AF (1995) Maintenance of protective immunity against malaria by persistent hepatic parasites derived from irradiated sporozoites. Proc Natl Acad Sci U S A 92:4066–4068

93. Schofield L, Villaquiran J, Ferreira A, et al. (1987) Gamma interferon, CD8+ T cells and antibodies required for immunity to malaria sporozoites. Nature 330:664–666

94. Sedegah M, Finkelman F, Hoffman SL (1994) Interleukin 12 induction of interferon gamma-dependent protection against malaria. Proc Natl Acad Sci U S A 91:10700–10702

95. Seder RA, Ahmed R (2003) Similarities and differences in CD4+ and CD8+ effector and memory T cell generation. Nat Immunol 4:835–842

96. Seguin MC, Ballou WR, Nacy CA (1989) Interactions of *Plasmodium berghei* sporozoites and murine Kupffer cells in vitro. J Immunol 143:1716–1722

97. Seguin MC, Klotz FW, Schneider I, et al. (1994) Induction of nitric oxide synthase protects against malaria in mice exposed to irradiated *Plasmodium berghei* infected mosquitoes: involvement of interferon gamma and CD8+ T cells. J Exp Med 180:353–358
98. Sprent J, Surh CD (2002) T cell memory. Annu Rev Immunol 20:551–579
99. Sprent J, Tough DF (2001) T cell death and memory. Science 293:245–248
100. Steers N, Schwenk R, Bacom DJ et al. (2005) The immune status of Kupffer cells profoundly influences their responses to infections *Plasmodium berghei* sporozoites. Eur J Immunol 35 (in press)
101. Sun P, Schwenk R, White K, et al. (2003) Protective immunity induced with malaria vaccine, RTS,S, is linked to Plasmodium falciparum circumsporozoite protein-specific CD4+ and CD8+ T cells producing IFN-gamma. J Immunol 171:6961–6967
102. Tsuji M, Miyahira Y, Nussenzweig RS, et al. (1995) Development of antimalaria immunity in mice lacking IFN-gamma receptor. J Immunol 154:5338–5344
103. Usherwood EJ, Hogan RJ, Crowther G, et al. (1999) Functionally heterogeneous CD8(+) T-cell memory is induced by Sendai virus infection of mice. J Virol 73:7278–7286
104. van Leeuwen EM, Gamadia LE, Baars PA, et al. (2002) Proliferation requirements of cytomegalovirus-specific, effector-type human CD8+ T cells. J Immunol 169:5838–5843
105. Waldmann TA, Dubois S, Tagaya Y (2001) Contrasting roles of IL-2 and IL-15 in the life and death of lymphocytes: implications for immunotherapy. Immunity 14:105–110
106. Weiss WR, Mellouk S, Houghten RA, et al. (1990) Cytotoxic T cells recognize a peptide from the circumsporozoite protein on malaria-infected hepatocytes. J Exp Med 171:763–773
107. Weiss WR, Sedegah M, Beaudoin RL, et al. (1988) CD8+ T cells (cyto-toxic/suppressors) are required for protection in mice immunized with malaria sporozoites. Proc Natl Acad Sci U S A 85:573–576
108. Weiss WR, Sedegah M, Berzofsky JA, et al. (1993) The role of CD4+ T cells in immunity to malaria sporozoites. J Immunol 151:2690–2698
109. Wherry EJ, Teichgraber V, Becker TC, et al. (2003) Lineage relationship and protective immunity of memory CD8 T cell subsets. Nat Immunol 4:225–234
110. White KL, Snyder HL, Krzych U (1996) MHC class I-dependent presentation of exoerythrocytic antigens to CD8+ T lymphocytes is required for protective immunity against *Plasmodium berghei*. J Immunol 156:3374–3381
111. Wizel B, Houghten R, Church P, et al. (1995) HLA-A2-restricted cytotoxic T lymphocyte responses to multiple *Plasmodium falciparum* sporozoite surface protein 2 epitopes in sporozoite-immunized volunteers. J Immunol 155:766–775
112. Zechini B, Cordier L, Ngonseu E, et al. (1999) *Plasmodium berghei* development in irradiated sporozoite-immunized C57BL6 mice. Parasitology 118 (Pt 4):335–338
113. Zhu J, Hollingdale MR (1991) Structure of *Plasmodium falciparum* liver stage antigen-1. Mol Biochem Parasitol 48:223–226
114. Zinkernagel RM, Bachmann MF, Kundig TM, et al. (1996) On immunological memory. Annu Rev Immunol 14:333–367

CTMI (2005) 297:25–70

Early Interactions Between Blood-Stage *Plasmodium* Parasites and the Immune System

B. C. Urban[1] (✉) · R. Ing[2] · M. M. Stevenson[2]

[1]Centre for Clinical Vaccinology and Tropical Medicine, Nuffield Department of Clinical Medicine, Oxford University, Churchill Hospital, Old Road, Oxford OX3 7LJ, UK
britta.urban@ndm.ox.ac.uk

[2]Centre for the Study of Host Resistance and Centre for Host Parasite Interactions, McGill University Health Centre Research Institute, 1650 Cedar Avenue, Montreal Quebec, H3G 1A4, Canada

Abstract Accumulating evidence provides strong support for the importance of innate immunity in shaping the subsequent adaptive immune response to blood-stage *Plasmodium* parasites, the causative agents of malaria. Early interactions between blood-stage parasites and cells of the innate immune system, including dendritic cells, monocytes/macrophages, natural killer (NK) cells, NKT cells, and γδ T cells, are important in the timely control of parasite replication and in the subsequent elimination and resolution of the infection. The major role of innate immunity appears to be the production of immunoregulatory cytokines, such as interleukin (IL)-12 and interferon (IFN)-γ, which are critical for the development of type 1 immune responses involving $CD4^+$ Th1 cells, B cells, and effector cells which mediate cell-mediated and antibody-dependent adaptive immune responses. In addition, it is likely that cells of the innate immune system, especially dendritic cells, serve as antigen-presenting cells. Here, we review recent data from rodent models of blood-stage malaria and from human studies, and outline the early interactions of infected red blood cells with the innate immune system. We compare and contrast the results derived from studies in infected laboratory mice and humans. These host species are sufficiently different with respect to the identity of the infecting *Plasmodium* species, the resulting pathologies, and immune responses, particularly where the innate immune response is concerned. The implications of these findings for the development of an effective and safe malaria vaccine are also discussed.

1
Introduction

Infection with *Plasmodium falciparum*, one of four human *Plasmodium* species, causes considerable morbidity and mortality mainly in children living in endemic areas [181]. Disease occurs during the asexual phase when blood-stage parasites replicate within red blood cells for approximately 48 h. After subsequent rupture of the infected red blood cells, 6–32 merozoites are released which, in turn, invade fresh red blood cells. Malarial disease ranges from life-threatening illness, characterized by one or more clinical syndromes such as coma, hyperparasitaemia, hypoglycaemia or anaemia, to mild febrile illness. Asymptomatic infections are also common especially in older children and adults. The age range of severe malarial disease and death is dependent on transmission intensity. In hyperendemic areas with more than 100 infectious bites per person per year, severe disease occurs in children under the age of 1 year. Severe malarial anaemia is the dominant clinical syndrome, whereas cerebral malaria is relatively unusual. In areas with infectious bite rates between 10 and a 100, severe malarial disease affects mainly children between the ages of 1 and 5 years and cerebral malaria is a common clinical complication [138, 155]. Yet, relative to the proportion of *P. falciparum*-infected individuals in an endemic area, severe malarial disease and death are actually rare events occurring in about 1% of cases, which nevertheless kills more than 1 million children per year [181]. For instance, in an endemic area in Kenya, almost all children and approximately 30% of adults carry *P. falciparum* blood stages but show only mild or no clinical symptoms [154]. Based on these observations, mathematical modelling suggests that clinical immunity to severe, non-cerebral falciparum malaria occurs after one or two infections, while the development of clinical immunity against mild disease takes much longer [58]. Although exposed to infection, infants are protected against severe disease for about 6 months after birth by maternal antibodies [156]. During this time, their immune system is primed and they start to build up a repertoire of specific humoral and cellular immune responses against infecting parasite variants, which, as protection by maternal antibodies wanes, allows most children to cope with the infection without developing severe disease. However, superinfection onto an established chronic infection is common and, together with the host's genetic make-up, parasite properties and exposure may determine whether or not a child develops severe malarial disease [153].

P. falciparum differs from other species infecting humans in that it achieves higher parasitaemias and the mature forms of the asexual blood stages sequester in postcapillary venules. Sequestration ensures that at least a proportion of infected red blood cells mature without passage through the spleen where they are removed by cordal macrophages due to their reduced deformability and opsonization with antibodies and/or complement [6, 25, 26]. Sequestration of infected red blood cells is mediated by a family of parasite-derived variant surface antigens, *Plasmodium falciparum* erythrocyte membrane protein 1 (PfEMP1), inserted into the membrane of infected red blood cells approximately 18 h after invasion [84]. PfEMP1 is encoded by 59 *var* genes; expression of these genes is mutually exclusive. In laboratory parasite lines, on and off switching rates differ for different *var* genes [69]. Antigenic variation of PfEMP-1 is an important mechanism of evasion of the host's humoral immune response. In addition, PfEMP-1 mediates adhesion of mature infected red blood cells to diverse host receptors expressed on endothelial cells, red blood cells and leucocytes. Almost all infected red blood cells isolated from children with malaria analysed so far bind to CD36 but with varying avidity. Individual isolates may also bind to a variety of other host receptors such as CD31, CD35, CD51 or CD54, and glycosaminoglycans [84]. Receptor-specific cytoadhesion has been associated with various clinical syndromes of the disease. Thus, CD54 (ICAM1)-binding infected red blood cells are more frequently isolated from children who suffer from cerebral malaria [171]. Likewise, rosetting of uninfected erythrocytes by infected erythrocytes and clumping of infected red blood cells with platelets are both associated with severe disease [118, 134]. Whether blocking of capillaries locally or the induction of inflammatory cytokines, or both, causes organ-specific pathology is not quite clear but these mechanisms are under active investigation. The best example of an association between organ-specific pathology and cytoadhesive properties of mature infected red blood cells comes from placental malaria in primigravidae women [12], which is reviewed elsewhere in this volume. By contrast, high avidity for CD36 in field isolates is associated with mild malarial disease [110, 133, 169]. In addition, selection of laboratory parasite isolates with immune sera from children with severe disease resulted in parasites with lower avidity to CD36 compared to the parental line [157]. Adhesion to CD36 is a feature of almost all PfEMP-1 variants expressed on infected erythrocytes from field isolates, suggesting that adhesion to CD36 may have a role beyond sequestration of infected erythrocytes to endothelial cells.

2
Immune Responses to Blood-Stage *Plasmodium* Infection

Humoral immune responses are critical for clinical immunity as has been shown by classical transfer experiments of adult hyperimmune serum into children with acute malaria [100]. In these children, parasitaemia was suppressed for prolonged periods of time although circulating blood-stage parasites were not permanently cleared. Many targets of the humoral immune response are polymorphic or clonally variant antigens exposed on the surface of merozoites or infected red blood cells, respectively [84, 131]. During acute infection, individuals develop specific antibody responses to antigens of the parasite variant to which they are exposed [1, 16]. These antibody responses are often, but not always, highly specific but may show some cross-reactivity to other variants of the same antigen [23, 51, 113, 129]. Hence, clinical immunity to blood-stage malaria evolves with the acquisition of a repertoire of antibodies to different variants of parasite antigens and is related to exposure and age of the host [17, 38]. Protective antibody responses have been associated with the development of IgG1 and IgG3 subclasses, the two main cytophilic antibodies that allow opsonization and clearance of merozoites or infected erythrocytes by macrophages and neutrophils [108, 167]. These antibody responses follow a classic pattern of primary and secondary responses

in most individuals, but a proportion of non-responders has also been identified in longitudinal studies [80]. However, an increasing number of studies
report that antibody responses against specific antigens are short-lived and
dependent on the presence of circulating parasites [18, 21, 31], suggesting
that memory formation and longevity of either B- and T-cell responses or
both are perturbed in falciparum malaria (reviewed in this volume). Both immunopathology and adaptive immune responses are critically dependent on
the early events in the host–parasite interaction and the resulting cytokine balance. Infected red blood cells directly interact with leucocytes such as natural
killer (NK) cells, monocytes/macrophages, and dendritic cells (DCs). These
interactions may depend on the infecting parasite phenotype and host genotype and, together with previous exposure and age, influence the balance of
immune responses. Pro-inflammatory cytokines, especially tumour necrosis
factor (TNF)-α, interferon (IFN)-γ and lymphotoxin (LT), have been associated with severe disease, yet are crucial for the initial control of parasitaemia
both in mice and in humans. The mechanisms are not yet well understood,
but secretion of IFN-γ by NK, NKT and γδ T cells may have cytotoxic effects on
parasite growth as well as activate monocytes and macrophages and enhance
non-opsonic phagocytosis of infected red blood cells. The concentrations of
anti-inflammatory cytokines, such as interleukin (IL)-10 and transforming
growth factor (TGF)-β, concurrent with those of pro-inflammatory cytokines
appear to have a balancing effect. Such cytokines are also important growth
factors for B-cell responses.

In this review, we outline the interactions of infected red blood cells with
cells of the innate immune system and their consequences for adaptive immune responses in rodent and human malaria. We deliberately differentiate
between results from rodent models and human studies because these systems are sufficiently different with respect to the infecting parasite species, the
resulting pathologies, and the cellular responses, particularly where innate
immune responses are concerned. However, we cross-reference between the
sections and where available point out the similarities and differences.

3
Overview of Innate Immunity

3.1
Dendritic Cells

DCs are important for the activation of immune responses and they provide
a vital link between innate and adaptive immunity. They reside in almost all
tissues where they constantly screen their environment by pinocytosis and

phagocytosis of protein and cellular debris. When they encounter foreign antigen, DCs are activated by either the pathogens themselves or cytokines and stress signals secreted by surrounding cells. They leave the tissue via the lymph or blood and migrate to the draining lymph node and the spleen. During migration, DCs become mature in that they down-regulate phagocytosis but up-regulate human leucocyte antigen (HLA) molecules and adhesion and co-stimulatory molecules, which allow them to present MHC:peptide complexes to and interact efficiently with T cells. Interaction with T cells further matures DCs and enhances their secretion of cytokines, which are important for the polarization of CD4$^+$ T helper (Th) cells and for activation of other leucocytes, such as NK cells, monocytes/macrophages, and B cells [10].

In humans, there are two major DC subsets that have overlapping functions but can be distinguished by their difference in localization. Myeloid DCs are lineage marker negative, HLA DR positive, and express CD11c and CD1c, also known as blood dendritic cell antigen-1 (BDCA1) [40, 81, 121]. They can be found in nearly all tissues and migrate preferentially via the lymph to the draining lymph node, although a proportion migrate via the blood into the spleen. However, they are also abundant in the marginal zone and perifollicular zone of the spleen, hence, in those regions where blood enters the open circulation of the spleen. Myeloid DCs are the major source of IL-12 [66].

Plasmacytoid DCs on the other hand are lineage marker negative, HLA DR positive, and express CD123 and BDCA2 [40, 81, 121]. They reside mainly in the extranodular compartment and around high endothelial venules (HEV) of lymph nodes, but are rarely found in the spleen [43]. They are the major source of IFN-α and their basal secretion of this cytokine is further enhanced by maturation [22, 42]. Activated plasmacytoid DCs also secret IL-12 [83]. Plasmacytoid and myeloid DCs differ in their locations and their expression of pattern recognition receptors (PRRs) and Fc receptors, thus allowing them to respond to a distinct but overlapping repertoire of pathogens [146]. Therefore, myeloid DCs are more likely to mature in response to pathogens that enter the body via the skin or mucosal surfaces or are disseminated through blood, whereas plasmacytoid DCs respond to systemic viral infection and blood-borne antigens.

Both DC subsets are important for the maintenance of peripheral tolerance [158]. It has been assumed that in the steady state, DCs recirculate from blood and tissues carrying self-derived antigens from the periphery into lymph nodes and spleen. Whether or not these cells undergo a partial maturation is not quite clear, but they can present MHC:peptide complexes to T cells. Secretion of anti-inflammatory cytokines, such as IL-10, differential expression of co-stimulatory molecules, and the expression of inhibitory receptors lead to the deletion of or anergy induction in autoreactive T cells.

In addition, both mature and tolerogenic DCs can activate regulatory T cells which, in turn, suppress activation and expansion of autoreactive T cells, either during steady-state conditions or during the resolution of inflammation [96].

In the mouse, four subsets of DCs have been distinguished. Spleen DCs can be divided into MHC class II positive, CD11c$^+$ DCs, which express either CD4 or CD8α or are double negative [36, 146]. In addition, the rodent counterpart of plasmacytoid DCs has recently been identified. These cells are CD11c$^+$, B220$^+$, and Gr1$^+$. Myeloid CD11c$^+$ CD8$^+$ DCs reside in the T-cell areas of the spleen and are the sole producers of IL-12, whereas the CD11c$^+$ CD4$^+$ DCs are found mainly in the marginal zone and do not produce IL-12. Unlike human DCs, both mouse plasmacytoid and CD11c$^+$ DC can secrete high levels of IFN-α following activation. Mouse and human DCs also differ in their expression of PRRs [36, 146].

3.2
Monocytes/Macrophages

Monocytes, precursors of macrophages and potentially DCs, circulate in the peripheral blood for approximately 3 days before migrating into tissue and differentiating into macrophages. There, they have an important scavenging function, removing cellular debris, apoptotic cells, and proteinaceous particles during the steady state. They are activated by pro-inflammatory cytokines, such as IFN-γ, TNF-α, IL-1 and IL-6, or by ligation of PRRs, which allows them to resist the cytopathic effects of intracellular pathogens and can induce production of oxygen radicals and nitric oxide (NO). Once activated, these cells display co-stimulatory molecules and MHC:peptide complexes on their surface and can efficiently activate memory T cells, although they may be unable to prime naïve T cells. In addition, they secrete growth factors important for survival and differentiation of B cells [55].

Although monocytes and macrophages are rapidly activated by the pro-inflammatory cytokines IFN-γ and TNF-α, an alternatively activated state has been described [56]. These macrophages respond to IL-4 and IL-13 and up-regulate MHC class II molecules and the mannose receptor. It has been suggested that they may play an important immunoregulatory role in some parasitic infections and allergy.

In the spleen, the marginal zone is equally rich in macrophages and DCs. In the mouse, the marginal zone contains metallophilic macrophages, which delineate the marginal sinus. Both are absent in human spleen and the capillaries end in the perifollicular zone surrounding the marginal zone. Macrophages and DCs in the marginal zone in mice and in the perifollicular zone in humans phagocytose cellular debris, pathogens, and other proteinaceous particles, thus, presenting an important barrier for blood-borne pathogens. Both DCs and macrophages activated by pathogens or their products can then interact with memory T and B cells located in the marginal zone. DCs also migrate deeper into the white pulp initiating innate and adaptive immune responses. The majority of macrophages are found in the red pulp in the splenic cords. There, they remove aged and antigenically altered red blood cells from the circulation and, therefore, have an important function in the filtration of blood [55, 56]. In addition, they phagocytose pathogens, which are not retained in the marginal or perifollicular zones.

3.3
NK Cells

NK cells are populations of lymphocytes that provide protection against infections and cancer through their cytotoxic activities and production of cytokines and chemokines. Rapid induction of NK cell responses (on the order of 2–6 days) limits an infection until adaptive immunity develops [13, 19]. NK cells do not express T-cell antigen receptors (TCR) and preferentially recognize and kill cells that express altered levels of MHC class I molecule, without the need for pre-activation or antibodies. To kill aberrant cells and avoid targeting of normal cells, NK cells use a complex repertoire of surface activation and inhibitory receptors. NK cell-activating receptors (e.g. human NKp30, NKp44 and NKp46; mouse Ly49D and Ly49H) bind a variety of ligands, including human MHC-I-related chain, pathogen-specific epitopes, and stress signals and inducible molecules expressed by infected or damaged cells. Alternatively, normal host cells present sufficient MHC class I molecules to MHC-I-sensing inhibitory receptors (e.g. human KIR and CD94/NKG2; mouse Ly49) resulting in down-regulation of NK cell function. Several NK cell receptors perform both activation and inhibition, depending on which isoforms are expressed; the activating isoforms lack inhibitory motifs in their short cytoplasmic domains and are able to associate with additional subunits that transduce activating signals to the cell nucleus. Therefore, the commitment to NK cell effector function is regulated by a fine balance in the expression of activating versus inhibiting receptors, the sequence of which can be influenced by the density and array of ligands, cytokine milieu, and class I and other surface molecules expressed by antigen-presenting cells (APCs), such as DCs (see below).

NK cells were discovered for their unique ability to spontaneously lyse tumour cell lines. This cytolytic capacity is mediated by several pathways and involves phenotypically distinct NK cell subsets. The main pathway is mediated by perforin and granzymes released by mature activated NK cells, although both immature and mature human NK cells employ Fas ligand (CD178) and/or TNF-related apoptosis-inducing ligand (TRAIL) to induce target cell death [184]. In addition, NK cells mediate antibody-dependent cellular cytotoxicity (ADCC) through an Fc-receptor complex (CD16) that recognizes the Fc portion of antibodies bound to target cell-associated antigens.

The production of immunoregulatory cytokines is an important mechanism by which NK cells direct haematopoietic cell differentiation and modulate other immune cells. In humans, subsets of CD56^{hi} NK cells with weak natural cytolytic capacity are able to produce high levels of IFN-γ, TNF-α, LT-α, GM-CSF, IL-10 and IL-13 following selective stimulation [29]. Based on their cytokine profiles, human NK cells have been categorized into NK1 and NK2 subsets [122]. More recent studies [91] showed that the maturation of human NK cells progresses sequentially from an early stage of proliferation and IL-13 production (type 2) to a late stage of terminal differentiation and IFN-γ production (type 1), suggesting that NK cell cytokine production may be developmentally regulated. However, mature CD56^{+} NK cells cultured in vitro and some CD56^{+} NK-cell clones have mixed type 0 profiles (IFN-γ, IL-4, IL-13), whereas CD56^{dim} NK cells produce low amounts of these cytokines but are highly cytolytic [28]. Given the need for efficient production of cytokines by NK cells early in the response to infection, the physiological relevance of cytokine production by clonal NK cells or following prolonged stimulation in vitro is presently unclear.

Murine NK cells are similar to their human counterparts in their ability to lyse target cells, produce cytokines, and express activating or inhibiting receptors. However, murine NK cells do not express a homologue of CD56 and, as a result, there are no comparative studies demonstrating functionally distinct subsets of NK cells in mice. Nonetheless, murine NK cells are potent producers of cytokines, particularly IFN-γ, following intracellular infection or stimulation with various combinations of cytokines. Specifically, NK cells derived from murine splenocytes stimulated by a combination of IL-12 and IL-18 secrete large amounts of IFN-γ compared to NK cells derived in IL-2 or IL-15 [87]. As the main producers of IFN-γ early after viral [13] or malaria infections [104], NK cells play a critical role in the innate immune response to stimulate Th1 cell development and induction of type 1 adaptive immune responses.

3.4
Natural Killer T Cells

Natural killer T, or NKT, cells are a heterogeneous population of lymphocytes with phenotypic and functional characteristics of both NK cells and classic

T cells. This cell type is especially abundant in the liver and is also found in the thymus, periphery, and spleen, but its presence is rare in lymph nodes. NKT cells express NK1.1 and an invariant $\alpha\beta$-TCR [59]. Murine NKT cells express a TCR α-chain (Vα14-Jα281, known now as Jα18) in association with Vβ2, Vβ7, or Vβ8 [54]. In humans, NKT cells express an invariant Vα24-Jα18 TCR α-chain in association with the Vβ11-TCR β-chain, the homologues of the mouse Vα14-Jα18 and Vβ8.2 chains, respectively. Because of their ability to rapidly secrete immunoregulatory cytokines, especially IFN-γ, IL-4 and TNF-α, following antigen-specific or polyclonal stimulation, NKT cells influence the polarization of CD4$^+$ Th cells [54, 139, 182]. NKT cells recognize glycolipid antigens via a repertoire of invariant VαVβ-TCR in the context of a non-classic, MHC class-I-like molecule, the CD1d molecule. Murine CD1d-restricted, Vα14-Jα18 expressing NKT cells and their human counterparts, Vα24-Jα18$^+$ NKT cells, are selectively activated in vitro and in vivo by exposure to the ligand α-galactosylceramide, either synthetically produced or derived from the marine sponge [54, 182].

The human CD1 system consists of five closely linked genes that map to chromosome 1. The five CD1 genes encode related but unique protein products designated as CD1a, b, c, d and e. Sequence analysis revealed that these proteins can be classified into two separate groups: group 1 consists of CD1a, b, c, and e, while the more divergent CD1d molecule belongs to group 2 [54]. Mice do not express group 1 molecules. Mice and other rodents, however, express CD1d molecules that have homology with human CD1d and thus belong to group 2 [148]. Human invariant TCR Vα24-JαQ/Vβ11 NKT cells are phenotypically and functionally homologous to murine NK1$^+$ T cells, and similar to their counterparts in mice, are CD1d-restricted and express the NK1.1 surface marker (Nkrplc or CD161c) [148]. Mouse CD1d-restricted NKT cells recognize human CD1d and vice versa. Such a remarkable degree of conservation between the two species makes mice an excellent experimental model to study the role of CD1d and NKT cells in immunity and immunopathogenesis in many diseases, including infections. Subsets of CD1d-dependent T cells, that either express or do not express the invariant Vα14-Jα18 (Vα24-Jα18 in humans) -TCR and/or NK1.1 (CD161 in humans), have been identified in both species and can be either CD4$^+$ or CD4$^-$ [54]. These subsets have been shown to produce unique patterns of cytokines. Together, these observations suggest distinct regulatory functions for subsets of CD1d-dependent NKT cells in vivo.

Although the contribution of NKT cells to immunity to infection has not been fully elucidated, recent studies suggest the importance of CD1d-restricted NKT cells in resistance to viral, bacterial, yeast, and parasitic infections, including malaria, as will be discussed in detail in Sect. 5.4 [59,

148]. There appear to be at least two possible mechanisms whereby NKT cells are involved in immunity to infection. NKT cells possess some of the machinery—including perforin, FAS ligand (CD95L), and receptors, such as NKG2D—required for cytotoxicity and have been found to be directly cytotoxic, particularly against virus-infected cells [59, 148]. A more likely role for NKT cells, however, is as immunoregulatory cells leading to activation of effector cells of the lymphoid series via a cytokine-dependent pathway [59, 148]. Rapid cytokine production, especially of IFN-γ, by NKT cells results in bystander activation of NK cells and conventional CD4$^+$ and CD8$^+$ T cells as well as macrophages.

3.5
$\gamma\delta$ T Cells

$\gamma\delta$ T cells are distinct from $\alpha\beta$ T cells due to their ability to recognize antigens in the absence of classic MHC antigen presentation. In comparison to T cells bearing the $\alpha\beta$-TCR which comprise the majority of peripheral blood lymphocytes, T cells bearing the $\gamma\delta$-TCR represent only a small fraction of circulating T cells. However, $\gamma\delta$ T cells make up the majority of intraepithelial lymphocytes in the gut and other mucosal tissue of adult humans and mice and function in maintaining the integrity of epithelial tissues [62, 63]. This cell type also plays an important role in innate immunity and may contribute to immunity in neonates [62]. $\gamma\delta$ T cells are recruited and expanded in response to a wide variety of infections and play both beneficial and pathological roles [15, 49, 62, 63]. Evidence has been documented to support a role for $\gamma\delta$ T cells in protective immunity to intracellular pathogens, including mycobacteria, salmonella, toxoplasma, and plasmodium parasites as well as to HIV [15, 37, 49].

4
Innate Immune Responses to *Plasmodium* Blood-Stage Infection in Mice

4.1
Mouse Models of Malaria

Infections of inbred mice with the rodent *Plasmodium* species, *P. chabaudi*, *P. berghei*, *P. yoelii* and *P. vinckei*, provide convenient and useful tools to investigate the immunobiology of blood-stage malaria. Although mouse models are widely used to mimic human malaria infections, the complete features of neither protection nor pathology associated with human malaria can be replicated in a single mouse model [86, 161]. One must also bear in mind that there are significant differences between the murine and human immune systems [101]. Some of these differences in terms of innate immunity have been highlighted in the preceding sections. Nevertheless, detailed studies of the host response to blood-stage malaria in laboratory mice have yielded tremendous insight into the biology of the human response to malaria. Areas of investigation which have been especially fruitful include elucidation of mechanisms of protective immunity as well as of immunopathogenesis and the identification of genes that regulate susceptibility to malaria [35, 50, 86]. Mouse models of malaria are also useful for vaccine development and for chemotherapy studies [86].

Various strains of rodent *Plasmodium* species cause blood-stage malaria in mice [161]. Dependent upon the parasite species and strain, a wide range of pathologies and outcomes are produced, including the level of blood parasitaemia and whether or not the host survives the infection [86, 161]. These differences are influenced not only by genetic variations among the *Plasmodium* parasites but also among inbred mouse strains [50, 86]. Whatever the host–parasite combination, however, a prominent feature of rodent malaria infections is that survival is linked to the ability to control the replication of blood-stage parasites during the first 7–14 days after infection [161].

Infections with strains of *P. chabaudi*, particularly the AS strain, have perhaps provided the most extensive dissection of the immune response to blood-stage malaria. The majority of these studies have been performed using *P. chabaudi* AS infection in C57BL/6 strain mice, which are resistant to infection with this parasite [50]. Evidence from the *P. chabaudi* AS model of blood-stage malaria highlights the importance of adaptive type 1 immune mechanisms that are dependent upon CD4$^+$ T cells and the cytokines IL-12, and IFN-γ for control of acute parasitaemia [163, 164]. Whether a type 1 or type 2 response is important for the elimination of blood-stage *P. chabaudi* AS during the chronic stage of infection is unclear. However, it is clear that this later stage requires B cells and antibody [103]. Studies from our laboratory [164] provide evidence that the Th1-associated antibody subclass IgG2a and possibly IgG3, rather than Th2-associated IgG1 as proposed in earlier studies [103], mediates the elimination and resolution of *P. chabaudi* AS infection. The *P. chabaudi* AS model has also been extremely useful in uncovering the importance of early innate interactions between blood-stage parasites and the immune system, as detailed elsewhere in this review.

4.2
Dendritic Cells

Over the past several years, there has been great interest in understanding the role of DCs in immunity to blood-stage malaria in mouse models. Some of the first observations derived from a study by Seixas et al. [145] showed that schizonts of *P. chabaudi* AS induced bone marrow-derived DCs to express the co-stimulatory molecules CD40, CD86, and MHC class II, and to produce the pro-inflammatory cytokines IL-12, TNF-α, and IL-6. Bone marrow-derived DCs from SCID mice and from gene-deficient Rag or CD40 knockout mice were also shown to be able to produce these cytokines in vitro, demonstrating that DC cytokine response to *P. chabaudi* AS schizonts is not dependent on the presence of T cells, NK cells, or CD40 expression. Interestingly, schizonts of *P. chabaudi* AS did not inhibit LPS-induced up-regulation of co-stimulatory and MHC molecule expression, contrary to findings with strains of the human parasite *P. falciparum* [172]. While these results obtained with DCs cultured from bone marrow precursors suggest APCs respond differently depending on the identity of *Plasmodium* species, it is the DC population in the spleen that is of major interest because of its central role in filtering parasitized red blood cells from the blood and in generating the immune response to blood-stage malaria.

Enlargement of the spleen or splenomegaly is a hallmark of malaria endemicity in humans and often serves as a phenotypic marker of host resistance in malaria-infected mice [159]. APCs isolated from spleens of *P. yoelii* 17X-infected mice have been observed to have increased expression of CD80 and MHC class II molecules and to stimulate high levels of IFN-γ production by naïve T cells [94]. Of the APC subsets, there is growing evidence that DCs are the cells primarily responsible for stimulating production of pro-inflammatory cytokines and activation of naïve CD4$^+$ T cells, leading to induction of protective type 1 responses to blood-stage malaria. Within 5 days of infection with *P. chabaudi* AS, CD11c$^+$ DCs migrate from the marginal zone of the spleen to the CD4$^+$ T-cell-rich periarteriolar lymphoid sheath [89]. In contrast, macrophage and B-cell populations expand but remain confined to the red pulp area. Concurrent with their migration within the spleen, CD11c$^+$ DCs have up-regulated expression of CD40, CD54, and CD86 as well as increased production of IFN-γ [89]. These observations are consistent with those of Perry et al. [124], who showed that splenic CD11c$^+$ DCs, but not CD11b$^+$ macrophages or B cells, from *P. yoelii* 17X-infected mice stimulate high levels of IL-2, IFN-γ and TNF-α production by naïve CD4$^+$ T cells. These responses were found to be antigen-specific as demonstrated by the ability of purified CD11c$^+$ DCs from infected mice to stimulate a *P. yoelii* 17X-specific T-cell hybridoma to secrete high levels of IL-2. Furthermore, both myeloid and lymphoid CD11c$^+$ DCs from infected mice were found to produce IL-2, IFN-γ, TNF-α and IL-12 p40, and importantly, induced IFN-γ secretion by CD4$^+$ T cells through an IL-12-dependent mechanism. In addition to providing the requisite co-stimulation and cytokines to stimulate T cells, there is evidence that DCs secrete DC-derived CC chemokine 1 (DC-CK1) that acts preferentially on naïve T and B cells [14]. DC-CK1 treatment in vitro stimulates chemotaxis of T and B cells; in vivo, this chemokine induces a strong IFN-γ-producing CD8[+] T-cell response to liver-stage *P. yoelii* 17XNL and also acts as a vaccine adjuvant by increasing protection to liver-stage malaria mediated by immunization with irradiated *P. yoelii* 17XNL sporozoites. The role of DC-CK1 as a chemotactic or immunostimulatory factor in cell-mediated immunity to blood-stage malaria remains to be investigated.

These findings provide increasing evidence that, in contrast to some isolates of *P. falciparum*, the murine parasites *P. yoelii* and *P. chabaudi* AS do not inhibit DC function. Consistent with the model of DC–T cell interaction, DCs activated in vitro and in vivo in mouse models of malaria are capable of presenting *Plasmodium* antigens (Signal 1), expressing co-stimulatory molecules (Signal 2), and producing pro-inflammatory cytokines and chemokines (Signal 3) to stimulate antigen-specific T-cell-dependent immune responses (Fig. 1). A recent study showed that mice immunized with bone marrow-derived DCs pulsed with the respective intact parasitized red blood cells survive lethal infections with blood-stage *P. yoelii* YM or *P. chabaudi* AS [127]. Transfer of antigen-pulsed DCs also can induce cross-strain protection and is associated with malaria-specific production of IFN-γ and IL-4 as well as malaria-specific antibody following challenge infection.

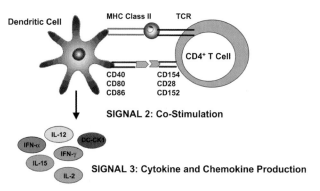

Fig. 1 DC-derived signals are required for T-cell priming. Based on data from mouse models of blood-stage malaria infection and consistent with the classic model of DC–T-cell interaction, DCs present *Plasmodium*-derived antigens (*Signal 1*) on MHC molecules, express high levels of co-stimulatory molecules such as CD40, CD80 and CD86 (*Signal 2*), and produce cytokines and chemokines (*Signal 3*) that promote and recruit antigen-specific CD4[+] T-cell responses

Moreover, no protection was observed in IL-12 p40$^{-/-}$ mice after lethal *P. yoelii* YM challenge, demonstrating that DC-induced immunity is dependent on host expression of IL-12. It is likely that T cells play an important role in mediating immunity conferred by transferred DCs, since splenic T cells isolated from mice immunized with antigen-pulsed DCs protected mice from *P. yoelii* YM challenge, although to a lesser degree compared to immunization by transfer of DCs. Despite these encouraging results, however, it is important to note that while antigen-pulsed DCs enhanced survival to lethal *Plasmodium* infections, the surviving mice continued to develop high levels of parasitaemia. Moreover, the high rates of mortality ($\geq$80%) reported in this study with *P. chabaudi* AS infections in C57BL/6 mice have not been observed in other laboratories, including those of the authors, using identical mouse and parasite strains [2]. Studies currently ongoing in our laboratory demonstrate that splenic CD11c$^+$ DCs purified from naïve mice and pulsed ex vivo with parasitized red blood cells can induce sterile immunity with 100% survival and 1% or less of parasitaemia following challenge infection with *P. chabaudi* AS in both genetically resistant C57BL/6 and susceptible A/J mice (R. Ing and M.M. Stevenson, unpublished observations/manuscript in preparation).

Contrary to reports that DCs are important mediators of protective immune responses to blood-stage malaria, Ocana-Morgner et al. [114] showed that *P. yoelii* 17XNL-infected red blood cells inhibit DC maturation and IL-12 secretion in response to LPS. Intriguingly, the parasite-induced modulation of DC functions was associated with suppressed protective CD8$^+$ T cell responses against liver-stage malaria. The ability of *P. yoelii* 17XNL-exposed DCs to inhibit immune responses to sporozoites was interpreted as a novel mechanism by which the *Plasmodium* parasite evades host immunity, leaving the host unprotected against reinfection. These results may help explain why naturally acquired resistance to malaria in humans develops very slowly, despite persistent exposure to *Plasmodium* parasites and intermittent episodes of infection in malaria-endemic areas.

4.3
Macrophages

The concept that macrophages suppress immune responses to blood-stage malaria has been documented extensively [2, 105, 142, 177]. Macrophages from mice infected with *P. chabaudi* AS [2, 142] or *P. yoelii* 17X [124] inhibit T-cell proliferation and production of the T-cell growth factor, IL-2. Phagocytosis of the malarial pigment, haemozoin, is associated with suppression of various monocyte and T-cell functions [105, 140, 141, 142], leading to the notion that phagocytic cells produce a soluble suppressive factor, such as NO, prostaglandin E_2 (PGE_2), or TGF-β. Haemozoin has been shown to increase NO synthesis by macrophages through an ERK/NFκB-dependent pathway [76]. Inhibition of both NO and PGE_2 reverses the suppressive effect of peritoneal macrophages from *P. chabaudi* AS-infected mice on mitogen-induced proliferation of normal splenocytes in vitro [2], whereas inhibition of NO alone did not restore IL-2 production by antigen-activated T-cell hybridomas cultured with macrophages from infected mice [142]. Recent studies [94, 124] provide further evidence that a soluble factor(s) produced by splenic CD11b$^+$ macrophages from *P. yoelii* 17X-infected mice inhibits T-cell proliferation and IL-2 production, but this factor does not appear to be NO, PGE_2 or TGF-β. Interestingly, CD11b$^+$ macrophages from infected mice are unable to inhibit IFN-γ or TNF-α production by naïve T cells, suggesting that macrophages play an important immunoregulatory function in limiting T-cell expansion to prevent malarial pathology while promoting high levels of IFN-γ production and, possibly as a result, Th1 cell differentiation during the acute stage of blood-stage malaria infection.

The suppressive effects of macrophages during malaria infection are not limited to T-cell responses. Following infection with *P. berghei* ANKA, peritoneal macrophages exhibit suppressed IL-12 p40, but not IL-12 p35, gene expression. Macrophages that had engulfed parasitized red blood cells in vitro were observed to be capable of inhibiting IL-12 p40 mRNA expression by uninfected macrophages, suggesting the presence of a soluble suppressive factor [183]. Indeed, this inhibition was found to be meditated by macrophage-produced IL-10, while PGE_2 and TGF-β do not seem to be involved. High levels of IL-12 p70 synthesis by splenic macrophages correlate with host resistance to *P. chabaudi* AS infection [136, 137], although the expression of both p40 and p35 mRNA is up-regulated in resistant C57Bl/6 as well as susceptible A/J mice during infection. Inhibition of IL-12, a key cytokine in the induction of protective type 1 immunity to blood-stage malaria, at the level of p40 gene expression or IL-12 p70 secretion, may be an important evasion strategy by the *Plasmodium* parasite. In addition, ingestion of *P. chabaudi* AS-infected red blood cells or haemozoin by peritoneal macrophages stimulates the release of macrophage migration inhibitory factor (MIF), a pro-inflammatory mediator that stimulates T-cell activation, antibody production, and delayed-type hypersensitivity reactions [99]. Martiney et al. [99] showed that MIF also can inhibit erythropoietin-dependent erythropoiesis in vitro, suggesting a potential role for macrophage-derived MIF in the pathogenesis of malarial anaemia.

Despite the immunosuppressive effects of macrophages on selective monocyte and T-cell functions during blood-stage malaria, phagocytosis of parasitized red blood cells is an important non-specific immune defence mechanism [147]. High levels of opsonin-independent phagocytosis of parasitized red blood cells and free merozoites were observed in mice that successfully control and resolve *P. chabaudi* AS infection [165]. Levels of opsonin-independent phagocytosis correlate with the ability of infected mice to produce IFN-γ and treatment of macrophages with IFN-γ enhances phagocytic activity, while treatment with IL-10 inhibits this activity. Thus, opsonin-independent phagocytosis by macrophages contributes to IFN-γ-dependent control of blood-stage malaria during the early stage of infection, prior to the development of antigen-specific adaptive immunity.

4.4
γδ T Cells

In vivo and in vitro studies have been performed to investigate the role of γδ T cells in immunity to blood-stage malaria. It is well established that there is expansion of the γδ T-cell population during infection with blood-stage parasites, a phenomenon that is evident in both mice and humans [103]. However, evidence from in vivo experiments using knockout mice lacking γδ T cells or mice depleted of γδ T cells by treatment with monoclonal antibody revealed that control and resolution of primary *P. chabaudi* AS, *P. chabaudi adami*, or *P. chabaudi chabaudi* CB occurred in the absence of these cells [103]. More recently, an important protective role for γδ T cells was revealed in mice genetically deficient in B cells and depleted of γδ T cells by monoclonal antibody treatment and in B-cell[-/-]TCRδ[-/-] double knockout mice [144, 176, 180]. Such experimental animals developed chronic, unremitting parasitaemia levels of more than 10% following infection with various strains of *P. chabaudi*. How γδ T cells contribute to controlling the replication of blood-stage malaria parasites has been the subject of investigation in mice and humans. Following stimulation with malaria antigens, γδ T cells from both species are capable of secreting pro-inflammatory cytokines critical for protective immunity to blood-stage parasites [103]. Analysis of the cellular source of IFN-γ and TNF-α at 24 h after infection with non-lethal *P. yoelii* 17X showed that both γδ T cells and NK cells contribute to early production of these cytokines and that this response is required for control of acute parasitaemia and subsequent resolution of infection [27]. The observation that γδ T cells secrete potentially harmful pro-inflammatory cytokines has also led to the hypothesis that these T cells play a role in malarial pathogenesis rather than protection [85]. The exact role of γδ T cells in immunity to blood-stage malaria is as yet unresolved and additional studies are, thus, warranted.

4.5
Interactions Between DC and NK Cells

DCs and NK cells are specialized cells of the innate immune system that perform distinct but mutually dependent functions in the innate immune response to infection. Both cell types are known to rapidly accumulate at the site of pathogen entry and in the marginal zone of the spleen, acting as sentinels against infection. DCs are the principal cells responsible for presenting antigen and activating an appropriate immune response, whereas NK cells are innate effector cells that through their cytolytic activity and secretion of pro-inflammatory cytokines, particularly IFN-γ, help control infection and augment downstream antigen-specific responses. Recent studies show that DCs and NK cells participate in bi-directional cross-talk which results in potent, reciprocal activation [47, 106]. Although much of the evidence for this cross-talk has been obtained from in vitro studies, NK cells have recently been shown to co-localize with DCs in lymph nodes during infection or antigen challenge [48, 106]. Thus, DC–NK cell interactions in the periphery as well as in secondary lymphoid organs may shape both the type and magnitude of innate as well as adaptive immune responses.

Upon contact with invading pathogens, DCs capture antigen for presentation and secrete chemokines, including CCL2 and IL-8, which recruit circulating NK cells to inflamed tissues. DCs then prime resting NK cells through cell–cell contact and release of soluble mediators, such as IFN-α, IL-2, IL-12, and IL-15 [4, 47, 57, 78, 125]. Some of these cytokines, notably IL-2 and IL-15, act as potent growth factors for NK cell development and proliferation. The specific mechanisms by which DCs activate NK cells are currently under intense investigation. Jinushi et al. [78] showed that DC-derived IL-15 and IFN-α induce autocrine expression of MHC class I-related chain A and B (MICA/B), ligands for the activating receptor, NKG2D, expressed on human resting NK cells, resulting in increased NK cytotoxicity. Studies in mice show that IL-2, secreted by DCs and T cells that possibly co-localize with NK cells in secondary lymphoid organs, acts directly on NK cells to promote optimal IFN-γ production and elicits effective anti-bacterial and anti-tumour NK cell activity [47, 57]. The maturation status of DCs is an important determinant of the ability of DCs to activate resting NK cells. Immature DCs are recognized via the NKp30 natural cytotoxicity receptor and TNF-related apoptosis-inducing ligand (TRAIL) and they become targeted for killing by NK cells. However, DCs matured by microbial stimuli, pro-inflammatory cytokines, or CD40 ligation are resistant to NK cell lysis [45, 46, 61]. Up-regulated expression of MHC class I molecules, such as HLA-E on human DCs, following antigen uptake by DCs, also confers protection against NK cell lysis [45, 46], thereby enabling mature DCs to survive and recruit and activate additional NK cells. A recent study showed that TGF-β significantly down-regulates NKp30 expression, rendering NK cells incapable of killing DCs [20]. This finding suggests a potential role for DC-derived cytokines in mediating DC–NK cell interactions that lead to either immune tolerance or activation, although TGF-β production by DCs in response to maturation signals has not yet been documented.

Reciprocally, NK cells have been to shown to induce DC maturation and cytokine production [53, 125]. Stimulation of DC responses by activated NK cells is critically dependent on cell–cell contact and, to a lesser extent, on TNF-α and IFN-γ secreted by NK cells [120, 125]. While it is unclear exactly how NK cell-derived TNF-α acts to stimulate DCs, IFN-γ secreted by NK cells has been shown to up-regulate expression of the co-stimulatory molecule inducible T cell antigen (4-IBB), which promotes autocrine/paracrine DC expansion, maturation, and migration [120]. As discussed above, NK cells lyse immature but not mature DCs using an array of cell surface receptors such as NKp30 and TRAIL. By recognizing and killing immature DCs, NK cells may play an immunoregulatory role in selecting an immunogenic DC population that could direct subsequent adaptive immune responses. In addition to their selective editing of DCs, NK cells may be the primary source of signals for type 1 polarization of DCs and T cells. Mailliard et al. [97] showed that DCs act as carriers of NK cell-derived signals that induce early polarization of Th cell responses. Following stimulation by NK cells, DCs carry NK cell-derived signals, including TNF-α and IFN-γ, into draining lymph nodes where DCs induce strong Th1 responses in naïve Th cells. Further research is required to determine the ability of NK cells to lyse endogenous DCs and to determine whether NK cells alter the numbers and functions of specific DC subsets in vivo.

To date, there are no published reports of DC–NK cell interactions in malaria infection, but there is preliminary evidence that such interactions occur in vivo and are important for directing immune responses and determining the outcome to blood-stage malaria. During the innate immune response to *Plasmodium* infection, DCs may express several cytokines, including IL-2, IL-12, IFN-γ and, in humans, IFN-α (Fig. 2) [47, 94, 124]. Some of these type 1 cytokines are known to activate macrophages and NK cells to secrete cytokines and to become phagocytic and/or cytolytic [4, 57, 165]. Activation of NK cells by DCs is potentially a critical event during the innate immune response because NK cells are one of the main producers of IFN-γ that is absolutely required for protective immunity to blood-stage malaria [102]. Recent work in our laboratory indicates that splenic CD11c$^+$ DCs purified from *P. chabaudi* AS-infected mice stimulate splenic DX-5$^+$ NK cells enriched from naïve mice to secrete high levels of IFN-γ in vitro (R. Ing and M.M. Stevenson, unpublished observations). The ability of DCs to stimulate Th1-type cytokine

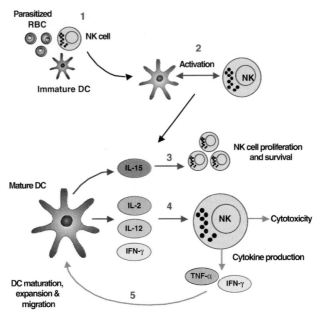

Fig. 2 Model of DC and NK cell interaction during blood-stage malaria infection. (*1*) During the early phase of the innate immune response, DCs and NK cells co-localize in the blood or secondary lymphoid organs, such as the spleen, and engage in recognition and uptake of *Plasmodium*-derived antigens expressed by parasitized red blood cells. To promote their co-localization, DCs secrete chemokines (e.g. CCL2 and IL-8) that recruit circulating NK cells to the site of infection. (*2*) Following antigen uptake, DCs and NK cells participate in bi-directional cross-talk that results in reciprocal activation. (*3*) DC-derived IL-15 promotes NK cell expansion and survival. (*4*) Other immunoregulatory cytokines, namely IL-2, IL-12 and IFN-γ, produced by mature DCs stimulate NK cell effector function such as cytotoxicity and cytokine production. (*5*) The production of the pro-inflammatory cytokines TNF-α and IFN-γ induces further maturation, expansion and migration of DCs

production by NK cells appears to correlate with host resistance, since DCs from genetically susceptible A/J mice induced NK cells to secrete high levels of IL-10, but only very low amounts of IFN-γ, compared with DCs from resistant C57BL/6 or H-2ᵃ congenic B10.A mice (R. Ing and M.M. Stevenson, unpublished observations). Given the importance of DC-derived IL-12 for induction of Th1-type responses and IL-15 for NK cell development, the relative contributions of IL-12 and IL-15 for DC responses and interactions with NK cells during blood-stage malaria were further delineated. Our unpublished studies showed that although IL-15 is important for NK cell function and can enhance DC cytokine production, IL-12 is necessary for up-regulated expression of co-stimulatory molecules and IFN-γ production by splenic CD11c$^+$ DCs during *P. chabaudi* AS infection. Importantly, IL-12, but not IL-15, is critically required for DC-mediated IFN-γ production by NK cells, whereas the role of IL-15 in DC–NK cell interactions is likely to promote NK cell growth and survival and to provide adjuvant support for IFN-γ production. Therefore, during the early innate immune response to blood-stage malaria, DCs may interact with NK cells through an IL-12-dependent mechanism to promote development of protective Th1-type immunity.

4.6
Cytokine Production by APC

A coordinated network of cytokine responses tightly regulates the innate immune response to infection in mice. DC-derived IL-15 stimulates DCs and macrophages to secrete IL-12 and IFN-γ [115], which in turn enables these cells to become further activated via a positive autocrine feedback loop. The type 1 cytokines produced by APCs also activate NK cells, NKT cells, CD8$^+$ T cells, and γδ T cells to produce large amounts of IFN-γ, which is crucial for priming CD4$^+$ T cells toward Th1 cell differentiation and subsequent development of type 1 adaptive immune responses required for control of blood-stage parasitaemia [34, 102, 144]. Moreover, IL-2 and IL-15 have been to shown to enhance CD154 (CD40 ligand) expression by activated CD4$^+$ T cells, thus prolonging T-cell stimulation even in the absence of cognate interaction with CD40-expressing APCs [150]. Activated Th1 cells, in the later phase of blood-stage malaria, would result in additional IFN-γ production, further APC and NK cell activation, and B-cell differentiation into plasma cells secreting Th1-dependent antibody isotypes. Therefore, multiple signals released during parasite–APC interactions influence CD4$^+$ Th cell differentiation and activation of downstream immune responses.

In addition to their coordinated interactions, some cytokines produced during the innate immune response also perform distinct, non-redundant functions. IL-12 is crucial for the development of type 1 immune responses, mainly due to its potent ability to induce IFN-γ production and Th1 cell differentiation. Moreover, high systemic IL-12 production and up-regulated expression of IL-12Rβ2, the receptor subunit mediating IL-12 signalling, correlate with resistance to *P. chabaudi* AS malaria [136]. IL-15, on the other hand, is important for NK cell development and function, and IL-15 has been shown to synergize with IL-12 to promote IFN-γ production and Th1 cell development. However, mice deficient in IL-15 show only slightly higher susceptibility during the chronic stage of *P. chabaudi* AS, suggesting that IL-15 probably plays a supporting but limited role in protective immunity to blood-stage malaria [74]. As discussed above, IL-15 functions mainly as a survival and proliferation factor for developing NK cells during both homeostasis and the immune response to infection [30, 74, 112, 128] The production of IFN-γ by APCs might effectively jump-start Th1 cell development by inducing autocrine APC activation as well as by priming commitment of other innate immune cells and CD4+ T cells toward type 1 responses. Although multiple cytokines may result in Th1 cell development, IFN-γ is considered to be the central effector cytokine mediating protective immunity to blood-stage malaria infection [160, 163].

5
Innate Immunity to *Plasmodium* Blood-Stage Infection in Humans

Innate immune responses are important for the control of initial parasitaemia both in rodents (see Sect. 4) and in humans [161]. These responses play a role not only in non-immune individuals infected for the first time but also in semi-immune individuals who may be infected with parasite variants they had not encountered before, necessitating the development of a new adaptive immune response. However, pre-existing memory T and B cells to conserved antigens may rapidly be activated and shift the cytokine environment in which innate and adaptive immune responses evolve.

5.1
Dendritic Cells

To date only very few studies have analysed the function of human DCs ex vivo in acutely infected individuals or in vitro using laboratory lines of infected red blood cells. Phenotypic analysis of DCs from patients who suffer from acute falciparum malaria gives some indication of DC function in vivo. In paraffin-fixed spleen sections from Vietnamese patients who died of falciparum malaria, we observed that myeloid DCs accumulate in the red pulp and in the marginal zone but not in the white pulp and T-cell areas. Furthermore, we noted a remarkable down-regulation of HLA DR molecules on myeloid cells, including cordal macrophages and DCs, but not sinusoidal lining cells [175]. This is in agreement with the observation that HLA DR expression is reduced on myeloid DCs in Kenyan children and Vietnamese adults suffering from acute malaria ([173] and B.C. Urban, unpublished observations).

Modulation of DC function by infected erythrocytes was also observed in vitro. Using monocyte-derived DCs, we have shown that CD36-adherent *P. fal-*

ciparum-infected erythrocytes or antibodies against CD36 modulate DC maturation and function [172, 174]. Parasite-modulated DCs fail to up-regulate the expression of MHC, co-stimulatory and adhesion molecules, fail to secrete IL-12 and to activate T cells but secrete IL-10 and TNF-α in response to stimulation with LPS, CD40-ligand, TNF-α or monocyte-conditioned medium ([172] and B.C. Urban, unpublished observations). Subsequently, both naïve and memory T cells co-cultured with parasite-modulated DCs are functionally unresponsive with respect to proliferation and secretion of IL-2. It has also been observed that differentiation of monocytes which have phagocytosed haemozoin have impaired differentiation into DCs and an impaired response to maturation signals [149]. Impairment was accompanied by increased expression of the peroxisome proliferator-activated receptor-γ, the up-regulation of which is known to interfere with DC maturation [5, 109]. The effect on differentiation of monocytes appears to be mediated by the same biochemical processes as haemozoin-induced changes in monocyte function (see Sect. 5.2).

Interestingly, a recent study on the frequency of DCs in peripheral blood from adults suffering from mild or severe falciparum malaria reported that the frequency of plasmacytoid DCs was reduced while the plasma levels of IFN-α were increased in individuals with both complicated and uncomplicated malaria [126]. In addition, this study demonstrated that mature schizonts and lysate thereof induced the expression of CD86, but not CD40, and the secretion of IFN-α by plasmacytoid DCs in vitro. Plasmacytoid DCs co-cultured with schizont lysate subsequently activated γδ T cells (see Sect. 5.5). These responses appear to be due to a soluble ligand of TLR9 in schizont lysate.

There are several possible explanations for the discrepancy between findings of functional DC responses observed in mice infected with some *Plasmodium* strains and those of studies with isolates of the human parasite, *P. falciparum*, and in one report of *P. yoelii* infection in mice, which were observed to inhibit LPS-induced DC maturation and stimulation of T-cell responses (Table 1). Following stimulation with LPS, DCs may enter a refractory period during which maturation and pro-inflammatory responses are down-regulated even in the presence of malarial antigens, as discussed by Stevenson and Riley [161]. Alternatively, DC maturation may be delayed, as discussed by Pouniotis et al. [127]. Furthermore, LPS is know to induce DC maturation without CD40 ligation, which has been shown to be required for maximal expression of a mature DC phenotype and cytokine production [41, 162]. It is also possible that *P. falciparum* may affect DC function through cytoadhesion via CD36 [172, 174]. Such a mechanism of immune evasion has not been observed with rodent *Plasmodium* species and may represent an

Table 1 Dendritic cell function in different models of *Plasmodium* infection

Model	Parasite	Assay	DC	Outcome	Reference
Human	*P. falciparum*	In vitro	mono-DC	Haemozoin modulates differentiation of monocytes to immature DC and subsequent maturation in response to LPS	149
Human	*P. falciparum*	Ex vivo	pDC	Schizont lysate activates pDC to secrete IFN-α, dependent on TLR9	126
				pDC frequency reduced in adults during acute malaria	
Human	*P. falciparum*	In vitro	mono-DC	Intact infected iRBC modulate DC maturation in response to LPS	172
				iRBC-modulated DC fail to secret IL-12 but produce TNF-α and IL-10	
				iRBC-modulated DC are poor stimulators of primary and secondary T-cell responses	
Human	*P. falciparum*	Ex vivo	pDC/mDC	Peripheral blood DC show reduced expression levels of HLA DR in children with acute malaria	173
Mouse	*P. chabaudi* AS	In vitro	bmDC	Schizonts directly induce DC maturation and secretion of TNF-α, IL-12 and IL-6	145
Mouse	*P. chabaudi* AS	In vivo	Splenic CD11c+	DC migrate from marginal zone into white pulp as early as day 5 after infection	89
				Surface expression of CD54, CD40 and CD86 increases from day 5 to day 7 after infection but returns to near pre-infection levels on day 9 for CD54 and CD86[a]	

Table 1 (continued)

Model	Parasite	Assay	DC	Outcome	Reference
Mouse	*P. yoelii* 17XNL	In vitro	bmDC	Intact iRBC co-cultured with DC inhibit maturation and subsequent T cell activation	114
	P. chabaudi AS *P. yoelii* YM	In vitro/ ex vivo	bmDC	Transfer of iRBC-pulsed DC into mice and subsequent blood-stage challenge with a lethal dose induce protection from death to homologous and heterologous strains	127
Mouse	*P. yoelii* 17X	Ex vivo	Splenic CD11c+	DC isolated from spleen on day 6 during acute malaria infection stimulate production of IL-2, IFN-γ and TNF-α in naïve and iRBC-specific T cells[b]	124
Mouse	*P. yoelii* YM	In vitro	bmDC	DC co-cultured with iRBC do not mature in response to LPS	127
	P. yoelii 17XNL	Ex vivo	Splenic CD11c+	DC show reduced surface expression of MHC and co-stimulatory molecules on day 7 after infection and fail to respond to LPS[c]	114
	P. yoelii 17XNL	In vitro/ in vivo	bmDC	DC co-cultured with iRBC suppress liver stage CD8+ T-cell responses when transferred into mice 7 days after immunization with irradiated sporozoites	114

mono-DC, human monocyte derived DC; pDC, human plasmacytoid DC; mDC, human myeloid DC; bmDC, mouse bone marrow-derived DC; iRBC, infected red blood cell

[a] Blood-stage infection induced with 10^5 infected red blood cells

[b] Blood-stage infection inoculation rate not known, parasitaemia on day 6:13%

[c] Blood-stage infection induced with 4×10^6 infected red blood cells

important difference between human and rodent malaria species. In studies with *P. falciparum*, DCs are usually derived from human peripheral blood cells and exposed to the parasite in vitro. Under such conditions, DCs develop and interact with *P. falciparum* in the absence of the cytokine milieu provided by NK cells, T cells, and other cell types normally present in vivo in the tissue microenvironment that support and promote DC maturation.

5.2
Monocytes/Macrophages

In vitro studies suggest that monocytes produce TNF-α within 24 h of exposure to live mature infected red blood cells in the presence of $\gamma\delta$ T cells [64, 143]. Furthermore, binding to CD36 expressed on monocytes and macrophages mediates non-opsonic phagocytosis of infected red blood cells, which is directly correlated with the expression level of CD36, but this interaction does not result in increased TNF-α secretion [147]. However, CD36-mediated phagocytosis leads to the accumulation of haemozoin in monocytes and macrophages. Haemozoin is the crystallized form of haeme, a by-product resulting from digestion of haemoglobin by the parasite in the red blood cell. When mature schizonts rupture, haemozoin, together with other debris, is released into the circulation and rapidly taken up by neutrophils and monocytes. In children and adults, the amount of pigment in peripheral blood monocytes is a marker for disease severity and, due to its long persistence, a marker for recent infection [32, 95, 111]. Haemozoin is not biochemically inert but reacts with membrane phospholipids and is transformed into hydroxy-polyunsaturated fatty acids, which cause membrane peroxidation. In addition, haemozoin catalysis induces the formation of prostaglandin PGE_2 and PGF_{2a}. While hydroxy-polyunsaturated fatty acids inhibit monocyte function such as phagocytosis, activation by inflammatory cytokines and generation of an oxidative burst, the release of PGE_2 and PGF_{2a} either by trophozoites or by monocytes, which have ingested pigment and/or trophozoites, alters T- and B-cell functions. Thus, haemozoin is directly as well as indirectly associated with the alteration of cellular responses observed during acute falciparum malaria.

5.3
NK Cells

NK cells are the earliest cells producing IFN-γ after encounter with live infected red blood cells in vitro [7]. Not surprisingly, IL-12 and to a certain extent IL-18 are critical for NK cell activation and IFN-γ production. Activated NK cells can kill *P. falciparum*-infected red blood cells; a study on experimentally infected volunteers reported elevated levels of granzyme A and B in peripheral blood just before infected red blood cells could be detected and before the onset of fever [65, 116]. Interestingly, recent reports by Artavanis-Tsakonas et al. [8] suggest that activation of NK cells is dependent on contact with infected red blood cells but varies between individuals. The same authors suggest that infected red blood cells may bind to the polymorphic KIR receptor family and lectin-like receptors CD94//NKG2A.

5.4
NKT Cells

The role of NKT cells in human falciparum malaria has not yet been studied in detail. Like NK cells, they are among the earliest producers of IFN-γ when exposed to live infected red blood cells, although activation occurs slightly later [9]. CD4$^+$ NKT cells produce not only IFN-γ but also large amounts of IL-4 and a subset of CD8α$^+$ NKT cells has cytolytic activity [68]. *P. falciparum* products which activate NKT cells are not known. However, work in mice infected with *P. berghei* ANKA suggests that malarial GPI presented by CD1d provides an activating stimulus for these cells [59, 60].

5.5
γδ T Cells

γδ T cells follow a similar kinetic profile as NKT cells and are rapidly activated by live infected red blood cells [178]. During acute malarial disease, the frequency of activated peripheral blood γδ T cells is increased and a further increase occurs after onset of chemotherapy [73]. γδ T cells inhibit the growth of infected red blood cells in vitro in a contact-dependent interaction, although the specific receptor–ligand interactions are not yet known [170]. A recent study suggests that γδ T cells secrete granulysin which acts on late-stage mature infected red blood cells or merozoites without lysing the cells [44, 72]. The dramatic increase in γδ T cells during recovery from acute falciparum malaria suggests that they might have an additional role in immunoregulation and the resolution of inflammation.

Interestingly, Hviid and colleagues [72] demonstrated that the frequency of CD3$^+$ cells expressing the γδ-TCR is over twice as high in healthy adults residing in Ghana compared to a similar Danish population. As many as half or more of the γδ T cells obtained from healthy Ghanaians, in general, and from children, in particular, express the Vδ1 chain as part of the TCR [72]. Most peripheral T cells from healthy Caucasians in contrast express a γδ-TCR composed of Vγ9 and Vδ2. It was not possible to formally exclude a relationship between the frequencies of either γδ-TCR$^+$ or Vδ1$^+$ T cells and HIV infection in this study, as HIV tests were not carried out as part of the clinical profiling of the subjects.

5.6
Cytokines

When analysing plasma cytokine levels or cytokines produced by peripheral blood mononuclear cells (PBMCs) from individuals acutely ill with malaria, one has to bear in mind that this approach can only give a rough indication of the processes occurring in the spleen and lymph nodes. The subjects under investigation in different studies are not necessarily comparable because they often differ in age and exposure to malaria. Infected individuals present at different times after initial infection or at the onset of symptoms. Furthermore, infection can occur on different backgrounds of pre-existing chronic infection. It is, therefore, not surprising that reports on plasma cytokine levels often seem to be contradictory, although parasitaemia and pigment in peripheral blood monocytes can give some indication of the history of infection within an individual.

Priming of T cells is dependent on IL-12 and mature, myeloid DCs are the main, if not sole, producer of this important immunoregulatory cytokine. In individuals experimentally infected with *P. falciparum*, low levels of IL-12 p40, one of two subunits of the biologically active IL-12 p70 molecule, can be detected in plasma 1 day before the volunteers become slide positive for infected erythrocytes, suggesting that DCs produce this cytokine early during blood-stage infection [65]. Many studies in children suffering from acute malaria readily detected IL-12 in plasma [93]. In these studies, IL-12 production was negatively associated with parasitaemia and tended to be lower in children suffering from severe disease. IL-18 is produced by activated macrophages and mature myeloid DCs. Like IL-12, IL-18 plasma levels were observed in several studies to be raised consistently in children suffering from acute malaria and correlate with disease severity but not with parasitaemia [98, 107, 168].

IL-12 and IL-18 are critical for the activation of NK and NKT cells to produce IFN-γ, although this cytokine can also be produced by monocytes and T cells later in infection. IFN-γ production was observed to be higher in children with mild disease than in children suffering from severe disease [92], and is associated with a reduced risk of subsequent presentation with malaria fever and a longer time to reinfection [39, 92]. However, other studies have reported that individuals suffering from severe disease have higher circulating plasma concentrations of IFN-γ, and PBMC from malaria immune donors produce less of this cytokine in vitro in response to live infected red blood cells [24, 130, 132]. By contrast, plasma levels of IL-10 generally seem to increase with increasing parasitaemia [71]. Some studies report that the concentration of IL-10 is much higher in children with severe malaria [93, 123] or symptomatic malaria [75], and in adults who died with falciparum malaria [33]. However, in the latter study, a high level of IL-6 and low level of IL-10 appeared to be equally devastating. The ratio of IFN-γ to IL-10 produced by PBMC stimulated with schizont extract is also higher in individuals from non-endemic or low-endemic regions. Results from all of these studies emphasize that cytokines, and particularly IFN-γ and IL-10, can have both detrimental and beneficial effects on the host's ability to cope with infection and combat disease.

6
Linking Innate and Adaptive Immune Responses

Both innate and adaptive immune responses are critical for establishing clinical immunity and control of parasitaemia to infection with *P. falciparum*. How then do these two arms work together both during the first infection and in subsequent infections? Early in infection, when parasitaemia is still low, both plasmacytoid and myeloid DCs may be activated directly by intact infected red blood cells or indirectly by their products, then mature and secrete IFN-α, IL-12 or TNF-α (Fig. 3). These cytokines support activation of NK cells, which produce the first wave of IFN-γ. Host genotype might determine whether a direct interaction of NK cells and infected red blood cells occurs, setting the first threshold for the level of IFN-γ production [9]. IFN-γ-induced activation of monocytes and macrophages could enhance non-opsonic phagocytosis of infected red blood cells as well as intraerythrocytic killing of the parasites via NO production, although the actual role of NO during malaria remains unresolved. Mature DCs and activated monocytes/macrophages may present parasite antigens to naïve and primed T cells, respectively, and within this inflammatory cytokine environment promote Th1 polarization of CD4$^+$ T cells. However, with increasing parasitaemia, monocytes/macrophages and DCs may become paralysed by the ingestion of malaria pigment. In addition, DCs may be modulated in the marginal zone of the spleen through adhesion of infected red blood cells via CD36. Subsequent production of IL-10, and possibly TGF-β, may counteract the initial pro-inflammatory cytokine cascade and shift the balance towards an anti-inflammatory response. Nevertheless, IL-10 is an important growth factor for B cells and may promote B-cell survival and differentiation, eventually leading to class switching towards cytophilic IgG1 and IgG3. Once humoral immune responses to the infecting parasite variant

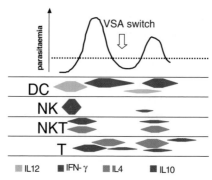

Fig.3 Hypothetical scenario of the possible sequence of leucocyte activation during the course of a self-limiting, mild *Plasmodium* blood-stage infection. Early in infection, DCs are activated, produce IL-12 and interact with NK cells and NKT cells, which in turn produce large amounts of IFN-γ (*NK*) and IFN-γ/IL-4 (*NKT*). CD4[+] T-cell activation by DCs occurs on the background of high levels of IFN-γ resulting in Th1 cell deviation. Activated T cells induce B-cell responses and the humoral immune response together with the growth-inhibiting effect of γδ T cells and increased opsonic phagocytosis of infected red blood cells by monocytes eventually leads to reduction in parasitaemia. In parallel with increasing parasitaemia, ingestion of haemozoin paralyses monocyte function and DC maturation, and in the case of *P. falciparum* infection, cytoadhesion of infected red blood cells to DCs modulates their function. Together, these events lead to reduced IL-12 and increased IL-10 secretion. IL-10 inhibits the effect of IFN-γ and TNF-α on other cells. When infected red blood cells switch surface expression of a different variant surface antigen (*Plasmodium* species infecting rodents have variant surface antigens although they do not seem to mediate cytoadhesion as is the case for *P. falciparum*), a second wave of infected red blood cells multiply. Activation of DCs, NK cells and NKT cells now occurs on a background of increased levels of IL-10 which counteract the effect of IFN-γ. Some DCs may still prime CD4[+] T-cell responses although they are now predominantly of a Th2 phenotype and parasite-modulated DCs may also induce regulatory T cells

are established, control of parasitaemia seems much more likely. However, antigenic variation of surface proteins such as PfEMP-1, which allows the parasite to escape the newly established immune response, initiates this scenario all over again, although on a quite different level of cellular activation and cytokine equilibrium.

Why then do some children cope with infection while others succumb to severe disease and why does immunity to severe disease occur relatively quickly, while cerebral malaria is experienced only after repeated exposure? In addition to differences in exposure and transmission rates in different endemic regions, it is likely that the genetic make-up of the host plays a role as already described for the activation of NK cells. It is well established that polymorphisms in red blood cell proteins are the most important factors protecting against severe malarial disease [179]. However, many polymorphisms in immune response genes such as MHC alleles as well as in the TNF-α and IL-12 promoters have been described and are associated with either protection or susceptibility to severe disease [67]. In addition, polymorphisms in adhesion molecules, such as CD36, CD35, ICAM-1 and CD31, may influence the degree of sequestration and vessel occlusion linked with organ-specific pathology [67].

One other factor influencing the outcome in humans, but often neglected when considering the heterogeneity of cellular immune responses to infected red blood cells, is the adhesion phenotype of the infecting parasite variant. The recent completion of the entire genome sequence of the laboratory *P. falciparum* line 3D7 allowed detailed analysis of its 59 *var* genes [52]. Despite considerable sequence heterogeneity, these *var* genes can be sub-grouped into different families according to their length and number of domains, their ability to bind to CD36, and their upstream 5'-prime promoter sequences (ups) [82, 88, 151, 152]. Thus, *var* genes with a type A ups tend not to bind to CD36, and are relatively long with more than five domains, while *var* genes with a type B or type C ups are more likely to bind to CD36, and are usually smaller and composed of five domains.

Although most studies on cytoadhesion of isolates from patients with acute malaria reported binding to CD36, with isolates from patients suffering from severe disease showing lower avidity for CD36 than isolates from patients with mild disease, lack of binding to CD36 has also been observed [11, 110, 133, 169]. Laboratory lines selected with acute immune serum from children experiencing severe malaria showed reduced adhesion to CD36 and preferentially expressed *var* genes with type A ups [77, 79, 157]. Furthermore, children with severe malaria carrying the 188G allele of CD36 [3, 119] were more likely to be infected with parasites expressing commonly recognized variant surface antigens, suggesting that adhesion to CD36 selects against their expression (P. Bull, manuscript submitted). Although these later data are based on experiments with very few parasite isolates, together they indicate that the immune status of the host and CD36 adhesion may influence selection of *var* genes expressed on field isolates.

It is conceivable that the ability of infected red blood cells to adhere to CD36 expressed on myeloid cells such as monocytes/macrophages and DCs may alter the immune response by modulating DC maturation, promoting secretion of anti-inflammatory cytokines, and inducing T-cell anergy. This scenario may still provide growth factors for B-cell differentiation into plasma cells but may not provide sufficient T-cell help, such as CD40 cross-linking, for the generation of long-lasting memory B cells. In a semi-immune host, parasites with immunomodulatory capacity as determined by their avidity for CD36 may have an advantage in that they can establish chronic infection. Clearly, the link between *var* gene expression, avidity for CD36, and immune responses needs to be established on a large number of samples from children with different degrees of malarial disease and asymptomatic infection. This issue is now under active investigation.

7
Strategies for Vaccine Development Based on Innate Immunity

Recent and compelling evidence reviewed here provides strong support for the importance of the cells comprising the innate immune system to shape the subsequent adaptive immune response to blood-stage malaria. Given the urgent need to develop an effective malaria vaccine to relieve the growing malaria burden, it is important that full consideration be directed to data emerging from studies of innate immunity to infection with blood-stage *Plasmodium* parasites conducted in both mice and humans. Field trials evaluating the efficacy of recombinant subunit vaccines based on protective antigens identified in the various stages of the *Plasmodium* life cycle, including the blood stage, have been disappointing leaving some to speculate that an effective malaria vaccine remains elusive.

Because of the plasticity associated with the response of many cell types of the innate immune system [70], a possible strategy for enhancing the immunogenicity of recombinant malaria antigens may be the inclusion of microbial products, recombinant cytokines, or synthetic compounds that activate innate immunity. Although the development of new adjuvants is an important area of research, many vaccine formulations still rely upon alum (aluminium hydroxide) as an adjuvant. This may be due to the fact that alum is one of few adjuvants approved for human use even though it is clear that this agent stimulates a type 2 immune response characterized by high levels of IgG1 in mice and an inability to induce macrophage activation or cytotoxic T-cell responses [166]. In contrast, microbial products, such as unmethylated CpG motifs recognized by TLR9, induce a type 1 pattern of cytokine production dominated by IL-12 and IFN-γ, with little secretion of type 2 cytokines [166]. CpG motifs have been found to be safe and useful as adjuvants for vaccines, including peptides vaccines, against various pathogens [166].

As reviewed in a recent publication [161], immunization with a combination of CpG oligodeoxynucleotides and the 19-kDa *P. yoelii* merozoite surface protein 1, recombinant MSP1$_{19}$, an important blood-stage vaccine candidate antigen, in alum resulted in a mixed Th1/Th2 cell response and improved vaccine efficacy. Recent studies by Su et al. [166] demonstrated that CpG motifs enhance the efficacy of a blood-stage vaccine in the model of *P. chabaudi* AS malaria in mice. In this study, the vaccine formulation consisted of a crude antigen preparation in alum. Furthermore, the type 1 pro-inflammatory cytokine IL-12 absorbed to alum was observed to enhance the efficacy of the same crude antigen vaccine by inducing a Th1 cell-mediated immune response [166]. Protection was found to be dependent on CD4$^+$ T cells, IFN-γ, and B cells and to be associated with high serum levels of malaria-specific IgG2a, the antibody subclass associated with a type 1 response. Other cytokines which regulate innate immune mechanisms involving DC and NK cells may potentially be useful for malaria vaccination and immunotherapy. On their own, early cytokines, such as IL-15, may not be critical for IFN-γ and antibody production. However, several in vitro and in vivo studies have provided intriguing results demonstrating the potential of IL-15 to function as an adjuvant in the induction of maximal IFN-γ and antibody responses [90, 117, 135]. As the mechanisms of innate immunity as well as the network of cytokines involved in the early response against blood-stage malaria parasites are delineated, additional factors will be identified which may have great potential as vaccine adjuvants.

8
Concluding Remarks

The cells comprising the innate immune system, namely, DCs, monocytes/macrophages, NK cells, NKT cells, and γδ T cells, play a fundamental role in shaping the adaptive immune response to blood-stage malaria. The most prominent result of the early interactions between *Plasmodium* parasites and the immune system appears to be the production of immunoregulatory cytokines, especially IL-12 and IFN-γ, which subsequently lead to the activation, in some cases bi-directional, of other cells of the innate immune system. These same cytokines, possibly amplified to higher concentrations during innate immunity, induce the activation of CD4$^+$ T cells and B cells that are ultimately required for the cell-mediated and antibody-dependent mechanism(s) leading to the control and resolution of infection. Innate immune responses are also likely to be necessary downstream for the generation of memory T-cell as well as B-cell responses leading to immunity against the clinical syndromes associated with malaria. Harnessing the information on innate immune responses to blood-stage malaria, which has recently been described in both *Plasmodium*-infected mice and humans, for the development of an effective malaria vaccine will require additional studies in several critical areas. These areas include the identification of host receptors and parasite ligands important in initiating these responses, the identification of host as well as parasite genetic factors influencing these responses, and the delineation of the network of cytokines involved in these responses. The information derived from studies on innate immunity to blood-stage malaria may also provide information for the development of novel immunotherapies to alleviate the tremendous burden of malaria in the developing world.

Acknowledgements B.C.U. holds a Career Development Fellowship in Basic Biomedical Research awarded by the Wellcome Trust. R.I. is supported by Studentships from the Department of Medicine and MUHCRI, McGill University. Support for the work in the laboratory of M.M.S. is provided by the Canadian Institutes of Health Research (MOP-14663 and MOP 57695) and the Fonds de recherche sur la nature et les technologies Québec. We thank Pete Bull, Sue Keyes, Paul Horrocks, Dragana Jankovic, Alan Sher, and Zhong Su for critical discussion. We gratefully acknowledge the assistance of M.F. Tam in the preparation of this manuscript.

References

1. Ahlborg N, Ling IT, Howard W, Holder AA, Riley EM (2002) Protective immune responses to the 42-kilodalton (kDa) region of *Plasmodium yoelii* merozoite surface protein 1 are induced by the C-terminal 19-kDa region but not by the adjacent 33-kDa region. Infect Immun 70:820–825
2. Ahvazi BC, Jacobs P, Stevenson MM (1995) Role of macrophage-derived nitric oxide in suppression of lymphocyte proliferation during blood-stage malaria. J Leukoc Biol 58:23–31
3. Aitman TJ, Cooper LD, Norsworthy PJ, Wahid FN, Gray JK, Curtis BR, McKeigue PM, Kwiatkowski D, Greenwood BM, Snow RW, Hill AV, Scott J (2000) Malaria susceptibility and CD36 mutation. Nature 405:1015–1016
4. Alli RS, Khar A (2004) Interleukin-12 secreted by mature dendritic cells mediates activation of NK cell function. FEBS Lett 559:71–76
5. Angeli V, Hammad H, Staels B, Capron M, Lambrecht BN, Trottein F (2003) Peroxisome proliferator-activated receptor gamma inhibits the migration of dendritic cells: consequences for the immune response. J Immunol 170:5295–5301
6. Angus BJ, Chotivanich K, Udomsangpetch R, White NJ (1997) In vivo removal of malaria parasites from red blood cells without their destruction in acute falciparum malaria. Blood 90:2037–2040
7. Artavanis-Tsakonas K, Riley EM (2002) Innate immune response to malaria: rapid induction of IFN-gamma from human NK cells by live *Plasmodium falciparum*-infected erythrocytes. J Immunol 169:2956–2963
8. Artavanis-Tsakonas K, Eleme K, McQueen KL, Cheng NW, Parham P, Davis DM, Riley EM (2003) Activation of a subset of human NK cells upon contact with *Plasmodium falciparum*-infected erythrocytes. J Immunol 171:5396–5405

9. Artavanis-Tsakonas K, Tongren JE, Riley EM (2003) The war between the malaria parasite and the immune system: immunity, immunoregulation and immunopathology. Clin Exp Immunol 133:145–152
10. Banchereau J, Briere F, Caux C, Davoust J, Lebecque S, Liu Y-J, Pulendran B, Palucka K (2000) Immunobiology of dendritic cells. Annu Rev Immunol 18:767–811
11. Beeson JG, Brown GV, Molyneux ME, Mhango C, Dzinjalamala F, Rogerson SJ (1999) *Plasmodium falciparum* isolates from infected pregnant women and children are associated with distinct adhesive and antigenic properties. J Infect Dis 180:464–472
12. Beeson JG, Rogerson SJ, Cooke BM, Reeder JC, Chai W, Lawson AM, Molyneux ME, Brown GV (2000) Adhesion of *Plasmodium falciparum*-infected erythrocytes to hyaluronic acid in placental malaria. Nat Med 6:86–90
13. Biron CA, Nguyen KB, Pien GC, Cousens LP, Salazar-Mather TP (1999) Natural killer cells in antiviral defense: function and regulation by innate cytokines. Ann Rev Immunol 17:71–76
14. Bruna-Romero O, Schmieg J, Del Val M, Buschle M, Tsuji M (2003) The dendritic cell-specific chemokine, dendritic cell-derived CC chemokine 1, enhances protective cell-mediated immunity to murine malaria. J Immunol 170:3195–3203
15. Bukowski JF, Morita CT, Brenner MB (1999) Human gamma delta T cells recognize alkylamines derived from microbes, edible plants, and tea: implications for innate immunity. Immunity 11:57–65
16. Bull PC, Lowe BS, Kortok M, Marsh K (1999) Antibody recognition of *Plasmodium falciparum* erythrocyte surface antigens in Kenya: evidence for rare and prevalent variants. Infect Immun 67:733–739
17. Bull PC, Kortok M, Kai O, Ndungu F, Ross A, Lowe BS, Newbold CI, Marsh K (2000) *Plasmodium falciparum*-infected erythrocytes: agglutination by diverse Kenyan plasma is associated with severe disease and young host age. J Infect Dis 182:252–259
18. Bull PC, Lowe BS, Kaleli N, Njuga F, Kortok M, Ross A, Ndungu F, Snow RW, Marsh K (2002) *Plasmodium falciparum* infections are associated with agglutinating antibodies to parasite-infected erythrocyte surface antigens among healthy Kenyan children. J Infect Dis 185:1688–1691
19. Carayannopoulos LN and Yokoyama WM (2004) Recognition of infected cells by natural killer cells. Curr Opin Immunol 16:26–33
20. Castriconi R, Della Chiesa M, Moretta A (2004) Shaping of adaptive immunity by innate interactions. C R Biol 327:533–537
21. Cavanagh DR, Elhassan IM, Roper C, Robinson VJ, Giha H, Holder AA, Hviid L, Theander TG, Arnot DE, McBride JS (1998) A longitudinal study of type-specific antibody responses to *Plasmodium falciparum* merozoite surface protein-1 in an area of unstable malaria in Sudan. J Immunol 161:347–359
22. Cella M, Jarrossay D, Facchetti F, Alebardi O, Nakajima H, Lanzavecchia A, Colonna M (1999) Plasmacytoid monocytes migrate to inflamed lymph nodes and produce large amounts of type I interferon. Nat Med 5:919–923
23. Chattopadhyay R, Sharma A, Srivastava VK, Pati SS, Sharma SK, Das BS, Chitnis CE (2003) *Plasmodium falciparum* Infection Elicits Both Variant-Specific and Cross-Reactive Antibodies against Variant Surface Antigens. Infect. Immun. 71:597–604

24. Chizzolini C, Grau GE, Geinoz A, Schrijvers D (1990) T lymphocyte interferon-gamma production induced by *Plasmodium falciparum* antigen is high in recently infected non-immune and low in immune subjects. Clin Exp Immunol 79:95–99

25. Chotivanich K, Udomsangpetch R, Dondorp A, Williams T, Angus B, Simpson JA, Pukrittayakamee S, Looareesuwan S, Newbold CI, White NJ (2000) The mechanisms of parasite clearance after antimalarial treatment of *Plasmodium falciparum* malaria. J Infect Dis 182:629–633

26. Chotivanich K, Udomsangpetch R, McGready R, Proux S, Newton P, Pukrittayakamee S, Looareesuwan S, White NJ (2002) Central role of the spleen in malaria parasite clearance. J Infect Dis 185:1538–1541

27. Choudhury HR, Sheikh NA, Bancroft GJ, Katz DR, de Souza JB (2000) Early non-specific immune response and immunity to blood-stage nonlethal *Plasmodium yoelii* malaria. Infect Immun 68:6127–6132

28. Colucci F, Caligiuri MA, Di Santo JP (2003) What does it take to make a natural killer? Nat Rev Immunol 3:413–425

29. Cooper MA, Fehniger TA, Turner SC, Chen KS, Ghaheri BA, Ghayur T, Carson WE, Caligiuri MA (2001) Human natural killer cells: a unique innate immunoregulatory role for the CD56[bright] subset. Blood 97:3146–3151

30. Cooper, MA, Bush JE, Fehniger TA, VanDeusen JB, Waite RE, Liu Y, Aguila HL, Caligiuri MA (2002) In vivo evidence for a dependence on interleukin 15 for survival of natural killer cells. Blood 100:3633–3638

31. Conway DJ, Cavanagh DR, Tanabe K, Roper C, Mikes ZS, Sakihama N, Bojang KA, Oduola AM, Kremsner PG, Arnot DE, Greenwood BM, McBride JS (2000) A principal target of human immunity to malaria identified by molecular population genetic and immunological analyses. Nat Med 6:689–692

32. Day N, Pham T, Phan T, Dinh X, Pham P, Lyy V, Tran T, Nguyen T, Bethell D, Nguyan H, Tran T, White N (1996) Clearance kinetics of parasites and pigment-containing leukocytes in severe malaria. Blood 88:4694–4700

33. Day NP, Hien TT, Schollaardt T, Loc PP, Chuong LV, Chau TT, Mai NT, Phu NH, Sinh DX, White NJ, Ho M (1999) The prognostic and pathophysiologic role of pro- and antiinflammatory cytokines in severe malaria. J Infect Dis 180:1288–1297

34. de Souza, JB, Williamson KH, Otani T, Playfair JH (1997) Early gamma interferon responses in lethal and nonlethal murine blood-stage malaria. Infect Immun 65(5): 1593–1598

35. de Souza JB, Riley EM (2002) Cerebral malaria: the contribution of studies in animals to our understanding of immunopathogenesis. Microbes Infect 4:297–300

36. Diebold SS, Montoya M, Unger H, Alexopoulou L, Roy P, Haswell LE, Al-Shamkhani A, Flavell R, Borrow P, Sousa CRe (2003) Viral infection switches non-plasmacytoid dendritic cells into high interferon producers. Nature 424:324–328

37. Dieli F, Troye-Blomberg M, Farouk SE, Sirecil G, Salerno A (2001) Biology of gammadelta T cells in tuberculosis and malaria. Curr Mol Med 1:437–446

38. Dodoo D, Theander TG, Kurtzhals JA, Koram K, Riley E, Akanmori BD, Nkrumah FK, Hviid L (1999) Levels of antibody to conserved parts of *Plasmodium falciparum* merozoite surface protein 1 in Ghanaian children are not associated with protection from clinical malaria. Infect Immun 67:2131–2137

39. Dodoo D, Omer FM, Todd J, Akanmori BD, Koram KA, Riley EM (2002) Absolute levels and ratios of proinflammatory and anti-inflammatory cytokine production in vitro predict clinical immunity to *Plasmodium falciparum* malaria. J Infect Dis 185:971–979

40. Dzionek A, Fuchs A, Schmidt P, Cremer S, Zysk M, Miltenyi S, Buck DW, Schmitz J (2000) BDCA-2, BDCA-3, and BDCA-4: Three markers for distinct subsets of dendritic cells in human peripheral blood. J Immunol 165:6037–6046

41. Edwards AD, Manickasingham SP, Sporri R, Diebold SS, Schulz O, Sher A, Kaisho T, Akira S, Reis e Sousa C (2002) Microbial recognition via Toll-like receptor-dependent and -independent pathways determines the cytokine response of murine dendritic cell subsets to CD40 triggering. J Immunol 169:3652–3660

42. Facchetti F, Candiago E, Vermi W (1999) Plasmacytoid monocytes express IL3-receptor alpha and differentiate into dendritic cells. Histopathology 35:88–89

43. Facchetti F, Vermi W, Mason D, Colonna M (2003) The plasmacytoid mono-cyte/interferon producing cells. Virchows Arch 443:703–717

44. Farouk SE, Mincheva-Nilsson L, Krensky AM, Dieli F, Troye-Blomberg M (2004) Gamma delta T cells inhibit in vitro growth of the asexual blood stages of *Plasmodium falciparum* by a granule exocytosis-dependent cytotoxic pathway that requires granulysin. Eur J Immunol 34:2248–2256

45. Ferlazzo G, Tsang ML, Moretta L, Melioli G, Steinman RM, Munz C (2002) Human dendritic cells activate resting natural killer (NK) cells and are recognized via the NKp30 receptor by activated NK cells. J Exp Med 195:343–351

46. Ferlazzo G, Morandi B, D'Agostino A, Meazza R, Melioli G, Moretta A, Moretta L (2003) The interaction between NK cells and dendritic cells in bacterial infections results in rapid induction of NK cell activation and in the lysis of uninfected dendritic cells. Eur J Immunol 33:306–313

47. Ferlazzo G, Munz C (2004) NK cell compartments and their activation by dendritic cells. J Immunol 172:1333–1339

48. Ferlazzo G, Thomas D, Lin S-L, Goodman K, Morandi B, Muller WA, Moretta A, Munz C (2004) The abundant NK cells in human secondary lymphoid tissues require activation to express killer cell Ig-like receptors and become cytolytic. J Immunol 172:1455–1462

49. Ferrick DA, King DP, Jackson KA, Braun RK, Tam S, Hyde DM, Beaman BL (2000) Intraepithelial gamma delta T lymphocytes: sentinel cells at mucosal barriers. Springer Semin Immunopathol 22:283–296

50. Fortin A, Stevenson MM, Gros P (2002) Susceptibility to malaria as a complex trait: huge pressure from a tiny creature. Hum Mol Genetics 11:2469–2478

51. Franks S, Baton L, Tetteh K, Tongren E, Dewin D, Akanmori BD, Koram KA, Ranford-Cartwright L, Riley EM (2003) Genetic diversity and antigenic polymorphism in *Plasmodium falciparum*: extensive serological cross-reactivity between allelic variants of merozoite surface protein 2. Infect Immun 71:3485–3495

52. Gardner MJ, Hall N, Fung E, White O, Berriman M, Hyman RW, Carlton JM, Pain A, Nelson KE, Bowman S, Paulsen IT, James K, Eisen JA, Rutherford K, Salzberg SL, Craig A, Kyes S, Chan MS, Nene V, Shallom SJ, Suh B, Peterson J, Angiuoli S, Pertea M, Allen J, Selengut J, Haft D, Mather MW, Vaidya AB, Martin DM, Fairlamb AH, Fraunholz MJ, Roos DS, Ralph SA, McFadden GI, Cummings LM, Subramanian GM, Mungall C, Venter JC, Carucci DJ, Hoffman SL, Newbold C, Davis RW, Fraser CM, Barrell B (2002) Genome sequence of the human malaria parasite *Plasmodium falciparum*. Nature 419:498–511

53. Gerosa F, Baldani-Guerra B, Nisii C, Marchesini V, Carra G, Trinchieri G (2002) Reciprocal activating interaction between natural killer cells and dendritic cells. J Exp Med 195:327–333

54. Godfrey DI, MacDonald HR, Kronenberg M, Smyth MJ, Van Kaer L (2004) NKT cells: what's in a name? Nat Rev Immunol 4:231–237

55. Gordon S (1998) The role of the macrophage in immune regulation. Res Immunol 149:685–688

56. Gordon S (2003) Alternative activation of macrophages. Nat Rev Immunol 3:23–35

57. Granucci F, Zanoni I, Pavelka N, Van Dommelen SL, Andoniou CE, Belardelli F, Degli Esposti MA, Ricciardi-Castagnoli P (2004) A contribution of mouse dendritic cell-derived IL-2 for NK cell activation. J Exp Med 200:287–295

58. Gupta S, Snow RW, Donnelly CA, Marsh K, Newbold C (1999) Immunity to non-cerebral severe malaria is acquired after one or two infections. Nat Med 5:340–343

59. Hansen DS, Siomos MA, Buckingham L, Scalzo AA, Schofield L (2003) Regulation of murine cerebral malaria pathogenesis by CD1d-restricted NKT cells and the natural killer complex. Immunity 18:391–402

60. Hansen DS, Siomos MA, De Koning-Ward T, Buckingham L, Crabb BS, Schofield L (2003) CD1d-restricted NKT cells contribute to malarial splenomegaly and enhance parasite-specific antibody responses. Eur J Immunol 33:2588–2598

61. Hayakawa Y, Screpanti V, Yagita H, Grandien A, Ljunggren HG, Smyth MJ, Chambers BJ (2004) NK cell TRAIL eliminates immature dendritic cells in vivo and limits dendritic cell vaccination efficacy. J Immunol 172:123–129

62. Hayday AC (2000) Gamma delta cells: a right time and a right place for a conserved third way of protection. Annu Rev Immunol 18:975–1026

63. Hedges JF, Graff JC, Jutila MA (2003) Transcriptional profiling of gamma delta T cells. J Immunol 171:4959–4964

64. Hensmann M, Kwiatkowski D (2001) Cellular basis of early cytokine response to *Plasmodium falciparum*. Infect Immun 69:2364–2371

65. Hermsen CC, Konijnenberg Y, Mulder L, Loe C, van Deuren M, van der Meer JW, van Mierlo GJ, Eling WM, Hack CE, Sauerwein RW (2003) Circulating concentrations of soluble granzyme A and B increase during natural and experimental *Plasmodium falciparum* infections. Clin Exp Immunol 132:467–472

66. Heufler C, Koch F, Stanzl U, Topar G, Wysocka M, Trinchieri G, Enk A, Steinman RM, Romani N, Schuler G (1996) Interleukin-12 is produced by dendritic cells and mediates T helper 1 development as well as interferon-gamma production by T helper 1 cells. Eur J Immunol 26:659–668

67. Hill AV (2001) The genomics and genetics of human infectious disease susceptibility. Annu Rev Genomics Hum Genet 2:373–400

68. Ho LP, Urban BC, Jones L, Ogg GS, McMichael AJ (2004) CD4-CD8alphaalpha subset of CD1d-restricted NKT cells controls T cell expansion. J Immunol 172:7350–7358

69. Horrocks P, Pinches R, Christodoulou Z, Kyes SA, Newbold CI (2004) Variable var transition rates underlie antigenic variation in malaria. Proc Natl Acad Sci U S A 101:11129–11134

70. Huang Q, Liu D, Majewski P, Schulte LC, Korn JM, Young RA, Lander ES, Hacohen N. (2001) The plasticity of dendritic cell response to pathogens and their components. Science 294:870–875

71. Hugosson E, Montgomery SM, Premji Z, Troye-Blomberg M, Bjorkman A (2004) Higher IL-10 levels are associated with less effective clearance of *Plasmodium falciparum* parasites. Parasite Immunol 26:111–117

72. Hviid L, Akanmori BD, Loizon S, Kurtzhals JA, Ricke CH, Lim A, Koram KA, Nkrumah FK, Mercereau-Puijalon O, Behr C (2000) High frequency of circulating gamma delta T cells with dominance of the v(delta)1 subset in a healthy population. Int Immunol 12:797–805

73. Hviid L, Kurtzhals JAL, Adabayeri V, Loizon S, Kemp K, Goka BQ, Lim A, Mercereau-Puijalon O, Akanmori BD, Behr C (2001) Perturbation and proinflammatory type activation of Vδ1+γδ T cells in african children with *Plasmodium falciparum* malaria. Infect. Immun. 69:3190–3196

74. Ing R, Gros P, Stevenson MM (2004) Interleukin 15 enhances innate and adaptive immune responses to blood-stage malaria infection in mice. (submitted)

75. Jakobsen PH, McKay V, N'Jie R, Olaleye BO, D'Alessandro U, Bendtzen K, Schousboe I, Greenwood BM (1996) Soluble products of inflammatory reactions are not induced in children with asymptomatic *Plasmodium falciparum* infections. Clin Exp Immunol 105:69–73

76. Jaramillo M, Plante I, Ouellet N, Vandal K, Tessier PA, Olivier M (2004) Hemozoin-inducible proinflammatory events in vivo: potential role in malaria infection. J Immunol 172:3101–3110

77. Jensen AT, Magistrado P, Sharp S, Joergensen L, Lavstsen T, Chiucchiuini A, Salanti A, Vestergaard LS, Lusingu JP, Hermsen R, Sauerwein R, Christensen J, Nielsen MA, Hviid L, Sutherland C, Staalsoe T, Theander TG (2004) *Plasmodium falciparum* associated with severe childhood malaria preferentially expresses PfEMP1 encoded by group A var genes. J Exp Med 199:1179–1190

78. Jinushi M, Takehara T, Tatsumi T, Kanto T, Groh V, Spies T, Suzuki T, Miyagi T, Hayashi N (2003) Autocrine/paracrine IL-15 that is required for type I IFN-mediated dendritic cell expression of MHC class I-related chain A and B is impaired in hepatitis C virus infection. J Immunol 171:5423–5429

79. Kaestli M, Cortes A, Lagog M, Ott M, Beck HP (2004) Longitudinal assessment of *Plasmodium falciparum* var gene transcription in naturally infected asymptomatic children in Papua New Guinea. J Infect Dis 189:1942–1951

80. Kinyanjui SM, Bull P, Newbold CI, Marsh K (2003) Kinetics of antibody responses to *Plasmodium falciparum*-infected erythrocyte variant surface antigens. J Infect Dis 187:667–674

81. Kohrgruber N, Halanek N, Groger M, Winter D, Rappersberger K, Schmitt-Egenolf M, Stingl G, Maurer D (1999) Survival, maturation, and function of CD11c- and CD11c+ peripheral blood dendritic cells are differentially regulated by cytokines. J Immunol 163:3250–3259

82. Kraemer SM, Smith JD (2003) Evidence for the importance of genetic structuring to the structural and functional specialization of the *Plasmodium falciparum* var gene family. Mol Microbiol 50:1527–1538

83. Krug A, Towarowski A, Britsch S, Rothenfusser S, Hornung V, Bals R, Giese T, Engelmann H, Endres S, Krieg AM, Hartmann G (2001) Toll-like receptor expression reveals CpG DNA as a unique microbial stimulus for plasmacytoid dendritic cells which synergizes with CD40 ligand to induce high amounts of IL-12. Eur J Immunol 31:3026–3037

84. Kyes S, Horrocks P, Newbold C (2001) Antigenic variation at the infected red cell surface in malaria. Annu Rev Microbiol 55:673–707

85. Langhorne J, Morris-Jones S, Casabo LG, Goodier M (1994) The response of γδ T cells in malaria infections Res Immunol 145:429–436

86. Langhorne J, Quin SJ, Sanne LA (2002) Mouse models of blood-stage malaria infections: immune responses and cytokines involved in protection and pathology. Chcm Immunol 80:204–228

87. Lauwerys BR, Garot N, Renauld J-C, Houssiau FA (2000) Cytokine production and killer activity of NK/T-NK cells derived with IL-2, IL-15, or the combination of IL-12 and IL-18. J Immunol 165:1847–1853

88. Lavstsen T, Salanti A, Jensen AT, Arnot DE, Theander TG (2003) Sub-grouping of *Plasmodium falciparum* 3D7 var genes based on sequence analysis of coding and non-coding regions. Malar J 2:27

89. Leisewitz AL, Rockett KA, Gumede B, Jones M, Urban B, Kwiatkowski DP (2004) Response of the splenic dendritic cell population to malaria infection. Infect Immun 72:4233–4239

90. Litinskiy MB, Nardelli B,, Hilbert DM, He B, Schaffer A, Casali P, Cerutti A. (2002) DCs induce CD40-independent immunoglobulin class switching through BlyS and APRIL. Nat Immunol 3:822–829

91. Loza MJ, Perussia B (2001) Final steps of natural killer cell maturation: a model for type1-type2 differentiation. Nat Immunol 2(10): 917–924

92. Luty AJ, Lell B, Schmidt-Ott R, Lehman LG, Luckner D, Greve B, Matousek P, Herbich K, Schmid D, Migot-Nabias F, Deloron P, Nussenzweig RS, Kremsner PG (1999) Interferon-gamma responses are associated with resistance to reinfection with *Plasmodium falciparum* in young African children. J Infect Dis 179:980–988

93. Luty AJ, Perkins DJ, Lell B, Schmidt-Ott R, Lehman LG, Luckner D, Greve B, Matousek P, Herbich K, Schmid D, Weinberg JB, Kremsner PG (2000) Low interleukin-12 activity in severe *Plasmodium falciparum* malaria. Infect Immun 68:3909–3915

94. Luyendyk J, Olivas OR, Ginger LA, Avery AC (2002) Antigen-presenting cell function during *Plasmodium yoelii* infection. Infect Immun 70:2941–2949

95. Lyke KE, Diallo DA, Dicko A, Kone A, Coulibaly D, Guindo A, Cissoko Y, Sangare L, Coulibaly S, Dakuo B, Taylor TE, Doumbo OK, Plowe CV (2003) Association of the intraleukocytic *Plasmodium falciparum* malaria pigment with disease severity, clinical manifestations, and prognosis in severe malaria. Am J Trop Med Hyg 69:253–259

96. Mahnke K, Qian Y, Knop J, Enk AH (2003) Induction of CD4+/CD25+ regulatory T cells by targeting of antigens to immature dendritic cells. Blood 101:4862–4869

97. Mailliard RB, Son YI, Redlinger R, Coates PT, Giermasz A, Morel PA, Storkus WJ, Kalinski P (2003) Dendritic cells mediate NK cell help for Th1 and CTL responses: two-signal requirement for the induction of NK cell helper function. J Immunol 171:2366–2373

98. Malaguarnera L, Pignatelli S, Simpore J, Malaguarnera M, Musumeci S (2002) Plasma levels of interleukin-12 (IL-12), interleukin-18 (IL-18) and transforming growth factor beta (TGF-beta) in *Plasmodium falciparum* malaria. Eur Cytokine Netw 13:425–430

99. Martiney JA, Sherry B, Metz CN, Espinoza M, Ferrer AS, Calandra T, Broxmeyer HE, Bucala R (2000) Macrophage migration inhibitory factor release by macrophages after ingestion of *Plasmodium chabaudi*-infected erythrocytes: possible role in the pathogenesis of malarial anemia. Infect Immun 68:2259–2267

100. McGregor IA (1964) The passive transfer of human malarial immunity. Am J Trop Med Hyg. 13:237–239.

101. Mestas J, Hughes CCW (2004) Of mice and not men: differences between mouse and human immunology J Immunol 172:2731–2738

102. Mohan K, Moulin P, Stevenson MM (1997) Natural killer cell cytokine production, not cytotoxicity, contributes to resistance against blood-stage *Plasmodium chabaudi* AS infection. J Immunol 159:4990–4998

103. Mohan K, Stevenson MM (1998) Acquired immunity to asexual blood-stages of malaria. In Malaria: Parasite Biology, Pathogenesis and Protection. (Ed. I.W. Sherman). ASM Press, Washington, DC, p. 467–493

104. Mohan K, Sam H, Stevenson, MM (1999) Therapy with a combination of low dose IL-12 and chloroquine completely cures primary blood-stage malaria, prevents severe anemia and induces immunity to reinfection. Infect. Immun. 67:513–519

105. Morakote N, Justus DE (1988) Immunosuppression in malaria: effect of hemozoin produced by *Plasmodium berghei* and *Plasmodium falciparum*. Int Arch Allergy Appl Immunol 86:28–34

106. Moretta A (2002) Natural killer cells and dendritic cells: rendezvous in abused tissues. Nat Rev Immunol 2:957–964

107. Nagamine Y, Hayano M, Kashiwamura S, Okamura H, Nakanishi K, Krudsod S, Wilairatana P, Looareesuwan S, Kojima S (2003) Involvement of interleukin-18 in severe *Plasmodium falciparum* malaria. Trans R Soc Trop Med Hyg 97:236–241

108. Ndungu FM, Bull PC, Ross A, Lowe BS, Kabiru E, Marsh K (2002) Naturally acquired immunoglobulin (Ig)G subclass antibodies to crude asexual *Plasmodium falciparum* lysates: evidence for association with protection for IgG1 and disease for IgG2. Parasite Immunol 24:77–82

109. Nencioni A, Grunebach F, Zobywlaski A, Denzlinger C, Brugger W, Brossart P (2002) Dendritic cell immunogenicity is regulated by peroxisome proliferator-activated receptor gamma. J Immunol 169:1228–1235

110. Newbold C, Warn P, Black G, Berendt A, Craig A, Snow B, Msobo M, Peshu N, Marsh K (1997) Receptor-specific adhesion and clinical disease in *Plasmodium falciparum*. Am J Trop Med Hyg 57:389–398

111. Nguyen P, Day N, Pram T, Ferguson D, White N (1995) Intraleukocytic malaria pigment and prognosis in severe malaria. Trans R Soc Trop Med Hyg 89:200–204

112. Nguyen KB, Salazar-Mather TP, Dalod MY, Van Deusen JB, Wie X-Q, Liew FY, Caligiuri MA, Durbin JE, Biron CA (2002) Coordinated and distinct roles for IFN-αβ, IL-12 and IL-15 regulation of NK cell responses to viral infection. J Immunol 169:4279–4287

113. Nielsen MA, Vestergaard LS, Lusingu J, Kurtzhals JA, Giha HA, Grevstad B, Goka BQ, Lemnge MM, Jensen JB, Akanmori BD, Theander TG, Staalsoe T, Hviid L (2004) Geographical and temporal conservation of antibody recognition of *Plasmodium falciparum* variant surface antigens. Infect Immun 72:3531–3535

114. Ocana-Morgner C, Mota MM, Rodriguez A (2003) Malaria blood stage suppression of liver stage immunity by dendritic cells. J Exp Med 197:143–151

115. Ohteki T, Suzue K, Maki C, Ota T, Koyasu S (2001) Critical role of IL-15: IL-15R for antigen-presenting cell functions in the innate immune response. Nat Immunol 2(12): 1138–1143

116. Orago AS, Facer CA (1991) Cytotoxicity of human natural killer (NK) cell subsets for *Plasmodium falciparum* erythrocytic schizonts: stimulation by cytokines and inhibition by neomycin. Clin Exp Immunol 86:22–29

117. Orengo AM, Carlo ED, Comes A, Fabbi M, Piazza T, Cilli M, Musiani P, Ferrini S (2003) Tumor cells engineered with IL-12 and IL-15 genes induce protective antibody responses in nude mice. J Immunol 171:569–575

118. Pain A, Ferguson DJ, Kai O, Urban BC, Lowe B, Marsh K, Roberts DJ (2001) Platelet-mediated clumping of *Plasmodium falciparum*-infected erythrocytes is a common adhesive phenotype and is associated with severe malaria. Proc Natl Acad Sci U S A 98:1805–1810

119. Pain A, Urban BC, Kai O, Casals-Pascual C, Shafi J, Marsh K, Roberts DJ (2001) A non-sense mutation in CD36 gene is associated with protection from severe malaria. Lancet 357:1502–1503

120. Pan PY, Gu P, Li Q, Xu D, Weber K, Chen SH (2004) Regulation of dendritic cell function by NK cells: mechanisms underlying the synergism in the combination therapy of IL-12 and 4–1BB activation. J Immunol 172:4779–4789

121. Patterson S, Robinson SP, English NR, Knight SC (1999) Subpopulations of peripheral blood dendritic cells show differential susceptibility to infection with a lymphotropic strain of HIV-1. Immunol Lett 66:111–116

122. Peritt D, Robertson S, Gri G, Showe L, Aste-Amezaga M, Trinchieri G (1998) Differentiation of human NK cells into NK1 and NK2 subsets. J Immunol 161:5821–5824

123. Perkins DJ, Weinberg JB, Kremsner PG (2000) Reduced interleukin-12 and transforming growth factor-beta1 in severe childhood malaria: relationship of cytokine balance with disease severity. J Infect Dis 182:988–992

124. Perry JA, Rush A, Wilson RJ, Olver CS, Avery AC (2004) Dendritic cells from malaria-infected mice are fully functional APC. J Immunol 172:475–482

125. Piccioli D, Sbrana S, Melandri E, Valiante NM (2002) Contact-dependent stimulation and inhibition of dendritic cells by natural killer cells. J Exp Med 195:335–341

126. Pichyangkul S, Yongvanitchit K, Kum-arb U, Hemmi H, Akira S, Krieg AM, Heppner DG, Stewart VA, Hasegawa H, Looareesuwan S, Shanks GD, Miller RS (2004) Malaria blood-stage parasites activate human plasmacytoid dendritic cells and murine dendritic cells through a Toll-like receptor 9-dependent pathway. J Immunol 172:4926–4933

127. Pouniotis DS, Proudfoot O, Bogdanoska V, Apostolopoulos V, Fifis T, Plebanski M (2004) Dendritic cells induce immunity and long-lasting protection against blood-stage malaria despite an in vitro parasite-induced maturation defect. Infect Immun 72:5331–5339

128. Prlic M, Blazar BR, Farrar MA, Jameson SC (2003) In vivo survival and homeostatic proliferation of natural killer cells. J Exp Med 197(8): 967–976

129. Recker M, Nee S, Bull PC, Kinyanjui S, Marsh K, Newbold C, Gupta S (2004) Transient cross-reactive immune responses can orchestrate antigenic variation in malaria. Nature 429:555–558

130. Rhee MS, Akanmori BD, Waterfall M, Riley EM (2001) Changes in cytokine production associated with acquired immunity to *Plasmodium falciparum* malaria. Clin Exp Immunol 126:503–510

131. Rich SM, Ayala FJ (2000) Population structure and recent evolution of *Plasmodium falciparum*. PNAS 97:6994–7001

132. Riley EM, Jakobsen PH, Allen SJ, Wheeler JG, Bennett S, Jepsen S, Greenwood BM (1991) Immune response to soluble exoantigens of *Plasmodium falciparum* may contribute to both pathogenesis and protection in clinical malaria: evidence from a longitudinal, prospective study of semi-immune African children. Eur J Immunol 21:1019–1025

133. Rogerson SJ, Tembenu R, Dobano C, Plitt S, Taylor TE, Molyneux ME (1999) Cytoadherence characteristics of *Plasmodium falciparum*-infected erythrocytes from Malawian children with severe and uncomplicated malaria. Am J Trop Med Hyg 61:467–472

134. Rowe A, Obeiro J, Newbold CI, Marsh K (1995) *Plasmodium falciparum* rosetting is associated with malaria severity in Kenya. Infect Immun 63:2323–2326

135. Rubinstein, MP, Kadima A.N, Salem ML, Nguyen CL, Gillanders WE, Cole DJ (2002). Systemic administration of IL-15 augments the antigen-specific primary CD8$^+$ T cell response following vaccination with peptide-pulsed dendritic cells. J. Immunol. 169:4928–4935

136. Sam H, Stevenson MM (1999) In vivo IL-12 production and IL-12 receptors beta1 and beta2 mRNA expression in the spleen are differentially up-regulated in resistant B6 and susceptible A/J mice during early blood-stage *Plasmodium chabaudi* AS malaria. J Immunol 162:1582–1589

137. Sam H, Stevenson MM (1999) Early IL-12 p70, but not p40, production by splenic macrophages correlates with host resistance to blood-stage *Plasmodium chabaudi* AS malaria. Clin Exp Immunol 117:343–349

138. Schellenberg JA, Newell JN, Snow RW, Mung'ala V, Marsh K, Smith PG, Hayes RJ (1998) An analysis of the geographical distribution of severe malaria in children in Kilifi District, Kenya. Int J Epidemiol 27:323–329

139. Schmieg J, Gonzalez-Aseguinolaza G, Tsuji M (2003) The role of natural killer T cells and other T cell subsets against infection by the pre-erythrocytic stages of malaria parasites. Microbes Infect 5:499–506

140. Schwarzer E, Turrini F, Ulliers D, Giribaldi G, Ginsburg H, Arese P (1992) Impairment of macrophage functions after ingestion of *Plasmodium falciparum*-infected erythrocytes or isolated malarial pigment. J Exp Med 176:1033–1041

141. Schwarzer E, Alessio M, Ulliers D, Arese P (1998) Phagocytosis of the malarial pigment, hemozoin, impairs expression of major histocompatibility complex class II antigen, CD54, and CD11c in human monocytes. Infect Immun 66:1601–1606

142. Scorza T, Magez S, Brys L, De Baetselier P (1999) Hemozoin is a key factor in the induction of malaria-associated immunosuppression. Parasite Immunol 21:545–554

143. Scragg IG, Hensmann M, Bate CA, Kwiatkowski D (1999) Early cytokine induction by *Plasomodium falciparum* is not classical endotoxin-like process. Eur J Immunol 29:2636–2644

144. Seixas EMG, Langhorne J (1999) γδ T cells contribute to control of chronic parasitemia in *Plasmodium chabaudi* infections in mice. J Immunol 162:2837–2841

145. Seixas E, Cross C, Quin S, Langhorne J (2001) Direct activation of dendritic cells by the malaria parasite, *Plasmodium chabaudi chabaudi*. Eur J Immunol 31:2970–2978

146. Shortman K, Liu YJ (2002) Mouse and human dendritic cell subtypes. Nat Rev Immunol 2:151–161

147. Serghides I, Smith TG, Pater SN, Kain KC (2003) CD36 and malaria: friends or foes? Trend Parasitol 19:461–469

148. Skold M, Bchar SM (2003) Role of CD1d-restricted NKT cells in microbial immunity. Infect Immun 71:5447–5455

149. Skorokhod OA, Alessio M, Mordmuller B, Arese P, Schwarzer E (2004) Hemozoin (malaria pigment) inhibits differentiation and maturation of human monocyte-derived dendritic cells: a peroxisome proliferator-activated receptor-gamma-mediated effect. J Immunol 173:4066–4074

150. Skov S, Bonyhadi M, Ødum N, Ledbetter JA (2000) IL-2 and IL-15 regulate CD154 expression on activated CD4 T cells. J Immunol 164:3500–3505

151. Smith JD, Subramanian G, Gamain B, Baruch DI, Miller LH (2000) Classification of adhesive domains in the *Plasmodium falciparum* erythrocyte membrane protein 1 family. Mol Biochem Parasitol 110:293–310

152. Smith JD, Gamain B, Baruch DI, Kyes S (2001) Decoding the language of var genes and *Plasmodium falciparum* sequestration. Trends Parasitol 17:538–545

153. Smith T, Felger I, Tanner M, Beck HP (1999) Premunition in *Plasmodium falciparum* infection: insights from the epidemiology of multiple infections. Trans R Soc Trop Med Hyg 93 Suppl 1:59–64

154. Snow RW, Schellenberg JR, Peshu N, Forster D, Newton CR, Winstanley PA, Mwangi I, Waruiru C, Warn PA, Newbold C, et al. (1993) Periodicity and space-time clustering of severe childhood malaria on the coast of Kenya. Trans R Soc Trop Med Hyg 87:386–390

155. Snow RW, Bastos de Azevedo I, Lowe BS, Kabiru EW, Nevill CG, Mwankusye S, Kassiga G, Marsh K, Teuscher T (1994) Severe childhood malaria in two areas of markedly different falciparum transmission in east Africa. Acta Trop 57:289–300

156. Snow RW, Nahlen B, Palmer A, Donnelly CA, Gupta S, Marsh K (1998) Risk of severe malaria among African infants: direct evidence of clinical protection during early infancy. J Infect Dis 177:819–822

157. Staalsoe T, Nielsen MA, Vestergaard LS, Jensen AT, Theander TG, Hviid L (2003) In vitro selection of *Plasmodium falciparum* 3D7 for expression of variant surface antigens associated with severe malaria in African children. Parasite Immunol 25:421–427

158. Steinman RM, Hawiger D, Nussenzweig MC (2003) Tolerogenic dendritic cells. Annu Rev Immunol 21:685–711

159. Stevenson MM, Skamene E (1985) Murine malaria: resistance of AXB/BXA recombinant inbred mice to *Plasmodium chabaudi*. Infect Immun 47:452–456

160. Stevenson MM, Su Z, Sam H, Mohan K (2001) Modulation of host responses to blood-stage malaria by interleukin-12: from therapy to adjuvant activity. Microbes and Infect 3:49–59

161. Stevenson MM, Riley EM (2004) Innate immunity to malaria. Nat Rev Immunol 4:169–180

162. Straw AD, MacDonald AS, Denkers EY, Pearce EJ (2003) CD154 plays a central role in regulating dendritic cell activation during infections that induce Th1 or Th2 responses. J Immunol 170:727–734

163. Su Z, Stevenson, MM (2000) The central role of endogenous IFN-γ in protective immunity against acute blood-stage *Plasmodium chabaudi* AS infection. Infect. Immun. 68:4399–4406

164. Su Z, Stevenson MM (2002) IL-12 is required for antibody-mediated protective immunity against blood-stage *Plasmodium chabaudi* AS malaria infection in mice. J. Immunol. 168:1348–1355

165. Su Z, Fortin A, Gros P, Stevenson MM (2002) Opsonin-independent phagocytosis: an effector mechanism against acute blood-stage *Plasmodium chabaudi* AS infection. J Infect Dis 186:1321–1329

166. Su Z, Tam MF, Jankovic D, Stevenson MM (2003) Vaccination against blood-stage malaria in mice using novel immunostimulatory adjuvants. Infect. Immun. 71:5178–5187

167. Taylor RR, Allen SJ, Greenwood BM, Riley EM (1998) IgG3 antibodies to *Plasmodium falciparum* merozoite surface protein 2 (MSP2): increasing prevalence with age and association with clinical immunity to malaria. Am J Trop Med Hyg 58:406–413

168. Torre D, Giola M, Speranza F, Matteelli A, Basilico C, Biondi G (2001) Serum levels of interleukin-18 in patients with uncomplicated *Plasmodium falciparum* malaria. Eur Cytokine Netw 12:361–364

169. Traore B, Muanza K, Looareesuwan S, Supavej S, Khusmith S, Danis M, Viriyavejakul P, Gay F (2000) Cytoadherence characteristics of *Plasmodium falciparum* isolates in Thailand using an in vitro human lung endothelial cells model. Am J Trop Med Hyg 62:38–44

170. Troye-Blomberg M, Worku S, Tangteerawatana P, Jamshaid R, Soderstrom K, Elghazali G, Moretta L, Hammarstrom M, Mincheva-Nilsson L (1999) Human gamma delta T cells that inhibit the in vitro growth of the asexual blood stages of the *Plasmodium falciparum* parasite express cytolytic and proinflammatory molecules. Scand J Immunol 50:642–650

171. Turner GD, Morrison H, Jones M, Davis TM, Looareesuwan S, Buley ID, Gatter KC, Newbold CI, Pukritayakamee S, Nagachinta B, et al. (1994) An immuno-histochemical study of the pathology of fatal malaria. Evidence for widespread endothelial activation and a potential role for intercellular adhesion molecule-1 in cerebral sequestration. Am J Pathol 145:1057–1069

172. Urban BC, Ferguson DJ, Pain A, Willcox N, Plebanski M, Austyn JM, Roberts DJ (1999) *Plasmodium falciparum*-infected erythrocytes modulate the maturation of dendritic cells. Nature 400:73–77

173. Urban BC, Mwangi T, Ross A, Kinyanjui S, Mosobo M, Kai O, Lowe B, Marsh K, Roberts DJ (2001) Peripheral blood dendritic cells in children with acute *Plasmodium falciparum* malaria. Blood 98:2859–2861

174. Urban BC, Willcox N, Roberts DJ (2001) A role for CD36 in the regulation of dendritic cell function. Proc Natl Acad Sci U S A 98:8750–8755

175. Urban BC, Hien TT, Day NP, Phu NH, Roberts R, Pongponratn E, Jones M, Mai NT, Bethell D, Turner GD, Ferguson D, White NJ, Roberts DJ (2005) Fatal Plasmodium falciparum malaria causes specific patterns of splenic architectural disorganization. Infect Immun 73:1986–1994

176. van der Heyde HC, Ellso MM, Chang W-L, Kaplan M, Manning DD, Weidanz WP (1995) Gamma delta T cells function in cell-mediated immunity to acute blood-stage *Plasmodium chabaudi adami* malaria. J Immunol 154:3985–3990

177. Warren HS, Weidanz WP (1976) Malarial immunodepression in vitro: adherent spleen cells are functionally defective as accessory cells in the response to horse erythrocytes. Eur J Immunol 6:816–819

178. Waterfall M, Black A, Riley E (1998) Gammadelta+ T cells preferentially respond to live rather than killed malaria parasites. Infect Immun 66:2393–2398

179. Weatherall DJ, Miller LH, Baruch DI, Marsh K, Doumbo OK, Casals-Pascual C, Roberts DJ (2002) Malaria and the red cell. Hematology (Am Soc Hematol Educ Program) 35–57

180. Weidanz WP, Kemp JR, Batchelder JM, Cigel FK, Sandor M, van der Heyde HC (1999) Plasticity of immune responses suppressing parasitemia during acute *Plasmodium chabaudi* malaria. J Immunol 154:3985–3990

181. World malaria situation in 1994. Part I. Population at risk. (1997) Wkly Epidemiol Rec 72:269–274

182. Yoshimoto T, Paul WE (1994) CD4$^+$, NK1.1$^+$ T cells promptly produce interleukin 4 in response to in vivo challenge with anti-CD3. J Exp Med 179:1285–1295

183. Xu X, Sumita K, Feng C, Xiong X, Shen H, Maruyama S, Kanoh M, Asano Y (2001) Down-regulation of IL-12 p40 gene in *Plasmodium berghei*-infected mice. J Immunol 167:235–241

184. Zamai L, Ahmad M, Bennett IM, Azzoni L, Alnemri ES, Perussia B (1998) Natural killer (NK) cell-mediated cytotoxicity: differential use of TRAIL and Fas ligand by immature and mature primary human NK cells. J Exp Med 188:2375–80

CTMI (2005) 297:71–102
© Springer-Verlag Berlin Heidelberg 2005

Longevity of the Immune Response and Memory to Blood-Stage Malaria Infection

A. H. Achtman[1] (✉) · P. C. Bull[2] · R. Stephens[3] · J. Langhorne[3]

[1]Molecular Tumor Genetics and Immunogenetics, Max-Delbrück-Center for Molecular Medicine, Robert-Rössle-Str. 10, 13092 Berlin, Germany
achtman@mdc-berlin.de

[2]Weatherall Institute of Molecular Medicine, Headington, Oxford OX39DS, UK

[3]Division of Parasitology, National Institute for Medical Research, The Ridgeway, Mill Hill, London NW7 1AA, UK

Abstract Immunity to malaria develops slowly with protection against the parasite lagging behind protection against disease symptoms. The data on the longevity of protective immune responses are sparse. However, studies of antibody responses associated with protection reveal that they consist of a short- and a long-lived component. Compared with the antibody levels observed in other infection and immunization systems, the levels of the short-lived antibody compartment drop below the detectable threshold with unusual rapidity. The prevalence of long-lived antibodies is comparable to that seen after bacterial and protozoan infections. There is even less available data concerning T cell longevity in malaria infection, but what there is seems to indicate that T cell memory is short in the absence of persistent antigen. In general, the degree and duration of parasite persistence represent a major factor determining how immune response longevity and protection correlate. The predilection for short-lived immune responses in malaria infection could be caused by a number of mechanisms resulting from the interplay of normal regulatory mechanisms of the immune system and immune evasion by the parasite. In conclusion, it appears that the parasite–host relationship has developed to favor some short-lived responses, which allow the host to survive while allowing the parasite to persist. Anti-malarial immune responses present a complex picture, and many aspects of regulation and longevity of the response require further research.

Abbreviations

CSP	Circumsporozoite protein
LSA-1	Liver-stage antigen
MSP-1	Merozoite surface protein-1
MSP-2	Merozoite surface protein-2
Pf155/RESA	Ring-infected erythrocyte surface antigen
PfEMP1	*P. falciparum* erythrocyte membrane protein-1
PIESA	*P. falciparum*-infected erythrocyte surface antigens
RAP1	Rhoptry-associated protein 1
TRAP	Thrombospondin-related protein

1
Introduction

For many pathogens, a single infection enables the immune system to protect the host from disease for the remainder of the host's life span. In contrast, malaria is contracted repeatedly under both endemic and epidemic conditions, and completely sterile immunity does not develop; longevity of a protective response, once elicited, can be of variable length and is generally not life-long in the absence of continuous or regular exposure to the parasite. However, some long-term immunity does exist. Although, emigrants from endemic areas, or previously exposed adults, frequently develop malaria when infected after several years of absence, they often have lower parasitemias and milder clinical disease than completely naive individuals (Deloron and Chougnet 1992; Di Perri et al. 1995). There is no consensus on how long immune responses are maintained after a malaria infection and to what extent short-lived responses are a sign of impaired immunological memory, nor do we know which arms of the immune response are responsible for long-term protection. This review seeks to address the issue of immune response longevity by analyzing the responses associated with protection.

We have chosen to focus mainly on the immune response to the blood stages of infection since these stages not only induce protective immune responses in natural infection but are also strongly associated with clinical protection. Although both B and T cells play a role in the immune response to *Plasmodium* parasites, the longevity of immunity will be discussed with a strong emphasis on antibody responses, as these represent the most commonly studied parameter in field studies. The available data on the longevity of malarial antibody responses will be presented and compared with the longevity of the humoral response seen in other immunization and infection systems. These data will be considered in the context of the current understanding of the immune response and we will discuss how the parasite may bias immune responses to its benefit.

2
Development of Immunity to Malaria

Clinical immunity to malaria, or protection against disease symptoms, develops more rapidly than anti-parasite immunity (protection against parasitemia) (Fig. 1). The development of clinical immunity is thought to depend on the generation of immune mechanisms which limit the inflammatory processes responsible for the pathology (reviewed in Marsh 1992; Artavanis-Tsakonas et al. 2003). This non-sterilizing form of immunity is frequently referred to as premunition and may be dependent on regular rechallenge with parasites (reviewed in Druilhe and Pérignon 1994). The term premunition was originally coined to describe the prevention of superinfections (reviewed in Smith et al. 1999) and the change in word usage emphasizes how closely parasite chronicity and anti-malarial immunity are linked.

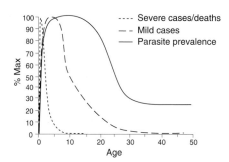

Fig. 1 Development of clinical immunity in comparison to anti-parasite immunity in Kilifi, Kenya

In areas of moderate to high malaria endemicity, children develop clinical immunity over the first 5 years of life in which they show reduced disease symptoms while retaining high parasite burdens. Mathematical modeling of infections in these areas suggest that protection against severe but non-cerebral malaria may be generated after only one to three episodes of disease (Gupta et al. 1999). The development of clinical immunity follows a somewhat different pattern when exposure begins in adulthood. Population relocation programs in Indonesia have revealed that roughly three to six infections at the hyperendemic level occur before malaria morbidity drops in adults (Baird et al. 1993; Baird 1998). In the transmigrant population, parasite prevalence drops more slowly in children than in adults, although the latter suffer more malarial morbidity.

Compared with clinical immunity, anti-parasite immunity is more difficult to assess in the field, as asymptomatic parasite carriers go undetected unless regular blood film analysis is carried out on all participants of a longitudinal study. However, some information can be gleaned from studies where controlled malaria infections were used to treat the neurological symptoms of syphilis. Retrospective analysis of infections performed in the USA shows that both clinical immunity and anti-parasite immunity are improved in the secondary infection, but that neither is complete (Collins and Jeffery 1999). A series of *P. falciparum* infections undertaken in Romania shows that all patients were free of fever by the fifth inoculation whereas 3%–5% of the patients still developed parasitemia in the eighth to tenth inoculations, clearly demonstrating the different development rates of clinical and anti-parasite immunity (Ciuca et al. 1934).

Thus, the development of immunity to malaria is a complex issue and any evaluation of experiments analyzing the longevity of anti-malarial immune responses requires the critical consideration of numerous factors: differentiation between anti-parasite and clinical immunity, the age of the study group and the degree and continuity of parasite exposure. Furthermore, the influence of infection with different strains and species of *Plasmodium* must also be taken into account.

3
Link Between Antibodies and Protection

Studies in a variety of experimental models of malaria support the view that B cells and antibody are crucial components of the protective immune response. (a) Transfer of immune serum or specific antibodies into naïve mice or monkeys can diminish or prevent infection in the recipient (Jarra et al. 1986; Berzins et al. 1991; Diggs et al. 1995; Gysin et al. 1996; Gozalo et al. 1998; Vukovic et al. 2000). (b) Mice lacking B cells develop a fluctuating chronic infection (Grun and Weidanz 1983; van der Heyde et al. 1994; von der Weid et al. 1996) which is only eliminated by transfer of B cells and/or antibody (Langhorne et al. 1998). (c) Immunization with various malarial antigens resulting in protection is also dependent on, or associated with, specific antibodies in mice (Daly and Long 1995; Ling et al. 1995; Calvo et al. 1996; Tian et al. 1996; Hirunpetcharat et al. 1997; Anders et al. 1998; Rotman et al. 1999) and monkeys (Siddiqui et al. 1987; Chang et al. 1996; Baruch et al. 1999; Donati et al. 2004).

Similarly, several lines of evidence support a role for antibodies in the development of immunity to the *Plasmodium* parasite in humans: (a) Passive transfer of immune serum into non-immune humans can diminish or prevent infection in the recipient (Cohen et al. 1961; Sabchareon et al. 1991). (b) Infants are protected against malaria during the first few months of life (Snow et al. 1998) possibly due to the transfer of maternal antibodies (Hviid L Staalsoe 2004; Branch et al. 1998), but this is not a universal observation (Dodoo et al. 1999). (c) In longitudinal studies, the prevalence and levels of antibodies against defined malarial antigens have been associated with resistance against disease (e.g., Riley et al. 1992; Egan et al. 1996; Metzger et al. 2003). (d) Among the studies which have tested cross-sectionally for a relationship between antibodies and parasites rather than malarial disease, a significant number have found an association between antibodies against ring-infected erythrocyte surface antigen (Pf155/RESA) and low levels of parasitemia (Chizzolini et al. 1988; Petersen et al. 1989; Hogh et al. 1992; Astagneau et al. 1994; Achidi et al. 1995) and a handful of studies have observed such an association for antibodies directed against the merozoite surface protein-1 (MSP-1) (Chizzolini et al. 1988; Riley et al. 1993; Egan et al. 1996). However, there are also studies reporting a positive association between parasitemia and antibodies for the sporozoite antigen circumsporozoite protein (CSP) (Achidi et al. 1995), MSP-1 (Terrientes et al. 1994; al-Yaman et al. 1995), MSP-2 (al-Yaman et al. 1994), glycophosphatidylinositol (Boutlis et al. 2002), rhoptry-associated protein 1 (RAP-1) (Jakobsen et al. 1997; Fonjungo et al. 1999) and the variant antigen *P. falciparum* erythrocyte membrane protein-1 (PfEMP-1) (Bull et al. 2002). This presents some problems in interpreting field data. While antibody levels may have a protective effect against future infection or disease, if they are short-lived, they may only be indicative of the recentness of past infections or to present infections. The importance of taking asymptomatic parasite infections into account when assessing the relationship between antibodies and infection or disease in longitudinal studies has been recognized previously (e.g., Brown et al. 1991) and has been incorporated into some recent studies (Bull et al. 2002; Kinyanjui et al. 2004; Polley et al. 2004).

Overall, data from field studies support an association between antibody responses and immunity to malaria. Variations between the results of different studies can be attributed to factors such as age, previous exposure to parasite, transmission rate, host genetic factors as well as the statistical power of the study. Furthermore, it is likely that multiple and diverse immune mechanisms functioning concurrently are required for full protection, making it difficult to dissect the individual effect of a particular antibody response. Since the prevalence or levels of antibodies against defined malarial antigens are frequently measured in both field studies and in experimental models, they will be used as indicators of the maintenance of host immunity and longevity of the immune response in the following sections, which will analyze the persistence of malaria-specific antibody following infection.

4
Antibody Persistence in Malaria

A frequent observation in the field is that malaria-specific antibody levels are diminished in the absence of parasite exposure. This could be attributed to a drop in the amount of antibody produced, resulting in lower titers and a smaller proportion of positive responders between the end of the rainy season and the end of the following dry season in areas of seasonal malaria transmission. However, the malarial antibody response also contains a long-lived component and the balance between these two types of response is shown by a number of field studies. Examples from the literature are summarized in Table 1. Frequently, the persistence of antibody is shorter in children, and in one study, it was shown that only children experienced fluctuations in antibody levels between the dry and rainy seasons, whereas antibody levels remained constant in adults (Taylor et al. 1996)

A major problem in interpreting these studies is that many of them did not include drug treatment for all subjects and therefore, the end of the transmission season does not necessarily correlate with a lack of parasites. It has been shown that 30%–40% of the study cohorts from areas of seasonal transmission actually had detectable parasitemia at the start of the transmission season (Ferreira and Katzin 1995; Metzger et al. 2003). Therefore, it is likely that chronic infections in some of the study participants will skew the overall trend in antibody level development.

Table 1 Examples of antibody development in areas of seasonal malaria transmission

Antigen	Study size/age	Transmission type	Interval between dry and rainy season	Drop in Ab prevalence	Drop in Ab level	Reference
MSP-1	61 Adults	Seasonal	9 Months	Not significant	Not significant	Riley 1993
MSP-1	52 Adults and children	Mesoendemic, unstable	8–9 Months	?	40%–45%	Cavanagh et al. 1998
MSP-1	37 Adults, 57 children	Hyperendemic, seasonal	7–8 Months	Significant in children but not in adults	Adults: 35–36% Children: 48–54%	Früh et al. 1991
P. vivax MSP-1	104 Adults and children	Seasonal	5 Months study interval	34%	About 50%	Soares et al. 1999b
MSP-1, MSP-2, CSP	96 Adults and children	Seasonal	3 Months study interval	22%–50%	6%–66%	Ramasamy et al. 1994
Liver-stage antigen	140 Adults and children (LSA-1)	Seasonal, episodic	4–5 Months	11.4%–30.5%	24% In children ≤ 6 years 53% In adults ≥ 18 years	John et al. 2002
RAP-1	53 Adults and children	Unstable, low intensity after drought	8–9 Months	Yes	Yes	Fonjungo et al. 1999

Additional studies show that the drop in antibody levels and prevalence also occurs after parasites have been eliminated. Antibody levels against total parasite antigen drop within the first few months after drug treatment (Brögger et al. 1978; Ferreira et al. 1996; Luty et al. 2000). Furthermore, both the prevalence and the levels of antibodies against the malarial antigens PfEMP-1, *P. vivax and P. falciparum* MSP-1 and RAP-1 drop soon after treatment (Cavanagh et al. 1998; Fonjungo et al. 1999; Giha et al. 1999; Soares et al. 1999a; Park et al. 2000; Braga et al. 2002). However, a few malarial antibody responses deviate from this trend. Antibody levels against rifin proteins remained constant over 2 years in four patients in the absence of re-infection, and antibodies against *P. falciparum*-infected erythrocyte surface antigens (PIESA) remained fairly constant over a period of 12 weeks in Kilifi, Kenya after a small initial drop (Abdel-Latif et al. 2003; Kinyanjui et al. 2003).

Analysis of longer intervals after infection shows that after the initial drop in prevalence and levels, anti-malarial antibodies can persist in the absence of patent infection. In a small study group, antibodies against sporozoite antigens were shown to persist 6–10 years after the hosts had left the malaria-endemic area (Druilhe et al. 1986). More surprisingly, a single 50-day outbreak of *P. vivax* in Brazil (followed by meticulous controls confirming the subsequent absence of parasites) resulted in antibodies against circumsporozoite protein and MSP-1 which could still be detected in 20% or 47% of the individuals after 7 years (Braga et al. 1998). On the Melanesian island Aneityum, IgG titers against total parasite antigen were determined 7 years after the initiation of a thorough eradication campaign. In 37% of the children and 80% of the adults, titers were higher than the cut-off point. However, a part of this response must be attributed to cross-reactivity with non-malarial antigen, as 19% and 29%, respectively, of the inhabitants of an island without malaria also had positive IgG titers (Kaneko 1999; Kaneko et al. 2000).

Overall, the data on antibody responses in humans suggest that some antibody responses to malarial antigens are relatively short-lived with the number of responders dropping up to 50% over a period of 3–9 months and antibody levels dropping up to 66% in the same time period. How far these observations reflect general characteristics of antibody responses following infection or immunization or real impairments in the maintenance of antibody levels remains to be determined. Data are lacking in experimental models. However, protection against lethal *P. berghei* decayed by about 60% over period of 1.3 years after the initial infection (Eling 1980). Since antibody-mediated mechanisms are thought to mediate protection in blood-stage infections, this can be taken as indirect evidence that anti-malarial antibody levels may also decay in mice. More precise studies in animal models are necessary to determine whether malaria parasites interfere with the generation of B cell memory and plasma cell generation or maintenance.

5
Antibody Persistence in Other Immunization and Infection Systems

The rapid loss of antibody prevalence in a large proportion of malaria- infected individuals is in contrast to many other infections and immunizations, where some drop in antibody titer is common, but is less rapid than that seen after malaria infections. In comparing different infection and immunization systems, it is important to consider the complexity of the immunogen or pathogen and the potential for re-exposure as well as chronicity.

The most readily available data for comparison are those that have determined the duration of antibody responses to common vaccines. While some anti-malarial antibody levels drop within 1 year after exposure, antibody against diphtheria and tetanus toxin takes decades rather than years to decay to non-protective levels (Maple et al. 2000). In this study, the percentage of vaccinees with non-protective antibody levels at 60 years of age is comparable to the number of malaria-infected individuals with undetectable levels of anti-malarial antibodies after 6 months. However, not all commonly used vaccines are this efficacious. Although over 95% of vaccinated children have protective antibody titers against tetanus, diphtheria and poliovirus 4 years after a booster immunization, levels of anti-pertussis antibodies are very low at this time point (Mallet et al. 2000). In the case of meningococcal vaccine, antibody levels drop strongly within the first 6 months after vaccination and have returned to pre-immunization levels by 4 years of age (Borrow et al. 2001; Richmond et al. 2001; Borrow et al. 2002; Goldblatt et al. 2002).

Attenuated viral vaccines also elicit very constant antibody responses. Antibody levels against *Varicella* were shown to remain constant over 3 years (after an initial drop) or even rise over a period of 5 years (LaRussa et al. 1990; Zerboni et al. 1998). An attenuated mumps vaccine induced antibody responses which persisted at least 4 years with a reduction in responders of only 15% (Davidkin et al. 1995) while antibody responses to *Rubella* were maintained over a period of 12–23 years in the absence of re-exposure to the virus or vaccine (Asahi et al. 1997). Antibody levels against the non-attenuated smallpox vaccine are also extremely stable over periods up to 75 years with only 4 out of 306 serum values negative at more than 30 years (Hammarlund et al. 2003) or 3 out of 27 values negative at 20–60 years after vaccination (Crotty et al. 2003).

Studies of natural viral infections in isolated populations have also shown that serum antibodies are produced for decades after a single infection. Some of the classic cases have demonstrated the presence of neutralizing antibodies 75 years after an outbreak of yellow fever and the maintenance of polio- and vaccinia-specific antibodies over 40 and 15 years, respectively, in the absence of re-exposure to antigen (reviewed in Ahmed and Gray 1996; Slifka and Ahmed 1996).

As befits the greater structural complexity of bacteria and parasites, they present a more diverse picture. Some salivary and serum IgG responses against the enteric bacterium *Campylobacter jejuni* can be detected up to 1 year after infection, albeit at reduced levels (Cawthraw et al. 2002) and the antibody response to *Bordetella pertussis* antigens declines to roughly background levels within 5 years in a semi-enclosed community (Tomoda et al. 1992). However, despite an equally low risk of re-exposure to the pathogen, 22% of people infected with the intracellular bacterium *Francisella tularensis* still had specific IgG levels above the detection limit after 25 years and at 11 years, six out of six individuals were seropositive (Ericsson et al. 1994). For parasites, it has been shown that infection of calves with the protozoan parasite *Neospora caninum*, which may cause persistent infections, results in continued antibody persistence albeit with some fluctuation (Maley et al. 2001). Mice infected with *Trypanosoma cruzi* are still seropositive 3–6 months after treatment and become seronegative after 10–12 months (Andrade et al. 1991). Regarding a larger time frame, a mathematical model suggests that the mean duration of seropositivity after human *Toxoplasma* infection is 40 years (van Druten et al. 1990). Perhaps the closest similarity to malaria infection is seen with *Leishmania donovani* infection, where antibody levels drop drastically (96%) by 75 days after drug treatment, but are still in the detectable range (Anam et al. 1999).

Most of the infections described are either not chronic or have been terminated by drug treatment, although some of the viral infections may persist longer than previously assumed (Zinkernagel 2002; discussed in Sect. 6). Therefore, it is necessary to look at persisting infections. Murine gammaherpesvirus 68 causes life-long latent infections and IgG titers which are very constant for up to 90 days (Sangster et al. 2000), and the potentially persisting infection of mice with lymphocytic choriomeningitis virus (LCMV) results in antibody titers that are stable for at least 300 days (Ochsenbein et al. 2000). However, as with the *N. caninum* infection described above, these observation intervals are short compared to the time scale required for assessing malaria immunity. On a longer note, antibody levels in cystic fibrosis patients chronically infected with *Pseudomonas* behaved differently from malarial antibodies by rising over the course of 11 years (Ciofu et al. 1999).

In summary, all other persisting infections discussed here induced high stable or rising antibody titers or levels. The level at which pathogens persist as well as the initial antigen dose seem to have an effect on long-term antibody levels (Ochsenbein et al. 2000). The main difference between the antibody responses to malaria infection and the infections and immunizations described in this section lies in the lower antibody responses, and the rapidity with which a large proportion of the *Plasmodium*-specific antibodies drop below the detectable threshold. The long-lived component of the antibody response to malaria is less than that observed in viral infections, but may be comparable to that seen after bacterial or other protozoan infection.

6
Theories on Antibody Maintenance

Before discussing how the malaria parasite could affect the B cell and antibody response, it is necessary to present the current theories on the maintenance of serum antibody levels. Figure 2 schematically shows how different B cells contribute to serum antibody levels. The first rapid response is based on the differentiation of recirculating naive B cells to plasma cells which can secrete over 5,000 immunoglobulin molecules per second (reviewed in Slifka and Ahmed 1996). The majority of these plasma cells are short-lived and die after a period varying between 8 h and 3–10 days (Jacob et al. 1991; Ochsenbein et al. 2000; Sze et al. 2000). The antibodies produced by these plasma cells are critical for controlling pathogens before B cells with higher affinity are generated in the germinal centers. Many of the short-lived plasma cells are of

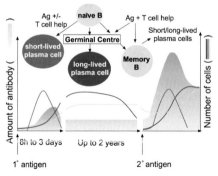

Fig. 2 Persistence of differentiated B cells and the maintenance of serum antibody levels after immunization or acute infection

the IgM isotype and the higher avidity of the pentameric IgM (as compared to monomeric IgG) can partially compensate for the poorer affinity.

Plasma cells are also generated as a consequence of the germinal center reaction where somatic hypermutation and affinity maturation combine to produce antibodies with improved binding characteristics. In mice, plasma cells have extended life spans of at least 90 days (Manz et al. 1997) or 8 months to over 1.5 years without memory restimulation (Slifka et al. 1995, 1998). They persist in the bone marrow and to a lesser extent in the spleen and may occupy an additional survival niche in chronically inflamed tissues (reviewed in Manz and Radbruch 2002). In these locations, the plasma cells continue to secrete antibodies and contribute to the maintenance of serum antibody levels after the termination of infection (Slifka and Ahmed 1996; Slifka et al. 1998). However, the actual life span of these plasma cells in mice and even more so in humans is still a matter of controversy.

The germinal center response also results in the generation of memory B cells, which are responsible for rapid secondary antibody responses comprising the IgG, IgA and IgE isotypes (reviewed in Ahmed and Gray 1996; MacLennan et al. 2000) and these cells have also undergone affinity maturation and selection and have lowered activation thresholds as well as an increased proliferative burst capacity (Martin and Goodnow 2002). Memory B cells have altered homing patterns leading to accumulation in particular locations (reviewed in MacLennan et al. 2000). There has been considerable debate about the ability of memory B cells to survive in the absence of stimulation by the appropriate antigen or a cross-reactive epitope. Current opinion is moving away from the view that antigen is required to maintain memory B cells (Gray and Skarvall 1988) to the idea that memory B cells are capable of persisting in a resting state in the absence of specific antigen (Vieira and Rajewsky 1990; Karrer et al. 2000; Maruyama et al. 2000). However, the involvement of antigen in long-term regulation of plasma cell and memory B cell maintenance is likely to be far more complex than a simple 'yes or no' answer as it is often difficult to determine levels of persisting antigen (reviewed in Zinkernagel and Hengartner 2001).

There is also considerable debate on how serum antibody levels are maintained, since secreted antibody has a limited half-life ranging from 2 days for IgA through 7 days for IgG3 to 21 days for IgG1 in humans (reviewed in Shakib 1990). Long-lived plasma cells are one possible source. However, it is difficult to envisage a limited niche in the bone marrow maintaining plasma cells of a given specificity for as long as 75 years after initial exposure in the face of growth of the repertoire due to new antigenic challenges. Therefore, restimulation of memory B cells to generate new antibody-producing plasma cells is likely to contribute to long-term antibody levels. This can occur by antigen-dependent or -independent restimulation. With respect to antigen-independent restimulation, it has been shown that memory B cells can be reactivated to produce fresh plasma cells via non-specific bystander activation (Bernasconi et al. 2002; Traggiai et al. 2003), but it seems unlikely that this could account for the steady antibody levels. Antigen-dependent activation of memory B cells as a mechanism for replenishing the serum antibody pool requires a source of persisting antigen. Antigen can persist in adjuvant depots after immunization or on follicular dendritic cells, but these options are of limited duration, i.e., the antigen–antibody complexes on follicular dendritic cells display an average half-life of only 8 weeks (Tew and Mandel 1979). However, it has been suggested that many of the classic results on persistence of antibody levels in the absence of the infecting agent need to be reconsidered in the light of previously undetected low-grade persistent infections, e.g., measles virus in neuronal tissues (Zinkernagel 2002). So far, there is no consensus on the relative contribution of these mechanisms to the maintenance of serum antibody levels in malaria, but it will be important to determine parasite status of exposed individuals by sensitive methods in order to determine whether parasite persistence is important for longevity of the response.

7
Effects of the *Plasmodium* Parasite on the Immune Network

Memory B cells, short- and long-lived plasma cells and helper T cells all form part of the immune response to malaria, and there are a number of ways in which the *Plasmodium* parasite could affect the immune network through these individual components. The persistence of malarial antibodies for long periods after the termination of infection (Sect. 4) may be due either to continued secretion of antibody by long-lived plasma cells or to continued activation of memory cells and differentiation into plasma cells. However, antibody levels against malarial antigens fall more rapidly and reach the detection limit sooner than in viral infections and immunizations. This could be because fewer long-lived plasma cells or memory B cells capable of full-scale restimulation are being generated during infection or because they do not survive as long as in other infections.

All immune responses are controlled by homeostatic mechanisms, which ensure that the host is not overburdened with maintaining the response to one pathogen to the exclusion of all others or even at the cost of other metabolic processes. The necessity of regulating the malarial antibody response is clear, as human malaria infection causes pronounced hypergammaglobulinemia

(Greenwood 1974). In mice, it has been shown that polyclonal B cell activation occurs during infection (Rosenberg 1978; Langhorne et al. 1985; Anders 1986) and that there is an unusually high splenic plasma cell response during acute infection (Achtman et al. 2003). Homeostatic mechanisms function at multiple levels of the antibody response, affecting serum antibody levels, plasma cell longevity, and memory B cell maintenance. Serum immunoglobulin levels are in part dependent on the half-lives of the individual isotypes, but their life span can also be regulated by the MHC class I-related receptor, FcRn (Ward et al. 2003; Akilesh et al. 2004; Ober et al. 2004). In situations of hypergammaglobulinemia such as in malaria, these processes could cause accelerated turnover of antibody in the serum, and together with the short life span of many of the *Plasmodium*-specific antibody-producing cells this can account for the rapid decline in malarial antibody levels after termination of infection.

The lifetime of plasma cells is also homeostatically regulated and the pool of long-lived plasma cells is strictly limited by the availability of a supportive microenvironment. Plasma cells represent only 0.5% of the mononucleated cells in the bone marrow translating into a total bone marrow capacity of about 400,000 plasma cells (reviewed in Manz and Radbruch 2002; O'Connor et al. 2003). In the long term, the splenic environment supports only 20–100 long-lived plasma cells per mm^2 (Sze et al. 2000) and over 80% of serum antibody stems from long-lived cells of the bone marrow (reviewed in O'Connor et al. 2003). It is unknown whether the splenomegaly common in malaria-endemic areas results in an increased support capacity for long-lived plasma cells, but even so, the niche size for these cells there or in bone marrow would be limited.

We do not know whether the polyclonal B cell activation in malaria gives rise to long-lived plasma cells, but infection with a complex protozoan parasite gives rise to many more antibody specificities than the hapten immunizations or viral infections commonly used to study plasma cell longevity. In addition, individuals living in malaria-endemic areas are host to numerous other pathogens whose antigens induce further plasma cell responses. Therefore, the competition for microenvironmental niches supporting plasma cell longevity will be high and the number of long-lived plasma cells specific for any given malarial antigen will be accordingly low. In light of this, it is of special interest that the rapid drop in antibody levels in drug-treated *Leishmania donovani* patients in India (Anam et al. 1999) bore the closest resemblance to malarial antibody kinetics of all the studies discussed in the previous section. None of these homeostatic regulatory mechanisms have been investigated in malaria infections. However, every pathogen-specific antibody response has a cut-off level below which the titers are considered insufficient for protection.

Thus, low antibody titers first caused by rapid turnover of serum antibody and then by homeostatic limitation of long-lived plasma cell numbers represent one attractive explanation for the contradictory results concerning the protectivity of antibody responses (Sect. 3).

A characteristic of long-term B cell-mediated protection is the potential for fast and high-affinity secondary antibody responses through reactivation of memory B cells. There is evidence in human malaria for the generation and reactivation of memory B cells and by implication for the activity of T helper cells required for the B cell response. Memory response patterns in form of increased antibody responses have been observed during re-infection in humans for MSP-1 and RAP-1 (Fonjungo et al. 1999; Soares et al. 1999a). In addition, *Plasmodium*-specific B cells from peripheral blood can be activated to produce antibody in vitro both from individuals living in endemic areas and from people who had probably last encountered malaria 8 years prior to analysis, suggesting that specific B cell memory is generated in the infection (Migot et al. 1995; Garraud et al. 2002). Further studies in humans and experimental models are clearly required to assess the extent of memory B cell generation and survival.

The homeostatic regulation described for plasma cells also applies to memory B cells, but there are additional ways in which memory B cell production or maintenance could differ between malaria and other infections. One possibility is that the shedding of large quantities of soluble antigen, which occurs during merozoite invasion, causes deletion of potential memory B cells as they leave the germinal centers. It has been shown in the mouse, using model antigens, that B cells leaving the germinal centers are deleted or anergised if they encounter large quantities of soluble antigen at this stage (Brink et al. 1992; MacLennan 1995; Pulendran et al. 1995; Shokat and Goodnow 1995). We have shown that the amplitude of the secondary antibody response in mice may be reduced when low numbers of parasites from a primary infection are still present compared to the secondary antibody response in mice after complete clearance by drug treatment (A.H. Achtman, R. Stephens, E. Cadman, V. Harrison, J. Langhorne, unpublished observations). Though it would appear from the studies cited above (Migot et al. 1995; Fonjungo et al. 1999; Soares et al. 1999a; Garraud et al. 2002) that in humans, long-lived, specific B cells are produced in malaria infection and survive in the absence of re-infection, there are no definite data on persistence of the parasite. This leaves open the possibility that chronic antigen stimulation either deletes or anergises malaria-specific B cells, or causes a defect in their reactivation and differentiation into antibody-producing cells in a second infection during this chronic phase. If any of these hypotheses are experimentally confirmed, it would be of utmost importance to ensure that all participants in malaria vaccine programs are free of parasites before vaccination, as the development of memory B cells might otherwise be impaired.

Conversely, chronic infection may also protect individuals living in endemic areas from severe sequelae. For example, a cohort of individuals living in a holoendemic area was significantly more susceptible to clinical malaria in the year following radical drug treatment than a comparable cohort which had not been treated (Owusu-Agyei et al. 2002). In another study, where children were treated prophylactically for 5 years, the rate of admission for clinical malaria was higher in the following year although neither mortality nor the parasite-positive rate were altered during the 5 years after termination of treatment (Greenwood et al. 1995).

The protective effect of an ongoing low-grade infection is also demonstrated by the fact that patients with several concurrent infections with different strains of *Plasmodium* are less likely to develop clinical malaria (al-Yaman et al. 1997; Smith et al. 1999). Taken together, these data support the hypothesis that short-lived effector cells (which could be plasma cells, T cells, or components of the innate immune system) maintained by the chronic infection have an anti-parasite effect in addition to the long-lived immune response generated by long-lived plasma cells, memory B cells, and memory T cells. Thus, these results would imply that short-lived effector cells stimulated by chronically persisting parasites or persisting antigen may be the mediators of premunition in endemic areas.

8
Memory T Cells

As antigen-specific T cells are required for activation of B cells, the generation of plasma cells and production, selection and reactivation of memory B cells, the longevity of protective immunity to malaria can also be affected by the nature and duration of the helper T cell response. Both antibody and the T cell cytokine interferon (IFN)-γ have been shown to correlate with protection in human studies. In rodent malaria infections, it has been shown that T cells have antibody-independent effector functions for reducing blood-stage parasitemia via cytokines and cytotoxicity (Weidanz et al. 1990; Stevenson and Tam 1993; von der Weid et al. 1996), but it is largely through their B cell helper function that they aid in final clearance of parasite (van der Heyde et al. 1994; von der Weid et al. 1996).

There are only few data on the persistence of T cell responses in either human malaria or experimental models, and fewer still that relate longevity of the response to resistance to infection or disease. In rodent malaria infections, there is some evidence that malaria-specific CD4 T cells undergo extensive apoptosis after the acute stage of a blood-stage infection, suggesting that subsequent generation of memory cells may be impaired (Xu et al. 2002), although direct evidence is still lacking. However, CD4 T cell responses in the form of B cell help and IL-4 production can be detected 3–6 months after a primary *P. chabaudi* infection (Quin and Langhorne 2001; J. Langhorne, unpublished observations).

Unlike antibody studies, interpretation of human T cell responses is limited to some extent by the limited access to T cells, which can only be obtained in humans from peripheral blood. The absence of a T cell response in a single sample taken at one time point may not indicate lack of memory or effector T cells, as the specific T cells could be in the lymphoid organs or in other organs or tissues as effector cells (Langhorne and Simon-Haarhaus 1991; Hviid et al. 1997) Longitudinal studies on individuals with known episodes of infection over the transmission and dry seasons must be carried out to address these problems.

Peterson and colleagues have identified T cell responses to several peptides of the blood-stage antigen Pf155/RESA in Liberians. Interestingly, although people who were not currently infected had significant responses to this antigen, which would be indicative of some form of surviving T cell memory, there did not appear to be an increase in the prevalence of T cell responsiveness with age (less than or greater than 30 years old) or exposure (Petersen et al. 1989). Studies using antigens of the pre-erythrocytic stages of the parasite, CSP and thrombospondin-related protein (TRAP) show that T cell proliferation and IFN-γ secretion to specific peptides can be measured during a transmission season and also that the small and variable proportion of exposed people who respond to a given peptide may have a short-lived protective advantage (Flanagan et al. 2003). However, it appears that malaria-exposed T cells may have a short half-life, and protection does not even last a whole transmission season, suggesting that perhaps T cell memory to these antigens does not develop in *P. falciparum* infection (Flanagan et al. 2003).

Interestingly, there may be a difference in generation of long-lived malaria-specific T cells between *P. falciparum* and *P. vivax*. Consistent with the studies of Flanagan and colleagues, CSP-specific proliferative responses in *P. falciparum* CD4 cells from exposed patients uncovered only a few epitopes which appeared to be specifically recognized in exposed donors and not in malaria-naïve individuals (Zevering et al. 1994). In contrast, in *P. vivax* infections specific responders to a similar array of CSP peptides were easily detected using the same assays. Furthermore, the longevity of T cell responses to *P. falciparum* CSP was shown to be about 2 years after exposure to the parasite

(Zevering et al. 1994), whereas in *P. vivax*, some individuals still show T cell responsiveness to CSP even 40 years after exposure (Bilsborough et al. 1993). It was hypothesized that the long-term presence of *P. vivax* as hypnozoites in the liver was responsible for the persistence of T cell responsiveness long after the termination of patent infection. These experiments therefore highlight a possible explanation for the decline of T cell memory and protection in *P. falciparum*: there is no recurrent parasitemia from latent liver forms, and therefore no long-term exposure to antigen after clearance of the blood stage parasites until re-infection occurs. This fits well with studies from other fields of infectious immunology which indicate that functional or protective CD4 and CD8 T cell memory may not last in the absence of antigen (Kundig et al. 1996; Uzonna et al. 2001; Kassiotis et al. 2002). However, some antigen-exposed CD4$^+$ T cells are thought to survive in the absence of antigen in mice (Garcia et al. 1999).

In summary, the little experimental evidence that exists suggests there may be a severe defect in prolonged T cell memory to malaria antigens, especially in *P. falciparum*. Longitudinal studies in humans and in experimental models are urgently required to determine the nature of this defect and the role of persistent antigen.

9
Longevity of Antibody Responses to Variant Antigens

This review began by discussing the development of protection in malaria and therefore it is fitting to conclude with some observations on how co-evolution of the *Plasmodium* parasite with its mammalian and avian hosts has led to the generation of fully functional immune responses which nevertheless do not lead to complete elimination of the parasite. This can be seen most clearly in the development of immune responses against polymorphic and variant antigens where immunity to one allele or variant antigen becomes irrelevant in controlling infection with a parasite expressing different alleleic forms of the antigen or variant antigens. Variant surface antigens (VSA) expressed on the surface of malaria-infected erythrocytes are encoded by multigene families (Brown and Brown 1965; Barnwell et al. 1982; McLean et al. 1982; Carlton et al. 2002). Some of these families, such as the *Vir* family, have homologs among different *Plasmodium* species (del Portillo et al. 2001; Carlton et al. 2002; Janssen et al. 2002) and others, such as *P. falciparum var* (Baruch et al. 1995; Pulendran et al. 1995; Newbold et al. 1997) and the *P. knowlesi SICAvar* (Barnwell et al. 1982; Galinski and Corredor 2004) gene families, are species-specific.

Several sets of observations suggest that VSA are likely to be targets of the protective immune response. (a) Antibodies to VSA such as the PfEMP-1 antigens encoded by the *var* gene family are associated with protection (Marsh et al. 1989; Carlson et al. 1990; Bull et al. 1998; Dodoo et al. 2001; Staalsoe et al. 2004). (b) Symptomatic infections including severe malaria can occur on the background of a pre-existing asymptomatic infection (Contamin et al. 1996; Bull et al. 2002), indicating that previously protective antibody responses can become ineffective due to rapid switching of surface antigens. (c) Parasite antigens that are likely to be exposed to the immune system while the parasite is still alive are highly polymorphic between different parasite genotypes and undergo positive immune selection (Hughes and Hughes 1995; Conway 1997; Polley and Conway 2001; Plotkin et al. 2004) or clonal antigenic variation (Roberts et al. 1992). In addition to rapid variation of surface antigen expression, which allows the parasite to persist in the presence of an immune response, the short-lived nature of the antibody to some of the epitopes of variant antigens may also contribute to chronicity of infection or lack of memory to re-infection with the same variant (Giha et al. 1998; Staalso and Hviid 1998; Smith et al. 1999; Bull et al. 2002). As a result, it is difficult to distinguish between the effect of the variability of these exposed targets on the surface of the parasite or infected erythrocyte and the longevity of immune responses to these antigens.

Probably both elements are important in explaining how chronic infections are maintained in the absence of transmission by mosquitoes, as seen, for example, during the dry season of areas with seasonal endemicity. Multiple genotype infections with highly complex dynamics have been observed in these situations (Daubersies et al. 1996; Farnert et al. 1997; Magesa et al. 2002). However, it is still unclear how sequential dominance of VSA variants is maintained without exhausting the repertoire given the rapid switch rate between variants (Robertset al. 1992). Explanations put forward for the maintenance of these dynamics have often emphasized the importance of short-lived responses to polymorphic targets of immunity allowing the same variants to be recycled several times during the dry season (Staalso and Hviid 1998; Smith et al. 1999).

A mathematical model by Recker and colleagues (Recker et al. 2004) suggests that the immune system may be partially responsible for the maintenance of chronic infections and shows how sequential dominance can potentially be maintained though a combination of specific long-lived responses and a network of short-lived, partially cross-reactive responses. Such a model would be compatible with existing field data which support the existence of both long-lived specific (Giha et al. 1999; Kinyanjui et al. 2003) and short-lived, partially cross-reactive responses (Giha et al. 1998; Bull et al. 2002). However, it is unlikely that immune responses to specific determinants fall neatly into these two categories. There appears to be considerable person-to-person variability in responses to PfEMP-1 (Giha et al. 1999; Kinyanjui et al. 2003). A key question that emerges from this is whether every host has the same capacity to sustain chronic infections and whether this is related to the dynamics of their immune response.

10
Conclusions

Chronicity of infection and incomplete immunity in malaria could be the result of not only the impairment of long-lived responses at the level of memory T cells, memory B cells, plasma cells, or antibody half-life, but can also be caused by rapid changes of important surface antigens by the parasite, which may not allow the generation of appropriate memory responses in the first place. There is an almost complete lack of information on the basic regulatory mechanisms responsible for generating B cell and antibody responses in malaria, and on the relative contribution of short-lived and long-lived responses to protective immunity. Clearly these are crucial areas of malaria immunology that must be understood if we are to develop successful long-term immune intervention strategies.

Acknowledgements We would like to thank Anja E. Hauser and Jeffrey R. Dorfman for supplying useful references and Kevin Marsh for providing Fig. 1.

References

Abdel-Latif MS, Dietz K, Issifou S, Kremsner PG, Klinkert MQ (2003) Antibodies to *Plasmodium falciparum* rifin proteins are associated with rapid parasite clearance and asymptomatic infections. Infect Immun 71:6229–6233

Achidi EA, Perlmann H, Berzins K (1995) Asymptomatic malaria parasitaemia and seroreactivities to *Plasmodium falciparum* antigens in blood donors from Ibadan, south-western Nigeria. Ann Trop Med Parasitol 89:601–610

Achtman AH, Khan M, MacLennan IC, Langhorne J (2003) *Plasmodium chabaudi chabaudi* infection in mice induces strong B cell responses and striking but temporary changes in splenic cell distribution. J Immunol 171:317–324

Ahmed R, Gray D (1996) Immunological memory and protective immunity: understanding their relation. Science 272:54–60

Akilesh S, Petkova S, Sproule TJ, Shaffer DJ, Christianson GJ, Roopenian D (2004) The MHC class I-like Fc receptor promotes humorally mediated autoimmune disease. J Clin Invest 113:1328-1333 al-Yaman F, Genton B, Anders RF, Falk M, Triglia T, Lewis D, Hii J, Beck HP, Alpers MP (1994) Relationship between humoral response to *Plasmodium falciparum* merozoite surface antigen-2 and malaria morbidity in a highly endemic area of Papua New Guinea. Am J Trop Med Hyg 51:593–602

al-Yaman F, Genton B, Kramer KJ, Taraika J, Chang SP, Hui GS, Alpers MP (1995) Acquired antibody levels to *Plasmodium falciparum* merozoite surface antigen 1 in residents of a highly endemic area of Papua New Guinea. Trans R Soc Trop Med Hyg 89:555–559

al-Yaman F, Genton B, Reeder JC, Anders RF, Smith T, Alpers MP (1997) Reduced risk of clinical malaria in children infected with multiple clones of *Plasmodium falciparum* in a highly endemic area: a prospective community study. Trans R Soc Trop Med Hyg 91:602–605

Anam K, Afrin F, Banerjee D, Pramanik N, Guha SK, Goswami RP, Saha SK, Ali N (1999) Differential decline in Leishmania membrane antigen-specific immunoglobulin G (IgG), IgM, IgE, and IgG subclass antibodies in Indian kala-azar patients after chemotherapy. Infect Immun 67:6663–6669

Anders RF (1986) Multiple cross-reactivities amongst antigens of *Plasmodium falciparum* impair the development of protective immunity against malaria. Parasite Immunol 8:529–539

Anders RF, Crewther PE, Edwards S, Margetts M, Matthew ML, Pollock B, Pye D (1998) Immunisation with recombinant AMA-1 protects mice against infection with Plasmodium chabaudi. Vaccine 16:240–247

Andrade SG, Freitas LA, Peyrol S, Pimentel AR, Sadigursky M (1991) Experimental chemotherapy of Trypanosoma cruzi infection: persistence of parasite antigens and positive serology in parasitologically cured mice. Bull World Health Organ 69:191–197

Artavanis-Tsakonas K, Tongren JE, Riley EM (2003) The war between the malaria parasite and the immune system: immunity, immunoregulation and immunopathology. Clin Exp Immunol 133:145–152

Asahi T, Ueda K, Hidaka Y, Miyazaki C, Tanaka Y, Nishima S (1997) Twenty-three-year follow-up study of rubella antibodies after immunization in a closed population, and serological response to revaccination. Vaccine 15:1791–1795

Astagneau P, Chougnet C, Lepers JP, Danielle M, Andriamangatiana-Rason MD, Deloron P (1994) Antibodies to the 4-mer repeat of the ring-infected erythrocyte surface antigen (Pf155/RESA) protect against *Plasmodium falciparum* malaria. Int J Epidemiol 23:169–175

Baird JK (1998) Age-dependent characteristics of protection *v.* susceptibility to *Plasmodium falciparum*. Ann Trop Med Parasitol 92:367–390

Baird JK, Purnomo, Basri H, Bangs MJ, Andersen EM, Jones TR, Masbar S, Harjosuwarno S, Subianto B, Arbani PR (1993) Age-specific prevalence of *Plasmodium falciparum* among six populations with limited histories of exposure to endemic malaria. Am J Trop Med Hyg 49:707–719.

Barnwell JW, Howard RJ, Miller LH (1982) Altered expression of Plasmodium knowlesi variant antigen on the erythrocyte membrane in splenectomized rhesus monkeys. J Immunol 128:224–226

Baruch DI, Ma XC, Pasloske B, Howard RJ, Miller LH (1999) CD36 peptides that block cytoadherence define the CD36 binding region for *Plasmodium falciparum*-infected erythrocytes. Blood 94:2121–2127

Baruch DI, Pasloske BL, Singh HB, Bi X, Ma XC, Feldman M, Taraschi TF, Howard RJ (1995) Cloning the P. falciparum gene encoding PfEMP1, a malarial variant antigen and adherence receptor on the surface of parasitized human erythrocytes. Cell 82:77–87

Bernasconi NL, Traggiai E, Lanzavecchia A (2002) Maintenance of serological memory by polyclonal activation of human memory B cells. Science 298:2199–2202

Berzins K, Perlmann H, Wahlin B, Ekre HP, Hogh B, Petersen E, Wellde B, Schoenbechler M, Williams J, Chulay J, al. e (1991) Passive immunization of Aotus monkeys with human antibodies to the *Plasmodium falciparum* antigen Pf155/RESA. Infect Immun 59: 1500–1506

Bilsborough J, Carlisle M, Good MF (1993) Identification of Caucasian CD4 T cell epitopes on the circumsporozoite protein of Plasmodium vivax. T cell memory. J Immunol 151:890–899

Borrow R, Goldblatt D, Andrews N, Richmond P, Southern J, Miller E (2001) Influence of prior meningococcal C polysaccharide vaccination on the response and generation of memory after meningococcal C conjugate vaccination in young children. J Infect Dis 184:377–380

Borrow R, Goldblatt D, Andrews N, Southern J, Ashton L, Deane S, Morris R, Cartwright K, Miller E (2002) Antibody persistence and immunological memory at age 4 years after meningococcal group C conjugate vaccination in children in the United kingdom. J Infect Dis 186:1353–1357

Boutlis CS, Gowda DC, Naik RS, Maguire GP, Mgone CS, Bockarie MJ, Lagog M, Ibam E, Lorry K, Anstey NM (2002) Antibodies to *Plasmodium falciparum* glycosylphosphatidylinositols: inverse association with tolerance of parasitemia in Papua New Guinean children and adults. Infect Immun 70:5052–5057

Braga EM, Barros RM, Reis TA, Fontes CJ, Morais CG, Martins MS, Krettli AU (2002) Association of the IgG response to *Plasmodium falciparum* merozoite protein (C-terminal 19 kD) with clinical immunity to malaria in the Brazilian Amazon region. Am J Trop Med Hyg 66:461–466

Braga EM, Fontes CJF, Krettli AU (1998) Persistence of humoral response against sporozoite and blood-stage malaria antigens 7 years after a brief exposure to *Plasmodium vivax*. J Infect Dis 177:1132–1135

Branch OH, Udhayakumar V, Hightower AW, Oloo AJ, Hawley WA, Nahlen BL, Bloland PB, Kaslow DC, Lal AA (1998) A longitudinal investigation of IgG and IgM antibody responses to the merozoite surface protein-1 19-kilodalton domain of *Plasmodium falciparum* in pregnant women and infants: associations with febrile illness, parasitemia, and anemia. Am J Trop Med Hyg 58:211–219

Brink R, Goodnow CC, Crosbie J, Adams E, Eris J, Mason DY, Hartley SB, Basten A (1992) Immunoglobulin M and D antigen receptors are both capable of mediating B lymphocyte activation, deletion, or anergy after interaction with specific antigen. J Exp Med 176:991–1005

Brögger LC, Mathews HM, Storey J, Ashkar TS, Molineaux L (1978) Changing patterns in the humoral immune response to malaria before, during, and after the application of control measures: a longitudinal study in the West African savanna. Bull World Health Organ 56:579–600

Brown AE, Webster HK, Krinchai K, Gordon DM, Wirtz RA, Permpanich B (1991) Characteristics of natural antibody responses to the circumsporozoite protein of Plasmodium vivax. Am J Trop Med Hyg 44:21–27

Brown KN, Brown IN (1965) Immunity to malaria: antigenic variation in chronic infections of Plasmodium knowlesi. Nature 208:1286–1288

Bull PC, Lowe BS, Kaleli N, Njuga F, Kortok M, Ross A, Ndungu F, Snow RW, Marsh K (2002) Plasmodium falciparum infections are associated with agglutinating antibodies to parasite-infected erythrocyte surface antigens among healthy Kenyan children. J Infect Dis 185:1688–1691

Bull PC, Lowe BS, Kortok M, Molyneux CS, Newbold CI, Marsh K (1998) Parasite antigens on the infected red cell surface are targets for naturally acquired immunity to malaria. Nat Med 4:358–360

Calvo PA, Daly TM, Long CA (1996) Both epidermal growth factor-like domains of the merozoite surface protein-1 from Plasmodium yoelii are required for protection from malaria. Ann N Y Acad Sci 797:260–262

Carlson J, Helmby H, Hill AV, Brewster D, Greenwood BM, Wahlgren M (1990) Human cerebral malaria: association with erythrocyte rosetting and lack of anti-rosetting antibodies. Lancet 336:1457–1460

Carlton JM, Angiuoli SV, Suh BB, Kooij TW, Pertea M, Silva JC, Ermolaeva MD, Allen JE, Selengut JD, Koo HL, Peterson JD, Pop M, Kosack DS, Shumway MF, Bidwell SL, Shallom SJ, van Aken SE, Riedmuller SB, Feldblyum TV, Cho JK, Quackenbush J, Sedegah M, Shoaibi A, Cummings LM, Florens L, Yates JR, Raine JD, Sinden RE, Harris MA, Cunningham DA, Preiser PR, Bergman LW, Vaidya AB, van Lin LH, Janse CJ, Waters AP, Smith HO, White OR, Salzberg SL, Venter JC, Fraser CM, Hoffman SL, Gardner MJ, Carucci DJ (2002) Genome sequence and comparative analysis of the model rodent malaria parasite Plasmodium yoelii yoelii. Nature 419:512–519

Cavanagh DR, Elhassan IM, Roper C, Robinson VJ, Giha H, Holder AA, Hviid L, Theander TG, Arnot DE, McBride JS (1998) A longitudinal study of type-specific antibody responses to Plasmodium falciparum merozoite surface protein-1 in an area of unstable malaria in Sudan. J Immunol 161:347–359

Cawthraw SA, Feldman RA, Sayers AR, Newell DG (2002) Long-term antibody responses following human infection with Campylobacter jejuni. Clin Exp Immunol 130:101–106

Chang SP, Case SE, Gosnell WL, Hashimoto A, Kramer KJ, Tam LQ, Hashiro CQ, Nikaido CM, Gibson HL, Lee-Ng CT, Barr PJ, Yokota BT, Hut GS (1996) A recombinant baculovirus 42-kilodalton C-terminal fragment of Plasmodium falciparum merozoite surface protein 1 protects Aotus monkeys against malaria. Infect Immun 64:253–261

Chizzolini C, Dupont A, Akue JP, Kaufmann MH, Verdini AS, Pessi A, Del Giudice G (1988) Natural antibodies against three distinct and defined antigens of Plasmodium falciparum in residents of a mesoendemic area in Gabon. Am J Trop Med Hyg 39:150–156

Ciofu O, Petersen TD, Jensen P, Hoiby N (1999) Avidity of anti-*P. aeruginosa* antibodies during chronic infection in patients with cystic fibrosis. Thorax 54:141–144

Ciuca M, Ballif L, Chelarescu-Vieru M (1934) Immunity in malaria. Trans R Soc Trop Med Hyg 27:619–622

Cohen S, McGregor IA, Carrington S (1961) Gamma-globulin and acquired immunity to human malaria. Nature 192:733–737

Collins WE, Jeffery GM (1999) A retrospective examination of secondary sporozoite- and trophozoite-induced infections with *Plasmodium falciparum*: development of parasitologic and clinical immunity following secondary infection. Am J Trop Med Hyg 61:20–35

Contamin H, Fandeur T, Rogier C, Bonnefoy S, Konate L, Trape JF, Mercereau-Puijalon O (1996) Different genetic characteristics of *Plasmodium falciparum* isolates collected during successive clinical malaria episodes in Senegalese children. Am J Trop Med Hyg 54:632–643

Conway DJ (1997) Natural selection on polymorphic malaria antigens and the search for a vaccine. Parasitol Today 13:26–29

Crotty S, Felgner P, Davies H, Glidewell J, Villarreal L, Ahmed R (2003) Cutting edge: long-term B cell memory in humans after smallpox vaccination. J Immunol 171:4969–4973

Daly TM, Long CA (1995) Humoral response to a carboxyl-terminal region of the merozoite surface protein-1 plays a predominant role in controlling blood-stage infection in rodent malaria. J Immunol 155:236–243

Daubersies P, Sallenave-Sales S, Magne S, Trape JF, Contamin H, Fandeur T, Rogier C, Mercereau-Puijalon O, Druilhe P (1996) Rapid turnover of *Plasmodium falciparum* populations in asymptomatic individuals living in a high transmission area. Am J Trop Med Hyg 54:18–26

Davidkin I, Valle M, Julkunen I (1995) Persistence of anti-mumps virus antibodies after a two-dose MMR vaccination. A nine-year follow-up. Vaccine 13:1617–1622

del Portillo HA, Fernandez-Becerra C, Bowman S, Oliver K, Preuss M, Sanchez CP, Schneider NK, Villalobos JM, Rajandream MA, Harris D, Pereira da Silva LH, Barrell B, Lanzer M (2001) A superfamily of variant genes encoded in the subtelomeric region of Plasmodium vivax. Nature 410:839–842

Deloron P, Chougnet C (1992) Is immunity to malaria really short-lived? Parasitol Today 8:375–378

Di Perri G, Bonora S, Vento S, Concia E (1995) Naturally acquired immunity to *Plasmodium falciparum*. Parasitol Today 11:346–347

Diggs CL, Hines F, Wellde BT (1995) *Plasmodium falciparum*: passive immunization of Aotus lemurinus griseimembra with immune serum. Exp Parasitol 80:291–296

Dodoo D, Staalsoe T, Giha H, Kurtzhals JA, Akanmori BD, Koram K, Dunyo S, Nkrumah FK, Hviid L, Theander TG (2001) Antibodies to variant antigens on the surfaces of infected erythrocytes are associated with protection from malaria in Ghanaian children. Infect Immun 69:3713–3718

Dodoo D, Theander TG, Kurtzhals JA, Koram K, Riley E, Akanmori BD, Nkrumah FK, Hviid L (1999) Levels of antibody to conserved parts of *Plasmodium falciparum* merozoite surface protein 1 in Ghanaian children are not associated with protection from clinical malaria. Infect Immun 67:2131–2137

Donati D, Zhang LP, Chen Q, Chene A, Flick K, Nystrom M, Wahlgren M, Bejarano MT (2004) Identification of a polyclonal B-cell activator in *Plasmodium falciparum*. Infect Immun 72:5412–5418

Druilhe P, Pérignon JL (1994) Immune mechanisms underlying the premunition against *Plasmodium falciparum* malaria. Mem Inst Oswaldo Cruz 89:51–53

Druilhe P, Pradier O, Marc JP, Miltgen F, Mazier D, Parent G (1986) Levels of antibodies to *Plasmodium falciparum* sporozoite surface antigens reflect malaria transmission rates and are persistent in the absence of reinfection. Infect Immun 53: 393–397.

Egan AF, Morris J, Barnish G, Allen S, Greenwood BM, Kaslow DC, Holder AA, Riley EM (1996) Clinical immunity to *Plasmodium falciparum* malaria is associated with serum antibodies to the 19-kDa C-terminal fragment of the merozoite surface antigen, PfMSP-1. J Infect Dis 173:765–769.

Eling WMC (1980) *Plasmodium berghei*: premunition, sterile immunity, and loss of immunity in mice. Exp Parasitol 49:89–96

Ericsson M, Sandstrom G, Sjostedt A, Tarnvik A (1994) Persistence of cell-mediated immunity and decline of humoral immunity to the intracellular bacterium Francisella tularensis 25 years after natural infection. J Infect Dis 170:110–114

Farnert A, Snounou G, Rooth I, Bjorkman A (1997) Daily dynamics of *Plasmodium falciparum* subpopulations in asymptomatic children in a holoendemic area. Am J Trop Med Hyg 56:538–547

Ferreira MU, Katzin AM (1995) The assessment of antibody affinity distribution by thiocyanate elution: a simple dose-response approach. J Immunol Methods 187:297–305

Ferreira MU, Kimura EA, De Souza JM, Katzin AM (1996) The isotype composition and avidity of naturally acquired anti-*Plasmodium falciparum* antibodies: differential patterns in clinically immune Africans and Amazonian patients. Am J Trop Med Hyg 55:315–323

Flanagan KL, Mwangi T, Plebanski M, Odhiambo K, Ross A, Sheu E, Kortok M, Lowe B, Marsh K, Hill AV (2003) Ex vivo interferon-gamma immune response to thrombospondin-related adhesive protein in coastal Kenyans: longevity and risk of *Plasmodium falciparum* infection. Am J Trop Med Hyg 68:421–430

Fonjungo PN, Elhassan IM, Cavanagh DR, Theander TG, Hviid L, Roper C, Arnot DE, McBride JS (1999) A longitudinal study of human antibody responses to *Plasmodium falciparum* rhoptry-associated protein 1 in a region of seasonal and unstable malaria transmission. Infect Immun 67:2975–2985

Früh K, Doumbo O, Muller HM, Koita O, McBride J, Crisanti A, Toure Y, Bujard H (1991) Human antibody response to the major merozoite surface antigen of *Plasmodium falciparum* is strain specific and short-lived. Infect Immun 59:1319–1324

Galinski MR, Corredor V (2004) Variant antigen expression in malaria infections: posttranscriptional gene silencing, virulence and severe pathology. Mol Biochem Parasitol 134:17–25

Garcia S, DiSanto J, Stockinger B (1999) Following the development of a CD4 T cell response in vivo: from activation to memory formation. Immunity 11:163–171

Garraud O, Perraut R, Diouf A, Nambei WS, Tall A, Spiegel A, Longacre S, Kaslow DC, Jouin H, Mattei D, Engler GM, Nutman TB, Riley EM, Mercereau-Puijalon O (2002) Regulation of antigen-specific immunoglobulin G subclasses in response to conserved and polymorphic *Plasmodium falciparum* antigens in an *in vitro* model. Infect Immun 70:2820–2827

Giha HA, Staalsoe T, Dodoo D, Elhassan IM, Roper C, Satti GM, Arnot DE, Theander TG, Hviid L (1999) Nine-year longitudinal study of antibodies to variant antigens on the surface of *Plasmodium falciparum*-infected erythrocytes. Infect Immun 67:4092–4098

Giha HA, Theander TG, Staalso T, Roper C, Elhassan IM, Babiker H, Satti GM, Arnot DE, Hviid L (1998) Seasonal variation in agglutination of *Plasmodium falciparum*-infected erythrocytes. Am J Trop Med Hyg 58:399–405

Goldblatt D, Borrow R, Miller E (2002) Natural and vaccine-induced immunity and immunologic memory to *Neisseria meningitidis* serogroup C in young adults. J Infect Dis 185:397–400

Gozalo A, Lucas C, Cachay M, Wellde BT, Hall T, Bell B, Wood J, Watts D, Wooster M, Lyon JA, Moch JK, Haynes JD, Williams JS, Holland C, Watson E, Kester KE, Kaslow DC, Ballou WR (1998) Passive transfer of growth-inhibitory antibodies raised against yeast-expressed recombinant *Plasmodium falciparum* merozoite surface protein-1(19). Am J Trop Med Hyg 59:991–997

Gray D, Skarvall H (1988) B-cell memory is short-lived in the absence of antigen. Nature 336:70–73

Greenwood BM (1974) Possible role of a B-cell mitogen in hypergammaglobulinaemia in malaria and trypanosomiasis. Lancet 1:435–436

Greenwood BM, David PH, Otoo-Forbes LN, Allen SJ, Alonso PL, Armstrong Schellenberg JR, Byass P, Hurwitz M, Menon A, Snow RW (1995) Mortality and morbidity from malaria after stopping malaria chemoprophylaxis. Trans R Soc Trop Med Hyg 89:629–633

Grun JL, Weidanz WP (1983) Antibody-independent immunity to reinfection malaria in B-cell-deficient mice. Infect Immun 41:1197–1204

Gupta S, Snow RW, Donnelly CA, Marsh K, Newbold C (1999) Immunity to non-cerebral severe malaria is acquired after one or two infections. Nat Med 5:340–343

Gysin J, Moisson P, Pereira da Silva L, Druilhe P (1996) Antibodies from immune African donors with a protective effect in *Plasmodium falciparum* human infection are also able to control asexual blood forms of the parasite in Saimiri monkeys. Res Immunol 147:397–401

Hammarlund E, Lewis MW, Hansen SG, Strelow LI, Nelson JA, Sexton GJ, Hanifin JM, Slifka MK (2003) Duration of antiviral immunity after smallpox vaccination. Nat Med 9:1131–1137

Hirunpetcharat C, Tian JH, Kaslow DC, van Rooijen N, Kumar S, Berzofsky JA, Miller LH, Good MF (1997) Complete protective immunity induced in mice by immunization with the 19-kilodalton carboxyl-terminal fragment of the merozoite surface protein-1 (MSP1[19]) of Plasmodium yoelii expressed in *Saccharomyces cerevisiae*: correlation of protection with antigen-specific antibody titer, but not with effector CD4[+] T cells. J Immunol 159:3400–3411

Hogh B, Petersen E, Dziegiel M, David K, Hanson A, Borre M, Holm A, Vuust J, Jepsen S (1992) Antibodies to a recombinant glutamate-rich *Plasmodium falciparum* protein: evidence for protection of individuals living in a holoendemic area of Liberia. Am J Trop Med Hyg 46:307–313

Hughes MK, Hughes AL (1995) Natural selection on Plasmodium surface proteins. Mol Biochem Parasitol 71:99–113

Hviid L, Kurtzhals JA, Goka BQ, Oliver-Commey JO, Nkrumah FK, Theander TG (1997) Rapid reemergence of T cells into peripheral circulation following treatment of severe and uncomplicated *Plasmodium falciparum* malaria. Infect Immun 65:4090–4093

Hviid L, Staalsoe T (2004) Malaria immunity in infants: a special case of a general phenomenon? Trends Parasitol 20:66–72

Jacob J, Kassir R, Kelsoe G (1991) In situ studies of the primary immune response to (4-hydroxy-3-nitrophenyl)acetyl. I. The architecture and dynamics of responding cell populations. J Exp Med 173:1165–1175

Jakobsen PH, Kurtzhals JA, Riley EM, Hviid L, Theander TG, Morris-Jones S, Jensen JB, Bayoumi RA, Ridley RG, Greenwood BM (1997) Antibody responses to Rhoptry-Associated Protein-1 (RAP-1) of *Plasmodium falciparum* parasites in humans from areas of different malaria endemicity. Parasite Immunol 19:387–393

Janssen CS, Barrett MP, Turner CM, Phillips RS (2002) A large gene family for putative variant antigens shared by human and rodent malaria parasites. Proc R Soc Lond B Biol Sci 269:431–436

Jarra W, Hills LA, March JC, Brown KN (1986) Protective immunity to malaria. Studies with cloned lines of *Plasmodium chabaudi chabaudi* and *P. berghei* in CBA/Ca mice. II. The effectiveness and inter- or intra-species specificity of the passive transfer of immunity with serum. Parasite Immunol 8:239–254

John CC, Ouma JH, Sumba PO, Hollingdale MR, Kazura JW, King CL (2002) Lymphocyte proliferation and antibody responses to *Plasmodium falciparum* liver-stage antigen-1 in a highland area of Kenya with seasonal variation in malaria transmission. Am J Trop Med Hyg 66:372–378

Kaneko A (1999). Malaria on islands: human and parasite diversities and implications for malaria control in Vanuatu. *In* "Department of Medicine, Unit of Infectious Diseases". Karolinska Institutet, Karolinska Hospital, Stockholm.

Kaneko A, Taleo G, Kalkoa M, Yamar S, Kobayakawa T, Björkman A (2000) Malaria eradication on islands. Lancet 356:1560–1564

Karrer U, Lopez-Macias C, Oxenius A, Odermatt B, Bachmann MF, Kalinke U, Bluethmann H, Hengartner H, Zinkernagel RM (2000) Antiviral B cell memory in the absence of mature follicular dendritic cell networks and classical germinal centers in TNFR1$^{-/-}$ mice. J Immunol 164:768–778

Kassiotis G, Garcia S, Simpson E, Stockinger B (2002) Impairment of immunological memory in the absence of MHC despite survival of memory T cells. Nat Immunol 3:244–250

Kinyanjui SM, Mwangi, T, Bull PC, Newbold CI, Marsh K (2004) Protection against clinical malaria by heterologous immunoglobulin G antibodies against malaria-infected erythrocyte variant surface antigens requires interaction with asymptomatic infections. J Infect Dis 190:1527–1533

Kinyanjui SM, Bull P, Newbold CI, Marsh K (2003) Kinetics of antibody responses to *Plasmodium falciparum*-infected erythrocyte variant surface antigens. J Infect Dis 187:667–674

Kundig TM, Bachmann MF, Oehen S, Hoffmann UW, Simard JJ, Kalberer CP, Pircher H, Ohashi PS, Hengartner H, Zinkernagel RM (1996) On the role of antigen in maintaining cytotoxic T-cell memory. Proc Natl Acad Sci U S A 93:9716–9723

Langhorne J, Cross C, Seixas E, Li C, von der Weid T (1998) A role for B cells in the development of T cell helper function in a malaria infection in mice. Proc Natl Acad Sci USA 95:1730–1734

Langhorne J, Kim KJ, Asofsky R (1985) Distribution of immunoglobulin isotypes in the nonspecific B-cell response induced by infection with Plasmodium chabaudi adami and Plasmodium yoelii. Cell Immunol 90:251–257

Langhorne J, Simon-Haarhaus B (1991) Differential T cell responses to Plasmodium chabaudi chabaudi in peripheral blood and spleens of C57BL/6 mice during infection. J Immunol 146:2771–2775

LaRussa PS, Gershon AA, Steinberg SP, Chartrand SA (1990) Antibodies to varicella-zoster virus glycoproteins I, II, and III in leukemic and healthy children. J Infect Dis 162: 627–633

Ling IT, Ogun SA, Holder AA (1995) The combined epidermal growth factor-like modules of *Plasmodium yoelii* Merozoite Surface Protein-1 are required for a protective immune response to the parasite. Parasite Immunol 17:425–433

Luty AJ, Ulbert S, Lell B, Lehman L, Schmidt-Ott R, Luckner D, Greve B, Matousek P, Schmid D, Herbich K, Dubois B, Deloron P, Kremsner PG (2000) Antibody responses to *Plasmodium falciparum*: evolution according to the severity of a prior clinical episode and association with subsequent reinfection. Am J Trop Med Hyg 62:566–572

MacLennan IC, Garcia de Vinuesa C, Casamayor-Palleja M (2000) B-cell memory and the persistence of antibody responses. Philos Trans R Soc Lond B Biol Sci 355:345–350

MacLennan ICM (1995) B cells. Avoiding autoreactivity. Nature 375:281

Magesa SM, Mdira KY, Babiker HA, Alifrangis M, Farnert A, Simonsen PE, Bygbjerg IC, Walliker D, Jakobsen PH (2002) Diversity of *Plasmodium falciparum* clones infecting children living in a holoendemic area in north-eastern Tanzania. Acta Trop 84:83–92

Maley SW, Buxton D, Thomson KM, Schriefer CE, Innes EA (2001) Serological analysis of calves experimentally infected with Neospora caninum: a 1-year study. Vet Parasitol 96:1-9

Mallet E, Fabre P, Pines E, Salomon H, Staub T, Schodel F, Mendelman P, Hessel L, Chryssomalis G, Vidor E, Hoffenbach A (2000) Immunogenicity and safety of a new liquid hexavalent combined vaccine compared with separate administration of reference licensed vaccines in infants. Pediatr Infect Dis J 19: 1119–1127

Manz RA, Radbruch A (2002) Plasma cells for a lifetime? Eur J Immunol 32:923–927

Manz RA, Thiel A, Radbruch A (1997) Lifetime of plasma cells in the bone marrow. Nature 388:133–134

Maple PA, Jones CS, Wall EC, Vyseb A, Edmunds WJ, Andrews NJ, Miller E (2000) Immunity to diphtheria and tetanus in England and Wales. Vaccine 19:167–173

Marsh K (1992) Malaria-a neglected disease? Parasitology 104: S53–S69

Marsh K, Otoo L, Hayes RJ, Carson DC, Greenwood BM (1989) Antibodies to blood stage antigens of *Plasmodium falciparum* in rural Gambians and their relation to protection against infection. Trans R Soc Trop Med Hyg 83:293–303

Martin SW, Goodnow CC (2002) Burst-enhancing role of the IgG membrane tail as a molecular determinant of memory. Nat Immunol 3:182–188

Maruyama M, Lam KP, Rajewsky K (2000) Memory B-cell persistence is independent of persisting immunizing antigen. Nature 407:636–642

McLean SA, Pearson CD, Phillips RS (1982) Plasmodium chabaudi: antigenic variation during recrudescent parasitaemias in mice. Exp Parasitol 54:296–302

Metzger WG, Okenu DM, Cavanagh DR, Robinson JV, Bojang KA, Weiss HA, McBride JS, Greenwood BM, Conway DJ (2003) Serum IgG3 to the *Plasmodium falciparum* merozoite surface protein 2 is strongly associated with a reduced prospective risk of malaria. Parasite Immunol 25:307–312

Migot F, Chougnet C, Henzel D, Dubois B, Jambou R, Fievet N, Deloron P (1995) Anti-malaria antibody-producing B cell frequencies in adults after a *Plasmodium falciparum* outbreak in Madagascar. Clin Exp Immunol 102:529–534

Newbold C, Warn P, Black G, Berendt A, Craig A, Snow B, Msobo M, Peshu N, Marsh K (1997) Receptor-specific adhesion and clinical disease in *Plasmodium falciparum*. Am J Trop Med Hyg 57:389–398

O'Connor BP, Gleeson MW, Noelle RJ, Erickson LD (2003) The rise and fall of long-lived humoral immunity: terminal differentiation of plasma cells in health and disease. Immunol Rev 194:61–76

Ober RJ, Martinez C, Vaccaro C, Zhou J, Ward ES (2004) Visualizing the site and dynamics of IgG salvage by the MHC class I-related receptor, FcRn. J Immunol 172:2021–2029

Ochsenbein AF, Pinschewer DD, Sierro S, Horvath E, Hengartner H, Zinkernagel RM (2000) Protective long-term antibody memory by antigen-driven and T help-dependent differentiation of long-lived memory B cells to short-lived plasma cells independent of secondary lymphoid organs. Proc Natl Acad Sci U S A 97:13263–13268

Owusu-Agyei S, Binka F, Koram K, Anto F, Adjuik M, Nkrumah F, Smith T (2002) Does radical cure of asymptomatic *Plasmodium falciparum* place adults in endemic areas at increased risk of recurrent symptomatic malaria? Trop Med Int Health 7:599–603

Park CG, Chwae YJ, Kim JI, Lee JH, Hur GM, Jeon BH, Koh JS, Han JH, Lee SJ, Park JW, Kaslow DC, Strickman D, Roh CS (2000) Serologic responses of Korean soldiers serving in malaria-endemic areas during a recent outbreak of *Plasmodium vivax*. Am J Trop Med Hyg 62:720–725

Petersen E, Hogh B, Perlmann H, Kabilan L, Troye-Blomberg M, Marbiah NT, Hanson AP, Bjorkman A, Perlmann P (1989) An epidemiological study of humoral and cell-mediated immune response to the *Plasmodium falciparum* antigen PF155/RESA in adult Liberians. Am J Trop Med Hyg 41:386–394

Plotkin JB, Dushoff J, Fraser HB (2004) Detecting selection using a single genome sequence of M. tuberculosis and P. falciparum. Nature 428:942–945

Polley SD, Conway DJ (2001) Strong diversifying selection on domains of the *Plasmodium falciparum* apical membrane antigen 1 gene. Genetics 158:1505–1512

Polley SD, Mwangi T, Kocken CHM, Thomas AW, Dutta S, Lanar DE, Remarque E, Ross A, Williams T, Mwambingu G, Lowe B, Conway DJ, Marsh K (2004) Human antibodies to recombinant protein constructs of *Plasmodium falciparum* Apical Membrane Antigen (AMA1) and their associations with protection from malaria. Vaccine 23:718–728

Pulendran B, Kannourakis G, Nouri S, Smith KG, Nossal GJ (1995) Soluble antigen can cause enhanced apoptosis of germinal-centre B cells. Nature 375:331–334.

Quin SJ, Langhorne J (2001) Different regions of the malaria merozoite surface protein 1 of *Plasmodium chabaudi* elicit distinct T-cell and antibody isotype responses. Infect Immun 69:2245–2251.

Ramasamy R, Nagendran K, Ramasamy MS (1994) Antibodies to epitopes on merozoite and sporozoite surface antigens as serologic markers of malaria transmission: studies at a site in the dry zone of Sri Lanka. Am J Trop Med Hyg 50:537–547

Recker M, Nee S, Bull PC, Kinyanjui S, Marsh K, Newbold C, Gupta S (2004) Transient cross-reactive immune responses can orchestrate antigenic variation in malaria. Nature 429:555–558

Richmond P, Borrow R, Goldblatt D, Findlow J, Martin S, Morris R, Cartwright K, Miller E (2001) Ability of 3 different meningococcal C conjugate vaccines to induce immunologic memory after a single dose in UK toddlers. J Infect Dis 183: 160–163

Riley EM, Allen SJ, Wheeler JG, Blackman MJ, Bennett S, Takacs B, Schonfeld HJ, Holder AA, Greenwood BM (1992) Naturally acquired cellular and humoral immune responses to the major merozoite surface antigen (PfMSP1) of *Plasmodium falciparum* are associated with reduced malaria morbidity. Parasite Immunol 14:321–337

Riley EM, Morris-Jones S, Blackman MJ, Greenwood BM, Holder AA (1993) A longitudinal study of naturally acquired cellular and humoral immune responses to a merozoite surface protein (MSP1) of *Plasmodium falciparum* in an area of seasonal malaria transmission. Parasite Immunol 15:513–524

Roberts DJ, Craig AG, Berendt AR, Pinches R, Nash G, Marsh K, Newbold CI (1992) Rapid switching to multiple antigenic and adhesive phenotypes in malaria. Nature 357:689–692

Rosenberg YJ (1978) Autoimmune and polyclonal B cell responses during murine malaria. Nature 274:170–172

Rotman HL, Daly TM, Long CA (1999) *Plasmodium*: immunization with carboxyl-terminal regions of MSP-1 protects against homologous but not heterologous blood-stage parasite challenge. Exp Parasitol 91:78–85

Sabchareon A, Burnouf T, Ouattara D, Attanath P, Bouharoun-Tayoun H, Chantavanich P, Foucault C, Chongsuphajaisiddhi T, Druilhe P (1991) Parasitologic and clinical human response to immunoglobulin administration in falciparum malaria. Am J Trop Med Hyg 45:297–308

Sangster MY, Topham DJ, D'Costa S, Cardin RD, Marion TN, Myers LK, Doherty PC (2000) Analysis of the virus-specific and nonspecific B cell response to a persistent B-lymphotropic gammaherpesvirus. J Immunol 164:1820–1828

Shakib F (1990). The human IgG subclasses: molecular analysis of structure, function and regulation. Pergamon Press, Oxford.

Shokat KM, Goodnow CC (1995) Antigen-induced B-cell death and elimination during germinal-centre immune responses. Nature 375:334–338

Siddiqui W, Tam L, Kramer K, Hui G, Case S, Yamaga K, Chang S, Chan E, Kan S (1987) Merozoite surface coat precursor protein completely protects Aotus monkeys against *Plasmodium falciparum* malaria. Proc Natl Acad Sci USA 84:3014–3018

Slifka MK, Ahmed R (1996) Long-term humoral immunity against viruses: revisiting the issue of plasma cell longevity. Trends Microbiol 4:394–400

Slifka MK, Antia R, Whitmire JK, Ahmed R (1998) Humoral immunity due to long-lived plasma cells. Immunity 8:363–372

Slifka MK, Matloubian M, Ahmed R (1995) Bone marrow is a major site of long-term antibody production after acute viral infection. J Virol 69:1895–1902

Smith T, Felger I, Tanner M, Beck HP (1999) Premunition in *Plasmodium falciparum* infection: insights from the epidemiology of multiple infections. Trans R Soc Trop Med Hyg 93 Suppl 1:59–64

Snow RW, Nahlen B, Palmer A, Donnelly CA, Gupta S, Marsh K (1998) Risk of severe malaria among African infants: direct evidence of clinical protection during early infancy. J Infect Dis 177:819–822

Soares IS, da Cunha MG, Silva MN, Souza JM, Del Portillo HA, Rodrigues MM (1999a) Longevity of naturally acquired antibody responses to the N- and C-terminal regions of *Plasmodium vivax* merozoite surface protein 1. Am J Trop Med Hyg 60:357–363

Soares IS, Oliveira SG, Souza JM, Rodrigues MM (1999b) Antibody response to the N and C-terminal regions of the *Plasmodium vivax* Merozoite Surface Protein 1 in individuals living in an area of exclusive transmission of *P. vivax* malaria in the north of Brazil. Acta Trop 72:13–24

Staalso T, Hviid L (1998) The role of variant specific immunity in asymptomatic malaria infections: maintaining a fine balance. Parasitol Today 14:177

Staalsoe T, Shulman CE, Bulmer JN, Kawuondo K, Marsh K, Hviid L (2004) Variant surface antigen-specific IgG and protection against clinical consequences of pregnancy-associated *Plasmodium falciparum* malaria. Lancet 363:283–289

Stevenson MM, Tam MF (1993) Differential induction of helper T cell subsets during blood-stage Plasmodium chabaudi AS infection in resistant and susceptible mice. Clin Exp Immunol 92:77–83

Sze DM, Toellner KM, Garcia de Vinuesa C, Taylor DR, MacLennan IC (2000) Intrinsic constraint on plasmablast growth and extrinsic limits of plasma cell survival. J Exp Med 192:813–821

Taylor RR, Egan A, McGuinness D, Jepson A, Adair R, Drakely C, Riley E (1996) Selective recognition of malaria antigens by human serum antibodies is not genetically determined but demonstrates some features of clonal imprinting. Int Immunol 8:905–915

Terrientes ZI, Kramer K, Herrera MA, Chang SP (1994) Naturally acquired antibodies against the major merozoite surface coat protein (MSP-1) of *Plasmodium falciparum* acquired by residents in an endemic area of Colombia. Mem Inst Oswaldo Cruz 89:55–61

Tew JG, Mandel TE (1979) Prolonged antigen half-life in the lymphoid follicles of specifically immunized mice. Immunology 37:69–76

Tian JH, Miller LH, Kaslow DC, Ahlers J, Good MF, Alling DW, Berzofsky JA, Kumar S (1996) Genetic regulation of protective immune response in congenic strains of mice vaccinated with a subunit malaria vaccine. J Immunol 157:1176–1183

Tomoda T, Ogura H, Kurashige T (1992) The longevity of the immune response to filamentous hemagglutinin and pertussis toxin in patients with pertussis in a semi-closed community. J Infect Dis 166:908–910

Traggiai E, Puzone R, Lanzavecchia A (2003) Antigen dependent and independent mechanisms that sustain serum antibody levels. Vaccine 21 Suppl 2: S35–37

Uzonna JE, Wei G, Yurkowski D, Bretscher P (2001) Immune elimination of Leishmania major in mice: implications for immune memory, vaccination, and reactivation disease. J Immunol 167:6967–6974

van der Heyde HC, Huszar D, Woodhouse C, Manning DD, Weidanz WP (1994) The resolution of acute malaria in a definitive model of B cell deficiency, the J_HD mouse. J Immunol 152:4557–4562

van Druten H, van Knapen F, Reintjes A (1990) Epidemiologic implications of limited-duration seropositivity after toxoplasma infection. Am J Epidemiol 132:169–180

Vieira P, Rajewsky K (1990) Persistence of memory B cells in mice deprived of T cell help. Int Immunol 2:487–494

von der Weid T, Honarvar N, Langhorne J (1996) Gene-targeted mice lacking B cells are unable to eliminate a blood stage malaria infection. J Immunol 156:2510–2516

Vukovic P, Hogarth PM, Barnes N, Kaslow DC, Good MF (2000) Immunoglobulin G3 antibodies specific for the 19-kilodalton carboxyl-terminal fragment of Plasmodium yoelii merozoite surface protein 1 transfer protection to mice deficient in Fc-gammaRI receptors. Infect Immun 68:3019–3022

Ward ES, Zhou J, Ghetie V, Ober RJ (2003) Evidence to support the cellular mechanism involved in serum IgG homeostasis in humans. Int Immunol 15:187–195

Weidanz WP, Melancon-Kaplan J, Cavacini LA (1990) Cell-mediated immunity to the asexual blood stages of malarial parasites: animal models. Immunol Lett 25:87–95

Xu H, Wipasa J, Yan H, Zeng M, Makobongo MO, Finkelman FD, Kelso A, Good MF (2002) The mechanism and significance of deletion of parasite-specific CD4(+) T cells in malaria infection. J Exp Med 195:881–892

Zerboni L, Nader S, Aoki K, Arvin AM (1998) Analysis of the persistence of humoral and cellular immunity in children and adults immunized with varicella vaccine. J Infect Dis 177:1701–1704

Zevering Y, Khamboonruang C, Rungruengthanakit K, Tungviboonchai L, Ruengpi-pattanapan J, Bathurst I, Barr P, Good MF (1994) Life-spans of human T-cell responses to determinants from the circumsporozoite proteins of Plasmodium falciparum and Plasmodium vivax. Proc Natl Acad Sci U S A 91:6118–6122

Zinkernagel RM (2002) On differences between immunity and immunological memory. Curr Opin Immunol 14:523–536

Zinkernagel RM, Hengartner H (2001) Regulation of the immune response by antigen. Science 293:251–253

CTMI (2005) 297:103–143
© Springer-Verlag Berlin Heidelberg 2005

Experimental Models of Cerebral Malaria

C. Engwerda[1] (✉) · E. Belnoue[2] · A. C. Grüner[2] · L. Rénia[2]

[1]Immunology and Infection Laboratory, Queensland Institute of Medical Research,
300 Herston Road, 4006 Herston, Queensland, Australia
chrisE@qimr.edu.au

[2]Département d'Immunologie, Institut Cochin, Hôpital Cochin, Bâtiment Gustave
Roussy, 27 rue du fg St Jacques, 75014 Paris, France

Abstract   Malaria remains a major global health problem and cerebral malaria is one of the most serious complications of this disease. Recent years have seen important advances in our understanding of the pathogenesis of cerebral malaria. Extensive analysis of tissues and blood taken from patients with cerebral malaria has been complimented by the use of animal models to identify specific components of pathogenic pathways. In particular, an important role for CD8[+] T cells has been uncovered, as well divergent roles for members of the tumor necrosis factor (TNF) family of molecules, including TNF and lymphotoxin alpha. It has become apparent that there may be more than one pathogenic pathway leading to cerebral malaria. The last few years have also seen the testing of vaccines designed to target malaria molecules that stimulate inflammatory responses and thereby prevent the development of cerebral malaria. In this review, we will discuss the above advancements, as well as other important findings in research into the pathogenesis of cerebral malaria. As our understanding of pathogenic responses to *Plasmodium* parasites gathers momentum, the chance of a breakthrough in the development of treatments and vaccines to prevent death from cerebral malaria have become more realistic.

Abbreviations

CM	Cerebral malaria
iRBC	Infected red blood cells
IL	Interleukin
MVEC	Microvascular endothelial cells
NO	Nitric oxide
NOS	Nitric oxide synthase
PbA	*Plasmodium berghei* ANKA
Pb K173	*Plasmodium berghei* Kyberg 173

1
Malaria, the Disease

Malaria is among the most important and oldest diseases of mankind having huge death and socio-economic tolls. Long before the discovery of the etiological agent, *Plasmodium* parasites, earliest descriptions of this disease have always been related to the particular pathology the parasites induce. Enlarged spleens and recurrent fevers have been reported in Vedic, Greek and Chinese writings. A large spectrum of clinical manifestations is observed, from asymptomatic infections to fulminant disease. The clinical characteristics of the infection depend on the *Plasmodium* species and on the age and immune status of the host. Clinical manifestations are linked to the replication cycles of the parasite. Rupture of infected red blood cells (iRBC) and release of toxic substances into the circulation are responsible for the repeated episode of chills, headaches and fevers, followed by profuse sweats (Maegraith and Fletcher 1972). The periodicity of this clinical presentation differs between species; either quartan cycle (*P.* malaria) or tertian cycle (*P. falciparum*, *P. vivax*, and *P. ovale*). The natural chronicity of these infections also leads to the development of splenomegaly, hepatomegaly, renal failure and severe anemia. Different factors, both parasitological and immunological, have been implicated in the development of these pathologies. However, a clear understanding of malaria pathogenesis is yet to be determined. Other complications, like acidosis, edema, respiratory problems, jaundice, hypoglycemia, and cerebral malaria (CM), can occur during a severe falciparum malaria episode (World Health Organization 1990). From these complications, hypoglycemia, severe anemia and cerebral malaria are the principal causes of death and thus represent a major public health problem.

2
Cerebral Malaria in Humans

CM is one of the most severe complications of *P. falciparum* infection, and has been extensively studied since the end of the nineteenth century (Marchiava and Bignami 1892). It can lead to death only 14 days after infection and the critical phase of this pathology may last as little as 48 h (Warrell et al. 1997). CM is a neurologic syndrome, described as a diffuse encephalopathy, associated with loss of conscience and of muscular tone. The degree of loss of conscience ranges from confusion to coma. In some instances, the coma can be reversible but CM is usually associated with a poor prognosis, as 20%–30% mortality is recorded even under active treatment (Brewster et al. 1990). Recent studies have shown that a large spectrum of neurological sequelae may be observed after a severe cerebral episode (Brewster et al. 1990; Schmutzard and Gerstenbrand 1984; Bondi 1992). Geographical differences, in terms of prevalence of the clinical syndrome and severity of the neurologic manifestations, exist. This might be due to differences in parasite and host genetic background, as well as epidemiological and socio-economic conditions.

The pathogenesis of CM is not fully understood and possibly results in part from the sequestration of iRBC and from pro-inflammatory cytokine responses. The first detailed histopathological description of brain capillary occlusion and sequestration of iRBC in the brain tissue of a patient who died of CM was made by Marchiava and Bignami (1900), an observation repeatedly confirmed by others through the twentieth century (Margulis 1914; Dürck 1917; Gaskell and Miller 1920; Rigdon and Fletcher 1944; Kean and Smith 1944; Spitz 1961). This phenomenon was accompanied by swelling of the endothelium, damage to the vessel wall, and cerebral hemorrhage. Reports have also described the presence of leukocytes in the brains of African children

(Grau et al. 2003; Clark et al. 2003) and in Indian adults with CM (Patnaik et al 1994). As a note of caution, it should be kept in mind that all histopathological data are derived from autopsy samples from patients who died of CM. Thus, this phenomenon may represent a terminal event. For obvious ethical reasons, the ongoing neuropathogenic processes cannot be studied.

The suggestion of a role for pro-inflammatory cytokines was originally put forward by Clark (1994) and Grau (Hunt and Grau 2003) and a large body of data have confirmed their part in CM pathogenesis. As for histopathological studies, ethical reasons limit the extent of cytokine studies in humans. Indeed, most of these studies have been performed with peripheral blood samples: serum or peripheral blood mononuclear cells for ex vivo and in vitro studies. These human studies together with the development of genetic studies on susceptibility have added to our knowledge, but have not allowed us to draw a firm conclusion on the pathogenesis of CM. Animal models, and in particular mouse models, though not perfect, have been instrumental in understanding certain aspects of CM (de Souza and Riley 2001; Lou et al. 2001).

3
Mouse Cerebral Malaria

The use of rodent malaria parasites in mice is the model of choice for studying the pathogenesis of CM. The availability of mice of defined genetic background, and the always-expanding numbers of transgenic or gene-deficient mice, has allowed a large variety of experiments. Moreover, using this model it is possible to perform kinetic experiments on whole organs (i.e., brain, spleen) in a strictly controlled manner. Four species and 13 subspecies of rodent *Plasmodium* exist (Landau and Boulard 1978), but only *P. berghei* and *P. yoelii* have been used consistently for CM studies. There has been some contention over the relevance of the rodent models, and it is evident that experimental models cannot reproduce all the features of CM. However, careful analysis of the data obtained and an in-depth knowledge of parasite biology and mouse physiology have allowed us to test hypotheses and establish new concepts of malaria pathogenesis for human CM.

Of all parasite species, *P. berghei* is the only one able to induce CM in mice, rats and hamsters (Mercado 1965; Bafort et al. 1980, Mackey et al. 1980; Rest 1982, 1983). *P. berghei* was first isolated from an infected *Anopheles dureni* in the Belgian Congo in 1948 (Vincke and Lips 1948). It was later shown that *Thamnomys surdaster* tree rats were the natural host of this parasite. A number of different strains of *P. berghei* were isolated in the same region of the Congo (Table 1) and four of them, *P. berghei* SP11, ANKA (PbA), NK65

Table 1 Rodent malaria parasites used for cerebral malaria studies

Species	Subspecies	Strain	Clones	Origin	Erythrocytic cycle	Rodent species used	Neurological signs
P. berghei		ANKA	1.49L, 1.94L, 4	Katanga, Congo	21 h	Mouse	Yes
			5, BdS, cl5, 15cy1	Katanga, Congo	21 h	Rat	Yes
						Golden Hamster	Yes
		NK65		Katanga, Congo	21 h	WM rat	Yes
		SP-11		Katanga, Congo	21 h	Mouse	Yes
		Keyberg 173		Katanga, Congo	21 h	Mouse	No
						Rat	Yes
P. yoelii	yoelii	17XL	1.1, YM	Centrafrican Republic	18 h	Mouse	No
	nigeriensis	N67		Nigeria	18 h	Mouse	No
P. chabaudi	chabaudi		AS	Centrafrican Republic	24 h	Mouse	No

and Kyberg 173 (K173), have been used to study CM. The neurovascular pathology induced by *P. berghei* was first reported for the K173 strain in rats by Mercado (1965). CM was later shown to occur in white mice with a pyrimethamine-resistant line of the SP11 strain (Jadin et al. 1975) and in rats with PbA (Bafort et al. 1980). The SP11 strain has not since been used in experiments. For a long time, only the ANKA strain was reported to induce neurological signs in mice. The NK65 strain was shown to induce CM in one occasion in WM rats (Kamiyama et al. 1987). The *P. berghei* K173 strain was sometimes used to study CM because histopathological analysis of the brains of infected mice showed cerebral involvement (Polder et al. 1983). Recently, low-dose injection of *P. berghei* K173 in mice was shown to induce CM-associated neurological signs (Ball et al. 2003). Most studies of CM have been performed using uncloned parasite lines. There is now increasing evidence that the ability of *P. berghei* to induce CM may vary between clones (Amani et al 1998).

Most strains of mice are susceptible to CM (CBA/ca, CBA/J, CBA/HN, C57BL/6J, C57BL/6N, SLJ/J, 129/Ola, Swiss and NMRI). However, there are contradictory reports on the resistance of certain strains, such as C3H, BALB/c, DBA/2 and 129Sv/ev (Mackey et al. 1980; Grau et al. 1990a; Amani et al. 1998; Bagot et al. 2002). Although the basis for this difference is unknown for 129Sv/ev and C3H mice, the susceptibility of BALB/c mice was shown to be dependent of the presence of a mouse mammary tumor virus (Gorgette et al. 2002), which modifies the repertoire of T cells present in infected animals. One report on DBA/2 mice described a resolving PbA-induced CM, while in another report DBA/2 mice were classified as resistant to the development of CM (Bagot et al. 2002). Variable susceptibility to PbA-induced CM has also been confirmed in congenic mice recently derived from wild mice (Bagot et al. 2002). Nevertheless, PbA in CBA/Ca and C57BL/6 mice and Pb K173 in C57BL/6 mice have been the most studied mouse/parasite combinations.

Most studies on murine CM have been performed through the direct inoculation of iRBC. Blood parasites were obtained from either an infected mouse or from frozen aliquots. Studies have shown that the age of the mouse has an inverse correlation with CM susceptibility (Hearn et al. 2000). The dose of inoculated iRBC is also likely to influence the development of CM (Schetters et al 1989; Amani et al. 1998; Ball et al. 2003). Another potential confounding factor in experiments using iRBC is the original source of the blood. It was shown in one study that propagation of a clonal PbA parasite through the different strains of mice could modify its ability to induce CM (Amani et al. 1998). This suggested that phenotypic alteration exists in PbA, similar to that demonstrated in *P. falciparum* (Roberts et al. 1992).

Recent studies have initiated infection using PbA sporozoites. In one study, the development of CM was dependent on the dose of sporozoites injected (Bagot et al. 2004). However, other studies have shown that CM was not reproducible and was independent of the sporozoite infective dose (L. Rénia and A.C. Grüner, unpublished results).

Susceptible mice infected with *P. berghei* ANKA develop a neurological syndrome characterized by paralysis, deviation of the head, ataxia, convulsions and coma. These symptoms occur 6–14 days after iRBC inoculation and lead to death in 60%–100% of mice with a relatively low parasitemia. Histopathological analysis of the brain shows a sequestration of leukocytes and to a lesser extent of iRBC (Polder et al. 1983, 1992; Neill and Hunt 1992, Neill et al. 1993; Hearn et al. 2000). Leukocyte infiltration between endothelial cells has been seldom observed, but in the majority of studies, leukocytes and iRBC accumulation was shown to occur intravascularly. Those mice that do not develop CM die during the second–third week post-infection from hyperparasitemia and severe anemia. One major difference from the human disease is that mice do not develop high fevers but instead develop a progressive hypothermia in the days prior to death (Cordeiro et al. 1983; Curfs et al. 1990; Amani et al. 1998). Mice deficient in a number of different molecules have been used to show the role of those proteins in CM pathogenesis (Table 2). Rats (Wistar, Osborn-Mendel, Sprague Dawley, and Holtzman strains) or Golden Hamster/*P. berghei* combinations have also been used but have received less attention than the PbA/mouse combination (Mercado 1965; Rest and Wright 1979; Bakker et al. 1992; Franz et al. 1987).

Alternative models of CM using *P. yoelii yoelii* 17XL or YM in CF1, Swiss and BALB/c mice, and *P. yoelii nigeriensis* N67 in Swiss mice have also been proposed (Yoeli and Heargraves 1974; Sharma et al. 1992). *P. yoelii* 17XL and YM as well as *P. yoelii nigeriensis* grow rapidly in these strains and mice usually die 6–9 days after a blood infection with very high parasitemia (up to 90%). Histopathological analysis of the brain of *P. yoelli*-infected mice showed moderate to heavy cerebral involvement. Capillaries were found partially or completely filled by sequestered red cells (mainly infected with schizont-stage parasites) in the relative absence of leukocytes (Yoeli and Heargraves 1974, Kaul et al. 1994; Sharma 1994). There has been one study reporting that BALB/c mice infected with *P. yoelii* 17XL can develop convulsions, ataxia and coma (Haque et al. 1999). We and others have observed such clinical signs in moribund mice with high parasitemia and severe anemia infected either with *P. yoelii* or *P. berghei*. However, these mice display different types of symptoms from those observed in mice with PbA-induced CM. Recently, Langhorne and collaborators have observed that infection with *P. chabaudi chabaudi* AS clone iRBC can induce cerebral vascular leakage, edema, and

Table 2 Cerebral malaria in deficient mice

Modified gene	Deficiency	Genetic background	CM[a]	References
Lymphocytes				
RAG-2	T and B cells	C57BL/6J	N	Nitcheu et al. 2003
SCID	T and B cells	C57BL/6	N	Yanez et al. 1996
T cells				
TCR αβ	αβ T cells	C57BL/6	N	Boubou et al. 1999
δ Chain	γδ T cells	129/Ola×C57BL/6		Boubou et al. 1999
		C57BL/6	R	Yanez et al. 1999
CD4	CD4[+] T cells	129/Sv/ev×C57BL/6	N	Boubou et al. 1999
		129/Sv/ev×C57BL/6	N	Belnoue et al. 2002
CD8	CD8[+] T cells	129Sv/ev×C57BL/6	N	Yanez et al 1996
		C57BL/6J	N	Belnoue et al. 2002
BALB.D2	Vβ6, Vβ7, Vβ8.1, Vβ9	BALB.D2	N	Boubou et al. 1999
BALBSW	Vβ6, Vβ7, Vβ8.1, Vβ9	BALBC AnN	N	Boubou et al. 1999
DBA/2	Vβ3, Vβ5, Vβ6, Vβ7	DBA/2N	N	Boubou et al. 1999
	Vβ8.1, Vβ9, Vβ11,Vβ12		Y*	Neill and Hunt 1992

Table 2 (continued)

Modified gene	Deficiency	Genetic background	CM[a]	References
MHC molecules				
Invariant chain	Invariant chain	129Sv/ev×C57BL/6	R	Yanez et al. 1996
	CD4$^+$ T cells			
I-A^b	I-A^b	129Sv/ev×C57BL/6	R	Yanez et al. 1996
	CD4$^+$ T cells			
β2Microglobulin	β$_2$M	129Sv/ev×C57BL/6	N	Yanez et al. 1996
	CD8$^+$ T cells	C57BL/6	N	Bagot et al. 2004
TAP-1	TAP-1, CD8$^+$ T cells	C57BL/6J	N	Belnoue et al. 2002
K^b	K^b	C57BL/6J	N	Bagot et al. 2004
D^b	D^b	C57BL/6J	N	Bagot et al. 2004
K^b/D^b	K^b/D^b, CD8$^+$ T cells	C57BL/6J	N	Bagot et al. 2004
CD1	CD1, NK T cells	C57BL/6	Y	Bagot et al. 2004
			Y	Hansen et al. 2003
Jα281	NK T cells	BALB/c	I	Hansen et al. 2003
		C57BL/6	Y	Hansen et al. 2003
B cells				
Chaîne J$_h$D	B cells	129Sv/ev×C57BL/6	R	Yanez et al. 1996
Chaîne μ	B cells	129Sv/ev×C57BL/6	R	Yanez et al. 1996

Table 2 (continued)

Modified gene	Deficiency	Genetic background	CM[a]	References
Costimulation molecules				
CD40	CD40	C57BL/6J	N	Piguet et al. 2001
CD54	ICAM-1	C57BL/6J	N	Favre et al. 1999
Cytokines				
TNF-αβ	TNF-αβ	129Sv/ev×C57BL/6	N	Rudin et al. 1997
TNF-α	TNF-α	C57B/6	Y	Engwerda et al. 2002
Lymphotoxin	Lymphotoxin	C57BL/6	N	Engwerda et al. 2002
TNFR1	TNFR1	129, B6	Y	Lucas et al. 1997
		C57BL/6	Y	Piguet et al. 2002
	TNFR2	129, B6	N	Lucas et al. 1997
		C57BL/6	N	Piguet et al. 2002
IFN-γ	IFN-γ	129, B6	N	Yanez et al. 1996
		C57BL/6	N	Sanni et al. 1998
		C57BL/6	N	van der Heyde 2001
IFN-γRa	IFN-γR	129Sv/ev	N	Amani et al. 2000
IL-2	IL-2	129, B6	N	Yanez et al. 1996
IL-4	IL-4	129, B6	R	Yanez et al. 1996
IL-10	IL-10	129, B6	Y	Yanez et al. 1996
IL-12	IL-12	C57BL/6	N	van der Heyde 2001

Table 2 (continued)

Modified gene	Deficiency	Genetic background	CM[a]	References
Mediators				
NOS2	NOS2	129Sv/ev×C57BL/6	Y	Favre et al. 1999
gp91^{phox}	NADPH oxydase, ROS	C57BL/6	Y	Potter et al. 1999
Perforin	Perforin	C57BL/6	N	Potter et al. 1999
			N	Nitcheu et al. 2003
Fas	Fas (lpr/lpr)	C57BL/6	Y*	Potter et al. 1999
		C57BL/6	Y	Nitcheu et al. 2003
Fas Ligand	Fas L (gld/gld)	C57BL/5	Y*	Nitcheu et al. 2003
Haptoglobin	Haptoglobin	C57BL/6	Y	Hunt et al. 2002
Adhesion molecules and associated molecules				
ICAM-1	ICAM-1	C57BL/6	N	Favre et al. 1999
P-selectin	P-selectin	C57BL/6J	D	Sun et al. 2003
			N	Combes et al. 2004
UPA	Urokinase plasminogen activator	129/Sv×C57BL/6	N	Piguet et al. 2000
uPAR	Urokinase plasminogen activator receptor	129/Sv×C57BL/6	D	piguet et al. 2000
tPA	tissue plasminogen activator	129×C57BL/6	Y	Piguet et al. 2000

Table 2 (continued)

Modified gene	Deficiency	Genetic background	CM[a]	References
Chemokine receptors				
CCR1	CCR1	C57BL/6J	N	L. Rénia, unpublished
CXCR3	CXCR3	C57BL/6J	N	L. Rénia, unpublished
CCR2	CCR2	129/Ola×C57BL/6	Y	Belnoue et al. 2003
CCR5	CCR5	129/Ola×C57BL/6	R	Belnoue et al. 2003 I
		C57BL/6J	D	Belnoue et al. 2003

[a]CM status: Y, 60–100% mice with CM; N, no CM; R, reduced proportion of CM; D, delayed development of CM
[b]Mice developed the neurological signs but did not die of CM I, increased proportion of CM

hemorrhage in the brain of interleukin (IL)-10-deficient C57BL/6 mice (Sanni et al. 2004). However, these mice did not display any clinical neurological symptoms, such as ataxia, paraplegia or coma.

4
Cerebral Malaria Pathogenesis

4.1
Sequestration of Malaria Parasites

4.1.1
P. falciparum

Sequestration of iRBC in brain capillaries from post-mortem tissue obtained from fatal *P. falciparum* cases has been commonly observed (Margulis 1914; Dürck 1917; Gaskell and Miller 1920; Rigdon and Fletcher 1944; Kean and Smith 1944; Spitz 1961). This is thought to be mediated by similar mechanisms as those that cause in vitro cytoadherence of iRBC to endothelial cells. It is has been proposed that cytoadherent iRBC reduce local blood flow and modify the integrity of endothelial barriers (Berendt et al. 1994; Adams et al. 2002). This then induces a local hypoxia and hemorrhagic necrosis. Further evidence for sequestration of *P. falciparum* iRBC in CM pathogenesis is the absence of *P. vivax* iRBC sequestration in the brain and associated inability of *P. vivax* to induce CM. However, *P. falciparum* iRBC sequestration has been observed in brain samples from infected patients who died from causes other than CM (Silamut et al. 1999).

Different molecules expressed by endothelial cells have been identified as ligands for iRBC in vitro. The binding phenotype to ICAM-1, VCAM-1, PECAM-1, ELAM-1, thrombospondin, CD36, chondroitin sulfate, P-selectin, E-selectin, integrin αvβ3, band 3 protein, hyaluronic acid (for review, see Heddini 2002) and membrane fractalkine (Hatabu et al. 2003) varies between *P. falciparum* clones and strains and may vary with time in culture (Roberts et al. 1992). Some of these ligands are positively regulated by proinflammatory cytokines (Dietrich 2002), and their expression is increased during *Plasmodium* infection (Grau 1990b). Platelets have also been shown to mediate adherence of iRBC to endothelial cells. The PfEMP1 multigene family is expressed by *P. falciparum* schizonts and interacts with endothelial cell adhesion molecules (Craig and Scherf 2001). Adherence of iRBC to endothelial cells was long thought to be unique to schizont lifecycle stage. However, ring-stage parasites have recently been shown to be adherent, but the relevance of this phenomenon to CM pathology is unclear (Pouvelle et al. 2000).

Other factors can contribute to capillary obstruction, such as the decreased deformability of iRBC, the formation of rosettes resulting from the interaction of iRBC with normal RBC (Udomsangpecth et al. 1987), and the formation of auto-agglutinates resulting from the interaction of iRBC with platelets (Roberts et al. 2000). The PfEMP1 and rifin multigene families are involved in rosetting (Rowe et al. 1997; Chen et al. 1998) and possibly in auto-agglutination (Pain et al. 2000).

4.1.2
Rodent Malaria

The relevance of rodent models, and in particular the PbA/mouse combination, has often been questioned in regard to the lack of parasite sequestration in the brain. Sequestration in a number of organs has been reported for different parasite species: *P chabaudi* AJ and AS has been shown to sequester preferentially in the mouse liver (Cox et al.1987; Gilks et al. 1990; Mota 2000), *P. berghei* NYU2 in the mouse liver and bone marrow (Alger 1963; Jacobs and Warren 1967; Miller and Fremont 1969) and in the heart and kidney of rat (Desowitz and Barnwell 1976), and *P. berghei* ANKA in the lungs (Coquelin et al. 1999). In the brain, the extent of sequestration varies between parasite species. In *P. yoelii yoelii* YM- or *P. yoelii nigeriensis*-infected mice, sequestration of schizonts is apparent within brain tissue sections (Yoeli and Heargraves. 1974; Kaul et al. 1994; Sharma et al. 1994). *P. chabaudi chabaudi* AS iRBC have been shown by electron microscopy to interact with brain endothelial cells in CBA/Ca mice (Mota et al. 2000), but in this study it was difficult to ascertain parasites actually sequestered in the brain. PbA and *P. berghei* K173 parasites have been observed in brain sections from animals with terminal CM (Rest 1982; Polder et al. 1983; Grau et al. 1987; Hearn et al. 2000, Jennings et al. 1998, Engwerda et al. 2002). One important drawback with these studies is that it is difficult to discriminate between iRBC located in the blood stream and iRBC bound to brain endothelial cells. However, recent studies of infected mice cleared of peripheral blood by intracardial perfusion have shown that PbA parasites do in fact sequester in the brain of infected mice (L. Rénia and B. Lucas, unpublished results).

4.2
Cytokines and Endothelial Cells in Cerebral Malaria

4.2.1
Cytokines

Cytokines are chemical messengers of the immune system. They are produced by many different cell types and signal via specific cell surface receptor complexes. They can be broadly divided into pro- and anti-inflammatory groups. Pro-inflammatory cytokines can induce cellular apoptosis, stimulate expression of adhesion molecules, chemokines and other pro-inflammatory cytokines, modulate the architecture of local tissue microenvironments and stimulate the production of microbicidal products, such as reactive nitrogen and oxygen intermediates. They can also cause substantial damage to host tissue when produced in excess or in inappropriate tissue sites. Many anti-inflammatory cytokines can counter the activities of pro-inflammatory cytokines, and are often produced during inflammatory immune responses as part of homeostatic mechanisms to prevent tissue damage. Recently, anti-inflammatory cytokines have also been found to play key roles in the initiation of cellular immunity. For example, IL-4 has been shown to play an important role in the generation of parasite-specific CD8[+] T cells following vaccination in experimental models of visceral leishmaniasis (Stager et al. 2003) and malaria (Carvalho et al. 2002). Thus, paradigms for the roles of pro- and anti-inflammatory cytokines in infectious diseases are undergoing continual modification and change.

CM is associated with relatively high levels of pro-inflammatory cytokines in the circulation (Clark et al. 1991). There is a growing body of evidence that these molecules directly contribute to the pathogenesis of CM. They can increase expression of adhesion molecules on microvascular endothelial cells (MVECs), thereby mediating the sequestration of iRBC to sensitive tissue sites, such as the brain, lungs and placenta. In addition, activated leukocytes may migrate to these sites in response to chemotactic signals and be retained by binding adhesion molecules, thereby placing them in a location where they can mediate pathology. In this section, we will discuss the roles of cytokines in the pathogenesis of CM. We will include the correlative studies conducted in malaria patients as well as studies performed in mouse models of experimental CM caused by *P. berghei* ANKA. These latter studies have enabled definitive investigations into the roles of various cytokines in CM pathogenesis through the use of blocking antibodies and gene-deficient mice.

4.2.1.1
Human Cerebral Malaria

As mentioned in the previous section, the vast majority of investigations on the role of cytokines in CM have analyzed serum or plasma cytokine levels and correlated these with incidences of CM. However, there is now increasing effort to analyze cytokine expression profiles in the brains of CM patients and to compare them with tissue samples taken from patients that have died from other causes.

4.2.1.2
Pro-inflammatory Cytokines

Elevated levels of tumor necrosis factor (TNF), IL-1β, IL-6 and interferon (IFN)γ have been reported in plasma and sera taken from CM patients (Grau et al. 1989b; Kwiatkowski et al.1990; Kern et al. 1989; Ho et al. 1995; Ringwald et al. 1991). Of these cytokines, TNF has been the most studied (Reviewed in Gimenez et al. 2003). TNF is a potent pro-inflammatory cytokine produced by macrophages, T and B cells and mast cells (Reviewed in Wallach 1999). It can exist as either a soluble or membrane-bound homotrimer, and it binds to two different receptors [TNFRI (CD120a) and TNFRII (CD120b)] with similar affinity. The TNFRI complex contains a death domain, and hence is able to mediate cellular apoptosis. No such domain exists in the TNFRII complex, and this receptor is thought to mediate proliferation, inflammation and lymph node organogenesis.

Studies in African children with malaria have shown a strong correlation between serum TNF levels and severity of disease (Grau et al. 1989b; Kwiatkowski et al. 1990). This has also been reported in non-immune adults with severe malaria (Kern et al. 1989). Studies of brain tissue taken from patients with CM have detected the presence of TNF protein and mRNA (Brown et al. 1999) as well as TNFRII on the surface of MVECs (Hunt and Grau 2003; Lou et al. 2001). Together, these data indicate that the TNF/TNFR2 pathway may be important in the pathogenesis of CM. However, blockade of this pathway using an anti-TNF monoclonal antibody (van Hensbroek et al. 1996) or pentoxifylline (Di Perri et al. 1995) failed to improve survival of African children with CM. Although these results do not exclude a role for TNF in the progression of malaria patients to CM, they do suggest that TNF may have a limited role in the terminal stages of CM pathology.

During the erythrocytic stage of *P. falciparum* infection, mature schizonts develop and rupture iRBC resulting in the release of host-reactive parasite molecules, such as the glycosylphosphatidylinositol (GPI)-anchor molecule of *P. falciparum* (Schofield and Hackett 1993). IL-1β, IL-6 and TNF are all produced when mononuclear cells recognize these parasite molecules via as-yet unidentified receptors (Clark et al. 1981; Kwiatkowski et al. 1989). The *P. falciparum* GPIs are now a major target for anti-pathology strategies. Mice immunized with synthetic *P. falciparum* GPI glycan conjugated to Keyhole limpet hemocyanin (KLH) produced antibodies capable of recognizing native GPI in *P. falciparum* trophozoites and schizonts. These antibodies could block *P. falciparum* GPI-induced TNF production by macrophages, and importantly, immunized mice were significantly protected from CM following *PbA* infection, compared with sham-immunized mice and naïve control mice (Schofield et al. 2002). No data are yet available on the efficacy of such a vaccine in humans.

Elevated serum IFNγ in CM patients (Ho et al. 1995; Ringwald et al. 1991) is likely to enhance the production of TNF, IL-1β and IL-6 by mononuclear cells. Both natural killer (NK) and γδ T cells have been identified as potential sources of IFNγ during *P. falciparum* infection by in vitro studies (Goodier et al. 1995; Hensmann and Kwiatkowski 2001; Artavanis-Tsakonas and Riley 2002), and it is likely that CD4$^+$ T cells are a significant source of this cytokine during malaria infection (Scragg et al. 1999). Studies aimed at blocking the function of this potent inflammatory cytokine have not been reported, and are unlikely to proceed because of the critical role IFNγ plays in host defense against pathogens. Nevertheless, strategies aimed at modulating IFNγ activity at specific stages of malaria infection or in particular tissue sites may be worth considering as a strategy to prevent CM.

Nitric oxide (NO) is a water- and lipid-soluble radical gas produced following oxidization of L-arginine in two sequential reactions catalyzed by nitric oxide synthase (NOS2) (Reviewed in MacMicking et al 1997). NO is able to react with oxygen in water to yield various reactive nitrogen intermediates that have multiple biological activities, including effects on cellular anti-microbial activity, smooth muscle contraction, neurotransmission, cytokine production and the expression of adhesion molecules on MVECs (MacMicking et al.1997). Given these different activities, it is not surprising that the role of NO in CM is controversial. Elevated levels of NOS2 in brain tissue taken from fatal cases of CM (Maneerat et al. 2000) support a role for NO in CM pathogenesis. The ability of NO to affect neurotransmission has also led Clark and colleagues to postulate that NO produced by cerebral MVECs in response to pro-inflammatory cytokines may cross the blood–brain barrier and disrupt neurotransmission during CM (Clark et al. 1991). Recently, NOS2 was found in the vessel walls of a subsample of brain tissue taken from patients with CM and this expression was closely associated with micro-hemorrhages (Clark and Cowden 2003), supporting a role for NO in the disruption of the blood–brain barrier (Clark and Cowden 2003). However, there are also data to suggest that NO may play a protective role in CM. This includes reports of low plasma arginine in Tanzanian children with CM, relative to healthy controls, leading to decreased NOS2 expression and low NO production (Anstey et al. 1996; Lopansri et al. 2003). Similar data were also reported in studies on plasma from Indonesian adults (Boutlis et al. 2003). In fact, NO generated by human monocytes has been shown to kill *P. falciparum* in vitro (Gyan et al. 1994). This has led Anstey and colleagues to propose that NO may protect against CM by decreasing production of pro-inflammatory cytokines, reducing expression of cell surface endothelial molecules, and thereby preventing iRBC sequestration (Boutlis et al. 2003). Given the complex interaction between NO and the immune system, it is possible that in some individuals NO may be protective against CM, while in others it is not. The ultimate role of NO in CM pathogenesis in any given individual may depend on many factors, including genetics, concurrent inflammatory status and the tissue site that pathology is manifested. Recently, Clark and colleagues (Clark et al. 2004) proposed that NO can reduce TNF production, thereby reducing the risk of CM, but that this ability is dependent of the rate at which NO is produced and that this is determined by polymorphisms in the *NOS2A* gene. Thus, severe malaria (including CM) would be less likely in individuals who are able to produce NO rapidly and quickly reduce systemic inflammation (Clark et al. 2004). Further studies are required to elucidate these factors and fully understand the role of NO in CM.

Recently, a potential role for macrophage inhibitory factor (MIF) in the pathogenesis of CM has been proposed (Clark and Cowden 2003). This molecule inhibits the functions of glucocorticoids, thereby allowing pro-inflammatory responses to progress (Calandra and Bucala 1997). Expression seems to co-localize with NOS2, except in the vascular endothelium and smooth muscle within the brain parenchyma (Clark and Cowden 2003). The modulation of MIF activity during CM is a potential treatment that warrants further testing.

Proponents of the cytokine theory of CM pathogenesis, whereby pro-inflammatory cytokines cause increased expression of adhesion molecules on endothelial cells, leading to tissue sequestration of iRBC and activated leukocytes, as well as direct physiological effects of the cytokines in particular tissue sites, such as the brain, might predict that decreased levels of anti-inflammatory cytokines would be found in *P. falciparum* -infected individuals with CM. However, there are few studies on anti-inflammatory cytokines in human CM. Although one study that analyzed serum IL-10 and TNF in children from Gabon with malaria found a reduced ratio of IL-10:TNF in those with CM (May et al. 2000), supporting a cytokine theory of CM pathogenesis. However, another study in children from Ghana failed to find any such difference (Kurtzhals et al. 1998), and a study of Vietnamese adults found that plasma IL-10 levels were higher in those that died with severe malaria than those that survived (Day et al. 1999), suggesting that high IL-10 levels are not protective against the development of CM. Transforming growth factor (TGF)β is another potent anti-inflammatory cytokine. However, its expression was detected in the brains of Malawian children that died with CM (Brown et al. 1999), and another study reported elevated levels of TGFβ in the brains of non-immune European patients that died with CM (Deininger et al. 2000), indicating a minor role for TGFβ in protection from CM. Together, these data provide little evidence that elevated levels of anti-inflammatory cytokines reduce the risk of CM in humans.

4.2.1.3
Experimental Cerebral Malaria

A number of inflammatory cytokines have also been implicated in the pathogenesis of experimental CM, and again TNF has been the subject of many studies. CBA/Ca mice infected with PbA had elevated serum TNF, compared with naïve controls, and antibody neutralization of TNF prevented the onset of CM symptoms (Grau et al.1987b). In addition, mice deficient in TNFR2, but not TNFR1, were resistant to CM (Lucas et al. 1997; Piguet et al. 2002), indicating that, similar to humans (see Sect. 4.2.2.2), the TNF/TNFR2 pathway is important in CM pathogenesis in mice. However, these latter experiments must be treated with some caution due to the 129/Sv and mixed C57BL/6×129/Sv mice used and the possible effects from genetic factors associated with 129/Sv mice.

TNF-mediated CM may also be confined to certain strains of mice, such as CBA, because C57BL/6 mice have been reported to have relatively low levels of serum TNF following *PbA* infection, and TNF blockade failed to prevent CM (Hermsen et al. 1997b). Furthermore, TNF-deficient C57BL/6 mice are as susceptible to CM as control animals (Engwerda et al. 2002). Instead, CM in C57BL/6 mice appears to involve the closely related TNF family member lymphotoxin (LT)α. LTα-deficient C57BL/6 mice failed to develop CM following PbA infection (Engwerda et al. 2002). They survived significantly longer than C57BL/6 controls and TNF-deficient mice, but ultimately died with hyperparasitemia and severe anemia. Interestingly, mice lacking either TNF or LTα had reduced serum IFNγ levels, low levels of ICAM-1 expression on cerebral endothelial cells and minimal leukocyte recruitment to the brain compared with C57BL/6 mice at the time the C57BL/6 and TNF-deficient mice developed CM (Engwerda et al. 2002). The one feature that distinguished TNF- and LTα-deficient mice was the accumulation of iRBC in the cerebral microvasculature (Engwerda et al. 2002), indicating that this event is important in CM pathogenesis in C57BL/6 mice.

IFNγ has also been shown to have an important role in the pathogenesis of CM. Neutralization of IFNγ in CBA mice prevented the development of CM (Grau et al. 1989a), and mice deficient in IFNγ (Yanez et al.1996) or IFNγR (Amani et al. 2000) were also protected from this condition. Again, however, the use of 129/Sv and mixed C57BL/6×129/Sv mice in these cytokine and receptor knockout studies means that other genetic factors cannot be excluded. Nevertheless, the IFNγ neutralization data in CBA mice (Grau et al. 1989a) support a model where IFNγ and TNF mediate increased expression of adhesion molecules on cerebral MVECs (see Sect. 4.3.2) that then mediate adhesion of activated leukocytes and iRBC. However, in C57BL/6 mice, evidence that IFNγ plays a role in CM induction is largely associative. A recent analysis of gene transcription in the brain, spleen and bone marrow of C57BL/6 mice infected with PbA reported that IFNγ-regulated gene transcripts were the most abundant of the inflammatory-related transcripts detected (Sexton et al. 2004).

Our understanding of the role of anti-inflammatory molecules in CM is relatively poor compared to that for pro-inflammatory cytokines, with IL-10 being the only cytokine that has undergone any serious investigation. When PbA-infected CBA mice were treated with IL-10, some protection against CM was observed (Eckwalanga et al. 1994; de Kossodo et al. 1997). In addition, treatment of resistant BALB/c mice following PbA infection with anti-IL-10 monoclonal antibody significantly increased the incidence of CM (de Kossodo et al. 1997). These data suggest that this cytokine may reduce the likelihood of CM. However, further studies are required to establish any protective role for IL-10 in the development of CM. Roles for other anti-inflammatory cytokines in CM, such as TGFβ, are unknown at present.

Use of NOS2-deficient mice or pharmacological intervention with specific NOS2 inhibitors showed that NO is not involved in the neuropathogenesis of experimental CM (Favre et al. 1999). Oxygen radicals or haptoglobin, an acute-phase protein that allows the elimination of heme, and a powerful oxidant, were also not involved in CM (Potter et al. 1999; Hunt et al. 2002).

4.3
Endothelial Cells

The endothelial cells in the brain form a vital component of the blood–brain barrier (Sedgwick et al. 2000), and their damage during PbA infection appears to be a critical event in CM pathogenesis (Grau et al 1993; Lou et al.

1997; Combes et al. 2004). Endothelial cells respond to a variety of cytokine signals following up-regulation of cytokine receptors on their surface and can also produce a range of cytokines when activated (Pober and Cotran 1990; Sedgwick et al. 2000).

4.3.1
Endothelial Cells and Adhesion Molecules

TNF activation of endothelial cells results in ICAM-1 up-regulation (Grau et al. 1991). LFA-1 expressed by leukocytes and platelets binds to ICAM-1, thereby mediating interactions between these cells and cerebral MVECs (Grau et al.1993). The importance of these cell adhesion interactions in CM pathogenesis was demonstrated by blocking either ICAM-1 or LFA-1 with antibody and preventing CM in susceptible mice (Grau et al. 1993; Falanga and Butcher 1993; Lou et al. 1997). Furthermore, mice deficient in ICAM-1 failed to develop CM (Favre et al. 1999). More recently, a role for CD62P (P selectin) in experimental CM pathogenesis has been established (Sun et al. 2003; Combes et al. 2004). Mice deficient in CD62P were relatively resistant to CM, and studies in radiation bone marrow chimeras indicated that CD62P expressed on MVECs plays an important role in CM pathogenesis.

4.3.2
Endothelial Cells and Cytokines

As mentioned, endothelial cells can produce pro-inflammatory cytokines under certain conditions. Most notably, TNF protein and mRNA have been detected in MVECs from mice with CM (de Kossodo and Grau 1993). More recently, we have detected LTα mRNA in MVECs isolated by laser microdissection from brain tissue taken from C57BL/6 mice with CM (C. Engwerda, unpublished data). The TNFR2 complex has also been found on MVEC in the brain from mice with CM (Lucas et al 1997; Stoelcker et al. 2002). Interestingly, a comparison between cerebral MVECs isolated from CM-susceptible CBA and resistant BALB/c mice found that TNF caused the up-regulation of ICAM-1, VCAM-1, TNFR1 and TNFR2 on cells from CBA mice, but not those from BALB/c mice. Furthermore, MVECs from CBA mice were significantly more sensitive to TNF-mediated cell lysis, compared to cells from BALB/c mice (Lucas et al. 1997). Together, these data indicate that cerebral MVECs are a primary site for CM pathogenesis, and are important targets for intervention to prevent the onset of CM.

4.4
Leukocytes

Although the role of leukocytes is well recognized in immunity against malaria, their role in CM remains controversial. The preponderance of iRBC, relative to leukocytes, in brain sections from human post-mortem tissues led to a belief that leukocytes played a minimal role in the pathogenesis of CM (MacPherson et al. 1985; White and Ho 1992). However, leukocytes are clearly observed in brain vessels in pediatric and adult CM in humans (Toro and Roman 1977; Patnaik et al. 1994; Grau et al. 2003; Clark et al. 2003). A detailed study to define the different cell populations present within the brain has yet to be performed, but lymphocytes and monocytes have been identified. In rodent CM induced by PbA or *Plasmodium berghei* K173, intravascular leukocyte sequestration is a common feature, but leukocyte infiltration across the blood–brain barrier is rare (Rest and Wright 1979; Rest 1983; Grau et al. 1987; Jennings et al. 1998; Hearn et al. 2000). In a recent quantitative study, sequestered monocytes/macrophages were predominant, but T cells, neutrophils and platelets were also present (Belnoue et al. 2002).

4.4.1
Monocytes/Macrophages

An accumulation of monocytes has been observed in cerebral vessels from mice with CM. These macrophages, often loaded with parasite-derived material, were frequently observed in intimate contact with endothelial cells (Rest 1982; Polder 1992). The binding of monocytes to endothelium has been described in regions of vascular destruction (Neill and Hunt 1992), where monocyte infiltration into the cerebral parenchyma is sometimes seen (Rest 1982; Polder 1992). Depletion of monocytes/macrophages by treatment with a liposome containing dichloromethylene diphosphonate, if administered before the day of infection, but not later, prevents the development of CM (Curfs 1993; Belnoue 2002). This suggests that monocytes/macrophages are important for the induction of CM, but not during the crisis phase. The role of macrophages is most likely related to the release of cytokines early in the infection.

4.4.2
Neutrophils

Small numbers of neutrophils have been observed in brain vessels in CBA/Ca mice with CM (Falanga 1991; Senaldi 1994). A recent quantitative study showed that neutrophil numbers increased in the brains of mice with CM (Belnoue 2002). Depletion of neutrophils with monoclonal antibodies has resulted in contradictory results. In one study, depletion the day before the infection prevented CM (Chen 2000). In addition, depletion at 5 days post-infection prevented CM in PBA-infected CBA/Ca mice (Senaldi et al. 1994). However, in another report, late depletion (at day 5 or 6 post-infection) did not prevent CM (Chen et al. 2000; Belnoue et al. 2003). Neutrophils may be involved directly in the development of CM by modulating cerebral sequestration of monocytes and leukocytes, perhaps through the regulation of cytokine and chemokine production early in infection (Chen and Sendo 2001). However, further work is required to define the role of this cell population in the pathogenesis of CM.

4.4.3
T Cells

Epidemiological observations have provided evidence for a role of T cells in CM. Children with Kwashiorkor, a syndrome due to malnutrition, have a severe thymic atrophy as shown by post-mortem studies (Trowell 1954) and rarely develop CM. Thus, Edington proposed that T cell deficiency was responsible for this observation (Edington 1967). Experiments in PbA-infected rodents have provided the first direct confirmation for a role for these cells in CM pathogenesis. Neonatal thymectomy or anti-thymocyte treatment prevented CM in rats and hamsters (Wright 1968, 1971; Rest 1983). Infections of nude or SCID mice have also indicated a role for T cells in CM (Finley et al. 1982; Yanez et al. 1996). However, infection of B cell-deficient mice has shown that B cells play a minor role in the development of CM (Yanez 1996). Antibody-depletion experiments and the use of T cell-deficient mice have clearly demonstrated a role for CD4[+] and CD8[+] T cells in murine CM (Grau et al. 1986; Yanez 1996; Hermsen et al. 1997, 1998; Boubou et al.1999; Belnoue et al. 2002).

Recently, different T cell subsets have been implicated in murine CM and their roles are currently being elucidated.

4.4.3.1
$\alpha\beta$T Cells

CD8[+] T Cells   Quantitative assessment of sequestered leukocytes in the brains of mice with and without CM has shown an increase in sequestered CD8[+] $\alpha\beta$ T cells in mice with CM. Despite only a relatively small increase in total brain CD8[+] T cells (50–100,000 cells), antibody depletion of CD8[+] T cells at day 6 post-infection, which is the day prior to the development of neurological signs in PbA-infected 129Sv/ev×C57BL/6 mice, prevented CM (Belnoue et al.

2002). This strongly suggested that brain-sequestered CD8$^+$ T cells played an important role in the development of CM. This was confirmed by adoptive transfer experiments where splenic CD8$^+$ T cells from mice with CM were administered to RAG-2-deficient mice and shown to migrate to the brain and induce CM (Nitcheu et al. 2003). A significant proportion of the CD8$^+$ T cells involved in CM development express the Vβ8.1,2 T cell receptor (Belnoue et al. 2002; Bagot et al. 2004). There are differing reports concerning the expression of other CD8$^+$ T cell surface markers. When CD8$^+$ T cells were purified after homogenization of brain tissues from mice with CM, followed by a percoll gradient purification step, CD8$^+$ T cells were shown to be CD44$^+$ CD62L$^-$ LFA-1$^+$ICAM-1$^+$ (Nitcheu et al. 2003; Bagot et al. 2004). However, CD8$^+$ T cells purified from collagenase-dissociated brain tissue removed from mice with CM that had been perfused intracardiacally were shown to be CD44^{low}CD62^{low}LFA-1^{low} and ICAM-1^{low}. It is possible that two populations of CD8$^+$ T cells with distinct phenotypes are present in the brains of mice with CM. The first cell subtype, which shows signs of activation (up-regulation of CD69 and CD44 markers), may be a recently arrived cell. The other population might be CD8$^+$ T cells which have arrived earlier and interacted with endothelial cells or monocytes and platelets, and have down-regulated activation markers, or which adhere to cerebral vasculature and other leukocytes via alternate ligands. Defining the exact phenotype of CD8$^+$ T cells involved in CM is of importance and requires further study.

The demonstration of a role for CD8$^+$ T cells in CM pathogenesis has led to the development of the hypothesis that these cells induce CM through direct damage of endothelium, leading to the loss of integrity of the blood–brain barrier and subsequent edema and hemorrhage (Yanez et al. 1996). Consistent with this hypothesis, antibody-mediated depletion of CD8$^+$ T cells was shown to reduce vascular permeability and cerebral edema (Chang et al. 2001). Moreover, PbA infection in susceptible mice induces the up-regulation of both MHC class I and class II on cerebral endothelial cells (Monso-Hinard 1997). The absence of CM in PbA-infected β2M- and TAP-double deficient K^b/D^b C57BL/6 mice, but not in single deficient C57BL/6 mice, has also indicated a requirement for MHC molecules and antigen presentation by endothelial cells for the development of CM (Bagot et al. 2004). However, these double-deficient mice have reduced numbers of peripheral blood CD8$^+$ T cells, and the absence of CM in these mice may be related to the lack of CD8$^+$ T cells rather than the absence of MHC class I molecules (Koller et al. 1990; van Kaer et al. 1992; Perarnau et al. 1999). Nevertheless, current data suggest that endothelial cells present MHC class I-restricted epitopes recognized by CD8$^+$ T cells in the brain. A major question is what type of antigen is presented by endothelial cells? Two possibilities exist. The more obvious is that endothelial cells present parasite-derived antigens. The other possibility is that parasite infection induces the expression of host antigens that are recognized by auto-reactive T cells.

Endothelial cells are not professional antigen-presenting cells (APC) and resting endothelial cells do not capture and present antigen efficiently. However, cytokine-activated endothelial cells can become phagocytic and efficient APC (Pober and Cotran 1991). In one report, *Saimiri*-derived brain endothelial cells were observed to take up *P. falciparum*-derived material (Robert et al. 1996). It is not yet known if this can also occur with human or mouse endothelial cells, but it clearly requires further investigation.

Different CD8$^+$ T cell-mediated mechanisms of target killing exist: the perforin pathway, the Fas/Fas ligand (CD95/CD95L) pathway, the TNF pathway and the TRAIL pathway. Perforin-deficient C57BL/6 mice infected with PbA parasites did not develop CM (Potter et al. 1999; Nitcheu et al. 2003). Studies in Fas-deficient (lpr/lpr) mice have yielded contradictory results. In two studies, lpr/lpr mice developed CM to the same degree as wild-type animals (Belnoue et al. 2002; Nitcheu et al. 2003), whereas in another study, these mice developed a reversible CM (Potter et al. 1999). This discrepancy may be related to the use of different PbA lines. However, Fas ligand-deficient gld/gld mice infected with PbA had no protection against CM. TNF and LT expressed on the surface of CD8$^+$ T cells do not seem to be involved in CM pathogenesis because TNF-deficient mice are fully susceptible to CM (Engwerda et al. 2002) and bone marrow engraftment experiments showed LT expression by non-bone marrow-derived cells is important for the development of CM. We have also shown that LTα is not expressed on the surface of CD8$^+$ T cells (L. Rénia and E. Belnoue, unpublished data). Malaria infection in humans has also been associated with an increase in the frequency of circulating CD8$^+$ T cells (Troye-Blomberg et al. 1983, 1984; Stach et al. 1986) and elevated plasma levels of soluble CD8 have been reported in acute *Plasmodium falciparum* patients (Kremsner et al. 1989). In light of the role of CD8$^+$ T cells in experimental CM, there is a need to elucidate their role in human CM.

CD4$^+$ T Cells   The numbers of this cell population increased in the brains of mice with CM, but not in those without CM (Belnoue et al. 2002). PbA-infection of CD4-deficient mice repeatedly demonstrated that CD4$^+$ T cells are involved in CM pathogenesis. This result was confirmed when mice infected with PbA or *P. berghei* K173 were treated with CD4-depleting monoclonal antibodies prior to infection or in the first days of the infection (Yanez et al. 1996; Hermsen et al. 1997; Belnoue et al. 2002). Conflicting results were observed when CD4$^+$ T cells were depleted later in infection (at day 6 post-infection). In one study, this treatment had no effect on CM (Belnoue et al. 2002), while in another study the treatment partially prevented CM (Hermsen et al. 1997). We recently demonstrated that these differences might have been caused by the specific parasite/mouse combinations used (L. Rénia and M. Kayibanda, unpublished data).

CD4$^+$ T cells could have two roles in CM pathogenesis. Firstly, CD4$^+$ T cells, through the secretion of IFN-γ, induce the secretion of TNF-α and chemokines and the up-regulation of adhesion molecules on endothelial cells (Hunt and Grau 2003). Secondly, in some parasite/mouse combinations they may also damage endothelial cells and participate in the destruction of the blood–brain barrier. MHC class II molecules have been shown to be up-regulated in susceptible, but not resistant mice after IFN-γ stimulation (Monso-Hinard et al. 1997). However, mice deficient for the MHC class II molecule A^b (the only class II molecule in C57BL/6 mice) were partially susceptible to CM. Complete abrogation of CM in these mice was only obtained after anti-CD4 antibody treatment. This suggests that the low number of CD4$^+$ T cells left in A^b-deficient mice were able to induce CM (Yanez et al.1996). Since MHC class II molecules are not expressed in this mouse strain, this suggests that these CD4$^+$ T cells were restricted by a non-MHC class II molecule. Thus, this particular CD4$^+$ T cell population might recognize alternative MHC molecules on endothelial cells and exert direct cytotoxicity.

NK T Cells   NK T cells are a population with unusual characteristics (Taniguchi et al. 2003). A subset of these cells recognizes glycolipid antigens presented by CD1 MHC molecules through an invariant T cell receptor. Depending on the nature of the stimulation, they produce IFN-γ, IL-4 or IL-13. The specific cytokine production patterns regulate cytokine secretion by other cells, such as conventional CD4$^+$ T cells (Lisbonne et al. 2003). CD1 deficiency had no effect on the development of CM in a genetically susceptible mouse strain (Hansen et al. 2003; Bagot et al. 2004). However, on a resistant background, CD1 deficiency increased susceptibility to CM (Hansen et al. 2003). This was associated with an increase in production of pro-inflammatory cytokines in vivo through modification of the Th1/Th2 balance. These results suggest a role for NK T cells in the development of murine CM. However, conventional αβ TCR CD8$^+$ T cells, as well as other cell populations, can also express the markers used to define the NK T cell subset bearing the invariant TCR. Therefore, further work is required to adequately ascribe a role for NK T cells in CM pathogenesis.

4.4.3.2
γδ T Cells

Depletion of γδ T cells with an anti-TCR γδ administered at day 0 or 3 after PbA infection, but not later, prevented the development of CM. However, around

50% of C57BL/6 mice deficient for the delta chain of the γδ receptor develop CM (Boubou et al. 1999; Yanez et al. 1999). This discrepancy is thought to be due to the development of compensatory cells responsible for CM pathology. The number of γδ T cells was increased in the brains of mice with CM (Belnoue et al. 2002). However, an effector function in CM for this population has been excluded because late depletion at day 5 post-infection did not prevent the development of CM (Yanez et al. 1999). Thus, the role of γδ T cells in CM might be through the release of pro-inflammatory cytokines and regulation of the expression of chemokines in the brain (Haas et al. 1993; Rzepczyk et al. 1997; Rajan et al. 2000). In humans, acute *P. falciparum* infection induces an increase in circulating γδ T cells (Hviid et al. 2001). Recent data point to a role for these cells in the early secretion of cytokines during malaria (Hensmann and Kwiatkowski 2001; Artavanis-Tsakonas et al. 2003; Stevenson and Riley 2004).

4.4.4
Platelets

Malaria infection, and in particular human CM, is frequently associated with thrombocytopenia (Horstmann et al. 1981). This led to the hypothesis that this deficiency was due to platelet sequestration in organs and disseminated intravascular coagulation (Devakul et al. 1966; Dennis et al. 1967). However, the importance of this condition to CM is unclear, and although thrombi can be seen in autopsy materials, it does not appear to be widespread (White and Ho 1992). In a seminal study on brain tissue taken from Thai adults that died with CM, it was noted that platelets were strikingly absent (MacPherson et al. 1985). Recent studies on brains from deceased African children with CM found platelets clustered with leukocytes and iRBC in the lumen of brain microvessels (Grau et al. 2003).

The role of platelets has been investigated in detail in PbA-induced CM. Platelets have been reported in the lumen of brain vessels from mice with CM, but not in those from mice without CM (Grau et al. 1993). Anti-platelet polyclonal or monoclonal antibody treatment prior to or at the time of infection was also shown to prevent CM (Grau 1993; Polack et al. 1992). In infected mice deficient for urokinase plasminogen activator (UPA) or its receptor (UPAR) and tissue plasminogen (TPA) activator, which are involved in platelet biology, CM was prevented in UPA and UPAR but not in TPA mice (Piguet et al 2000).

The role of platelets in CM pathogenesis remains to be fully ascertained, and they could be involved in many different ways. Platelets express adhesion molecules such as LFA-1and P selectin and costimulatory molecules like

CD40L may interact and/or adhere to endothelial cells. Mice deficient in P-selectin (Sun et al. 2003, Combes et al. 2004), CD40 or CD40L were shown to be protected from CM (Piguet et al. 2001). However, these molecules are also expressed by T cells and may be involved in T cell, but not platelet, activity. In murine CM, adherent platelets were found to fuse with endothelial cell, possibly contributing to their modification (Grau et al. 1993). Platelets may serve as a bridge between iRBC and endothelial cells, via adhesion molecules such as LFA-1 or CD36 (Wassmer et al. 2004). They may also release chemokines (Weyrich et al. 2002; Gear and Camerini 2003) after interaction with the endothelial cells, leading to the recruitment of leukocytes to the brain.

4.4.5
Migration of Leukocytes to the Brain: Role of Chemokine and Chemokine Receptors

Leukocyte accumulation in the brain strongly correlates with CM development in susceptible mice infected with PbA. It has been shown that this accumulation is especially observed when mice display neurological involvement (Belnoue et al. 2002). Chemokines and chemokine receptors are regulators of leukocyte trafficking, and it is likely that these molecules are involved in the pathogenesis of CM.

There are around 50 chemokines and 19 chemokine receptors reported to date. They provide necessary signals for the regulation of leukocyte trafficking in both homeostatic and inflammatory conditions. The redundancy and promiscuity of the chemokine/chemokine receptor system are a major characteristic. A chemokine may interact with different receptors, and a receptor may bind multiple chemokines (Rot and von Andrian 2004). Of all the chemokine receptors described so far, CCR5 and CCR2 have been the most extensively studied, as they act as co-receptors for the human immunodeficiency virus (O'Brien and Moore 2000). They have also been implicated in the migration of leukocytes to the brain in response to pathogens or in auto-immune disease (Huffnagle et al. 1999; Fife et al. 2000; Chen and Sendo 2001).

In PbA-infected mice with CM, brain sequestered-leukocytes, such as macrophages, T cells, and in particular CD8[+] T cells, were shown to express high levels of CCR2 or CCR5. When CM susceptible mice deficient for these chemokines (Kuziel et al. 1997, 2003) were infected with two different clones of PbA, it was observed that mice deficient for CCR5, but not CCR1, CCR2 and CXCR3, develop less CM or that CM development was delayed (Belnoue et al. 2003; Nitcheu et al. 2003; L. Rénia, unpublished results). In CCR5-deficient mice, which did not develop CM, there was a drastic reduction of leukocyte migration to the brain, particularly for CD8[+] T cells. CCR5 was also shown to influence cytokine production, since CCR5-deficient mice infected with PbA had decreased IFN-γ production. The expression of CCR5 on radio-resistant cells, possibly endothelial cells in the brain, was demonstrated in bone marrow engraftment experiments (Belnoue et al. 2003). Interaction between CCR5 and its ligands may induce the release of cytokines and cytokines by brain endothelial cells (Andjelkovic et al. 2000; Dorner et al. 2002) and contribute to the pro-inflammatory conditions in the brain during CM development. The incomplete protection of CCR5-deficient mice from the development of CM suggests that the absence of CCR5 function may be compensated for by one or more additional chemokine receptors. Knowledge on the repertoire of the chemokine receptors expressed by CD8$^+$ T cells in the brain of PbA-infected mice will shed light on the mechanism of migration of these cells during CM.

Little is known about the chemokines produced during CM. PbA infection caused increased accumulation of CXCL10 (γIP-10) and CCL2 (MCP-1) mRNA in the brains of both susceptible C57BL/6 and resistant BALB/c mice. However, the accumulation of CCL5 (RANTES) mRNA was only increased in the susceptible mouse strain (Hanum et al. 2003).

Recent histopathological data have shown that CCL5, a major CCR5 ligand, along with CCR5 and CCR3, was expressed in post-mortem brain tissue from patients who had died with CM (Sarfo et al. 2004). A number of polymorphisms and mutations in human CCR5 genes have been identified which alter, sometimes drastically, CCR5 functional activity and expression levels. For example, individuals homozygous for the delta32 mutation are deficient in CCR5 (Dean et al. 2002). It will be of interest to determine how natural CCR5 deficiency affects susceptibility to CM.

5
Conclusions

Experimental models of CM have been instrumental in identifying key molecules involved in the pathogenesis of CM. Evidence for a role for pro-inflammatory cytokines in human CM is strong. The role of iRBC and leukocytes sequestered in the brain for the pathogenesis of CM is still controversial, although the presence of both cell populations in the brain makes it likely that both are involved. Completion of the *Plasmodium* mouse and human genome and post-genomic techniques will help to uncover the mechanisms of CM pathogenesis.

References

Adams S, Brown H, Turner GDH (2002) Breaking down the blood-brain barrier: signaling a path to cerebral malaria? Trends Parasitol 18:348–351

Alger NE (1963) Distribution of schizonts of *Plasmodium berghei* in tissues of rats, mice and hamsters. J Protozool 10:6–10

Amani V, Boubou MI, Pied S, Marussig M, Walliker D, Mazier D, Rénia L (1998) Cloned lines of *Plasmodium berghei* ANKA differ in their abilities to induce experimental cerebral malaria1. Infect Immun 66:4093–4099

Amani V, Vigario AM, Belnoue E, Marussig M, Fonseca L, Mazier D, Renia L (2000) Involvement of IFN-gamma receptor-medicated signaling in pathology and anti-malarial immunity induced by *Plasmodium berghei* infection. Eur J Immunol 30:1646–1655

Andjelkovic AV, Pachter JS (2000) Characterization of binding sites for chemokines MCP-1 and MIP-1alpha on human brain microvessels. J Neurochem 75:1898–1906

Anstey NM, Weinberg JB, Hassanali MY, Mwaikambo ED, Manyenga D, Misukonis MA, Arnelle DR, Hollis D, McDonald MI, Granger DL (1996) Nitric oxide in Tanzanian children with malaria: inverse relationship between malaria severity and nitric oxide production/nitric oxide synthase type 2 expression. J Exp Med 184:557–567

Artavanis-Tsakonas K, Riley EM (2002) Innate immune response to malaria: rapid induction of IFN-gamma from human NK cells by live *Plasmodium falciparum*-infected erythrocytes. J Immunol 169:2956–2963

Artavanis-Tsakonas K, Eleme K, McQueen KL, Cheng NW, Parham P, Davis DM, Riley EM (2003) Activation of a subset of human NK Cells upon contact with *Plasmodium falciparum*-infected erythrocytes. J Immunol 171:5396–5405

Bafort JM, Pryor WH, Ramsey JM (1980) Immunization of rats against malaria: a new model. J Parasitol 66:337–338

Bagot S, Idrissa-Boubou M, Campino S, Behrschmidt C, Gorgette O, Guénet JL, Penha-Gonçalves C, Mazier D, Pied S, Cazenave PA (2002) Susceptibility to experimental cerebral malaria induced by *Plasmodium berghei* ANKA in inbred mouse strains recently derived from wild stock. Infect Immun 70:2049–2056

Bagot S, Nogueira F, Collette A, do Rosario VE, Lemonier F, Cazenave PA, Pied S (2004) Comparative Study of Brain CD8(+) T cells induced by sporozoites and those induced by blood-stage *Plasmodium berghei* ANKA involved in the development of cerebral malaria. Infect Immun 72:2817–2826

Bakker NPM, Eling WMC, De Groot AMTh, Sinkeldam EJ, Luyken R (1992) Attenuation of malaria infection, paralysis and lesions in the central nervous system by low protein diets in rats. Acta Trop 50:285–293

Ball HJ, MacDougall HG, McGregor IS, Hunt NH (2004) Cyclooxygenase-2 in the Pathogenesis of Murine Cerebral Malaria. J Infect Dis 189:751–758

Belnoue E, Kayibanda M, Vigario AM, Deschemin JC, van Rooijen N, Viguier M, Snounou G, Rénia L (2002) On the pathogenic role of brain-sequestered $\alpha\beta$ CD8$^+$ T cells in experimental cerebral malaria. J Immunol 169:6369–6375

Belnoue E, Costa FTM, Vigario AM, Voza T, Gonnet F, Landau I, van Rooijen N, Mack M, Kuziel WA, Rénia L (2003) Chemokine receptor CCR2 is not essential for the development of experimental cerebral malaria. Infect Immun 71:3648–3651

Belnoue E, Kayibanda M, Deschemin JC, Viguier M, Mack M, Kuziel WA, Rénia L (2003) CCR5 deficiency decreases susceptibility to experimental cerebral malaria. Blood 101:4253–4259

Berendt AR, Turner GDH, Newbold CI (1994) Cerebral malaria: the sequestration hypothesis. Parasitol Today 10:412–414

Bondi FS (1992) The incidence and outcome of neurological abnormalities in childhood cerebral malaria: a long-term follow-up of 62 survivors. Trans R Soc Trop Med Hyg 86:17–19

Boubou MI, Collette A, Voegtle D, Mazier D, Cazenave PA, Pied S (1999) T cell response in malaria pathogenesis: selective increase in T cells carrying the TCR V(beta)8 during experimental cerebral malaria. Int Immunol 11:1553–1562

Boutlis CS, Tjitra E, Maniboey H, Misukonis MA, Saunders JR, Suprianto S, Weinberg JB, Anstey NM (2003) Nitric oxide production and mononuclear cell nitric oxide synthase activity in malaria-tolerant Papuan adults. Infect Immun 71:3682–3689

Brewster DR, Kwiatkowski DP, White NJ (1990) Neurological Sequelae of Cerebral Malaria in Children. Lancet 336:1039–1043

Brown H, Turner G, Rogerson S, Tembo M, Mwenechanya J, Molyneux M, Taylor T (1999) Cytokine expression in the brain in human cerebral malaria. J Infect Dis 180:1742–1746

Calandra T, Bucala R (1997) Macrophage migration inhibitory factor (MIF): a glucocorticoid counter-regulator within the immune system. Crit Rev Immunol 17:77–88

Carvalho LH, Sano G, Hafalla JC, Morrot A, Curotto de Lafaille MA, Zavala F (2002) IL-4-secreting CD4+ T cells are crucial to the development of CD8+ T-cell responses against malaria liver stages. Nature Med 8:166–170

Chang WL, Jones SP, Lefer DJ, Welbourne T, Sun G, Yin L, Suzuki H, Huang J, Granger DN, van der Heyde HC (2001) CD8+-T-Cell Depletion Ameliorates Circulatory Shock in Plasmodium berghei-Infected Mice. Infect Immun 69:7341–7348

Chen Q, Barragan A, Fernandez V, Sundstrom A, Schlichtherle M, Sahlen A, Carlson J, Datta S, Wahlgren M (1998) Identification of Plasmodium falciparum erythrocyte membrane protein 1 (PfEMP1) as the rosetting ligand of the malaria parasite P. falciparum. J Exp Med 187:15–23

Chen L, Zhang Z, Sendo F (2000) Neutrophils play a critical role in the pathogenesis of experimental cerebral malaria. Clin Exp Immunol 120:125–133

Chen L, Sendo F (2001) Cytokine and chemokine mRNA expression in neutrophils from CBA/NSlc mice infected with Plasmodium berghei ANKA that induces experimental cerebral malaria. Parasitol Int 50:139–143

Clark IA, Virelizier JL, Carswell EA, Wood PR (1981) Possible importance of macrophage-derived mediators in acute malaria. Infect Immun 32:1058–1066

Clark IA, Rockett KA, Cowden WB (1991) Proposed link between cytokines, nitric oxide and human cerebral malaria. Parasitol Today 7:205–207

Clark IA, Awburn MM, Whitten RO, Harper CG, Liomba NG, Molyneux ME, Taylor TE (2003) Tissue distribution of migration inhibitory factor and inducible nitric oxide synthase in falciparum malaria and sepsis in African children. Malar J 2:6

Clark IA, Cowden WB (2003) The pathophysiology of falciparum malaria. Pharmacol Ther 99:221–260

Clark IA, Alleva LM, Mills AC, Cowden WB (2004) Pathogenesis of malaria and clinically similar conditions. Clin Microbiol Rev 17:509–539

Combes V, Rosenkranz AR, Redard M, Pizzolato G, Lepidi H, Vestweber D, Mayadas TN, Grau GE (2004) Pathogenic role of P-selectin in experimental cerebral malaria: importance of the endothelial compartment. Am J Pathol 164:781–786

Coquelin F, Boulard Y, Mora-Silvera E, Richard F, Chabaud AG, Landau I (1999) Final stage of maturation of the erythrocytic schizonts of rodent *Plasmodium* in the lungs 9075. C R Acad Sci (III) 322:55–62

Cordeiro RSB, Cunha FQ, Filho JA, Flores CA, Vasconcelos HN, Martins MA (1983) *Plasmodium berghei*: physiopathological changes during infections in mice. Ann Trop Med Parasitol 77:455–465

Cox J, Semoff S, Hommel M (1987) *Plasmodium chabaudi*: a rodent malaria model for *in vivo* and *in vitro* cytoadherence of malaria parasites in the absence of knobs. Parasite Immunol 9:543–561

Craig A, Scherf A (2001) Molecules on the surface of the *Plasmodium falciparum* infected erythrocyte and their role in malaria pathogenesis and immune evasion. Mol Biochem Parasitol 115:129–143

Curfs JHAJ, van Der Meer JWM, Sauerwein RW, Eling WMC (1990) IL-1 treatment inhibits parasitemia and protects against development of cerebral hemorrhages in *Plasmodium berghei* infected mice. The physiological and pathological effects of cytokines. Wiley-Liss, Inc., pp 331–337

Day NP, Hien TT, Schollaardt T, Loc PP, Chuong LV, Chau TT, Mai NT, Phu NH, Sinh DX, White NJ, Ho M (1999) The prognostic and pathophysiologic role of pro- and antiinflammatory cytokines in severe malaria. J Infect Dis 180:1288–1297

De Kossodo S, Grau GE (1993) Role of cytokines and adhesion molecules in malaria immunopathology. Stem Cells 11:41–48

De Kossodo S, Monso C, Juillard P, Velu T, Goldman M, Grau GE (1997) Interleukin-10 modulates susceptibility in experimental cerebral malaria. Immunology 91:536–540

De Souza JB, Riley EM (2002) Cerebral malaria: the contribution of studies in animal models to our understanding of immunopathogenesis. Microbes Infect 4:291–300

Dean M, Carrington M, O'Brien SJ (2002) Balanced polymorphism selected by genetic versus infectious human disease. Annu Rev Genomics Hum Genet 3:263–292

Deininger MH, Kremsner PG, Meyermann R, Schluesener HJ (2000) Differential cellular accumulation of transforming growth factor-beta1, -beta2, and -beta3 in brains of patients who died with cerebral malaria. J Infect Dis 181:2111–2115

Dennis LH, Eichelberger JW, Jr., Inman MM, Conrad ME (1967) Depletion of coagulation factors in drug-resistant *Plasmodium falciparum* malaria. Blood 29:713–721

Desowitz RS, Barnwell JW (1976) *Plasmodium berghei*: deep vascular sequestration of young forms in the heart and kidney of the white rat. Ann Trop Med Parasitol 70:475–476

Devakul K, Harinasuta T, Reid HA (1966) ^{125}I-labelled fibrinogen in cerebral malaria. Lancet 288:886–888

Di Perri G, Di Perri IG, Monteiro GB, Bonora S, Hennig C, Cassatella M, Micciolo R, Vento S, Dusi S, Bassetti D. (1995) Pentoxifylline as a supportive agent in the treatment of cerebral malaria in children. J Infect Dis 171:1317–1322

Dietrich JB (2002) The adhesion molecule ICAM-1 and its regulation in relation with the blood-brain barrier. J Neuroimmunol 128:58–68

Dorner BG, Scheffold A, Rolph MS, Huser MB, Kaufmann SHE, Radbruch A, Flesch IEA, Kroczek RA (2002) MIP-1α, MIP-1β, RANTES, and ATAC/lymphotactin function together with IFN-γ as type 1 cytokines. Proc Natl Acad Sci U S A 99:6181–6186

Durck H (1917) Uber die bei malaria comatosa aufretenden veranderungen des zentralnervensystems. Arch Schiff Tropenhygien 21:117–132

Eckwalanga M, Marussig M, Tavares MD, Bouanga JC, Hulier E, Pavlovitch JH, Minoprio P, Portnoi D, Rénia L, Mazier D (1994) Murine AIDS protects mice against experimental cerebral malaria: Down-regulation by interleukin 10 of a T-helper type 1 CD4+ cell- mediated pathology. Proc Natl Acad Sci USA 91:8097–8101

Edington GM (1967) Pathology of malaria in West Africa. Br Med J 1:715–718

Engwerda CR, Mynott TL, Sawhney S, De Souza JB, Bickle QD, Kaye PM (2002) Locally up-regulated lymphotoxin alpha, not systemic tumor necrosis factor alpha, is the principle mediator of murine cerebral malaria. J Exp Med 195:1371–1377

Falanga PB, Butcher EC (1991) Late treatment with anti-LFA-1 (CD11a) antibody prevents cerebral malaria in a mouse model. Eur J Immunol21:2259–2263

Favre N, Da Laperousaz C, Ryffel B, Weiss NA, Imhof BA, Rudin W, Lucas R, Piguet PF (1999) Role of ICAM-1 (CD54) in the development of murine cerebral malaria. Microbes Infect 1:961–968

Favre N, Ryffel B, Rudin W (1999) The development of murine cerebral malaria does not require nitric oxide production. Parasitology 118:135–138

Fife BT, Huffnagle GB, Kuziel WA, Karpus WJ (2000) CC chemokine receptor 2 is critical for induction of experimental autoimmune encephalomyelitis. J Exp Med 192:899–905

Finley RW, Mackey LJ, Lambert PH (1982) Virulent P. berghei malaria: prolonged survival and decreased cerebral pathology in cell-dependent nude mice. J Immunol 129:2213–2218

Franz DR, Lee M, Seng LT, Young GD, Baze WB, Lewis GEJ (1987) Peripheral vascular pathophysiology of Plasmodium berghei infection: a comparative study in the cheek pouch and brain of the golden hamster. Am J Trop Med Hyg 36:474–480

Gaskell SJ, Millar WL (1920) Studies on malignant malaria in Macedonia. Q J Med 24:317–322

Gear AR, Camerini D (2003) Platelet chemokines and chemokine receptors: linking hemostasis, inflammation, and host defense. Microcirculation 10:335–350

Gilks CF, Walliker D, Newbold CI (1990) Relationships between sequestration, antigenic variation and chronic parasitism in Plasmodium chabaudi chabaudi-a rodent malaria model. Parasite Immunol 12:45–64

Gimenez F, Barraud de Lagerie S, Fernandez C, Pino P, Mazier D (2003) Tumor necrosis factor alpha in the pathogenesis of cerebral malaria. Cell Mol Life Sci 60:1623–1635

Goodier MR, Lundqvist C, Hammarstrom ML, Troye-Blomberg M, Langhorne J (1995) Cytokine profiles for human V gamma 9+ T cells stimulated by Plasmodium falciparum. Parasite Immunol 17:413–423

Gorgette O, Existe A, Boubou MI, Bagot S, Guenet JL, Mazier D, Cazenave PA, Pied S (2002) Deletion of T cells bearing the Vβ8.1 T-cell receptor following mouse mammary tumor virus 7 integration confers resistance to murine cerebral malaria. Infect Immun 70:3701–3706

Grau GE, Piguet PF, Engers HD, Louis JA, Vassalli P, Lambert PH (1986) L3T4+ T lymphocytes play a major role in the pathogenesis of murine cerebral malaria. J Immunol 137:2348–2354

Grau GE, Del Giudice G, Lambert PH (1987a) Host immune response and pathological expression in malaria: possible implications for malaria vaccines. Parasitology 94:123–137

Grau GE, Fajardo LF, Piguet PF, Allet B, Lambert PH, Vassalli P (1987b) Tumor necrosis factor (cachectin) as an essential mediator in murine cerebral malaria. Science 237:1210–1212

Grau GE, Piguet PF, Gretener D, Vesin C, Lambert PH (1988) Immunopathology of thrombocytopenia in experimental malaria. Immunology 65:501–506

Grau GE, Heremans H, Piguet PF, Pointaire P, Lambert PH, Billiau A, Vassalli P (1989a) Monoclonal antibody against interferon gamma can prevent experimental cerebral malaria and its associated overproduction of tumor necrosis factor. Proc Natl Acad Sci USA 86:5572–5574

Grau GE, Taylor TE, Molyneux ME, Wirima JJ, Vassalli P, Hommel M, Lambert PH (1989b) Tumor necrosis factor and disease severity in children with falciparum malaria. N Engl J Med 320:1586–1591

Grau GE, Bieler G, Pointaire P, De Kossodo S, Tacchini-Cottier F, Vassalli P, Piguet PF, Lambert PH (1990a) Significance of cytokine production and adhesion molecules in malarial immunopathology. Immunol Lett 25:189–194

Grau GE (1990b) Implications of cytokines in immunopathology: experimental and clinical data. Eur Cyt Netw 1:203–210

Grau GE, Pointaire P, Piguet PF, Vesin C, Rosen H, Stamenkovic I, Takei F, Vassalli P (1991) Late administration of monoclonal antibody to leukocyte function-antigen 1 abrogates incipient murine cerebral malaria. Eur J Immunol 21:2265–2267

Grau GE, Tacchini-Cottier F, Vesin C, Milon G, Lou JN, Piguet PF, Juillard P (1993) TNF-induced microvascular pathology: active role for platelets and importance of the LFA-1/ICAM-1 interaction. Eur Cytokine Netw 4:415–419

Grau GE, Mackenzie CD, Carr RA, Redard M, Pizzolato G, Allasia C, Cataldo C, Taylor TE, Molyneux ME (2003) Platelet accumulation in brain microvessels in fatal pediatric cerebral malaria. J Infect Dis 187:461–466

Gyan B, Troye-Blomberg M, Perlmann P, Bjorkman A (1994) Human monocytes cultured with and without interferon-gamma inhibit *Plasmodium falciparum* parasite growth in vitro via secretion of reactive nitrogen intermediates. Parasite Immunol 16:371–375

Haas W, Pereira P, Tonegawa S (1993) γδ cells. Annu Rev Immunol 11:637–685

Hansen DS, Siomos MA, Buckingham L, Scalzo AA, Schofield L (2003) Regulation of murine cerebral malaria pathogenesis by CD1d-restricted NKT Cells and the natural killer complex. Immunity 18:391–402

Hanum PS, Hayano M, Kojima S (2003) Cytokine and chemokine responses in a cerebral malaria-susceptible or -resistant strain of mice to *Plasmodium berghei* ANKA infection: early chemokine expression in the brain. Int Immunol 15:633–640

Haque A, Graille M, Kasper LH, Haque S (1999) Immunization with heat-killed *Toxoplasma gondii* stimulates an early IFN- gamma response and induces protection against virulent murine malaria. Vaccine 17:2604–2611

Hatabu T, Kawazu SI, Aikawa M, Kano S (2003) Binding of *Plasmodium falciparum*-infected erythrocytes to the membrane-bound form of Fractalkine/CX3CL1. Proc Natl Acad Sci USA 100:15942–15946

Hearn J, Rayment N, Landon DN, Katz DR, De Souza JB (2000) Immunopathology of cerebral malaria: morphological evidence of parasite sequestration in murine brain microvasculature. Infect Immun 68:5364–5376

Heddini A (2002) Malaria pathogenesis: a jigsaw with an increasing number of pieces. Int J Parasitol 32:1587–1598

Hensmann M, Kwiatkowski D (2001) Cellular basis of early cytokine response to *Plasmodium falciparum*. Infect Immun 69:2364–2371

Hermsen C, van de Wiel T, Mommers E, Sauerwein R, Eling WMC (1997a) Depletion of CD4+ or CD8+ T-cells prevents *Plasmodium berghei* induced cerebral malaria in end-stage disease. Parasitology 114:7–12

Hermsen CC, Crommert JVD, Fredrix H, Sauerwein RW, Eling WMC (1997b) Circulating tumour necrosis factor α is not involved in the development of cerebral malaria in *Plasmodium berghei*-infected C57BL mice. Parasite Immunol. 19:571–577

Hermsen CC, Mommers E, van de Wiel T, Sauerwein RW, Eling WM (1998) Convulsions due to increased permeability of the blood-brain barrier in experimental cerebral malaria can be prevented by splenectomy or anti-T cell treatment. J Infect Dis 178:1225–1227

Ho M, Sexton MM, Tongtawe P, Looareesuwan S, Suntharasamai P, Webster HK (1995) Interleukin-10 inhibits tumor necrosis factor production but not antigen-specific lymphoproliferation in acute *Plasmodium falciparum* malaria. J Infect Dis 172:838–844

Horstmann RD, Dietrich M, Bienzle U, Rasche H (1981) Malaria-induced thrombocytopenia. Blut 42:157–164

Huffnagle GB, McNeil LK, McDonald RA, Murphy JW, Toews GB, Maeda N, Kuziel WA (1999) Role of C-C Chemokine Receptor 5 in Organ-Specific and Innate Immunity to *Cryptococcus neoformans*. J Immunol 163:4642–4646

Hunt NH, Driussi C, Sai-Kiang L (2002) Haptoglobin and malaria. Redox Rep 6:389–392

Hunt NH, Grau GE (2003) Cytokines: accelerators and brakes in the pathogenesis of cerebral malaria. Trends Immunol. 24:491–499

Hviid L, Kurtzhals JAL, Adabayeri V, Loizon S, Kemp K, Goka BQ, Lim A, Mercereau-Puijalon O, Akanmori BD, Behr C (2001) Perturbation and Proinflammatory Type Activation of Vδ1(+) γδ T Cells in African Children with *Plasmodium falciparum* Malaria. Infect Immun 69:3190–3196

Jacobs T, Graefe SE, Niknafs S, Gaworski I, Fleischer B (2002) Murine malaria is exacerbated by CTLA-4 blockade. J Immunol 169:2323–2329

Jadin J, Timperman G, De Ruysser F (1975) Comportement d'une lignée de *P. berghei* après préservation à basse température pendant plus de dix ans. Ann Soc Belge Med Trop 55:603–608

Jennings VM, Actor JK, Lal AA, Hunter RL (1997) Cytokine profile suggesting that murine cerebral malaria is an encephalitis. Infect Immun 65:4883–4887

Kamiyama T, Tatsumi M, Matsubara J, Yamamoto K, Rubio Z, Cortes G, Fujii H (1987) Manifestation of cerebral malaria-like symptoms in the WM/Ms rat infected with *Plasmodium berghei* strain NK65. J Parasitol 73:1138–1145

Kaul DK, Nagel RL, Llena JF, Shear HL (1994) Cerebral malaria in mice: demonstration of cytoadherence of infected red blood cells and microrheologic correlates. Am J Trop Med Hyg 50:512–521

Kean BH, Smith JA (1944) Death due to estivo-autumnal malaria. A resumé of one hundred autopsy cases, 1925–1942. Am J Trop Med 24:317–322

Kern P, Hemmer CJ, Van Damme J, Gruss HJ, Dietrich M (1989) Elevated tumor necrosis factor alpha and interleukin-6 serum levels as markers for complicated *Plasmodium falciparum* malaria. Am J Med 87:139–43

Koller BH, Marrack P, Kappler JW, Smithies O (1990) Normal development of mice deficient in β2 M, MHC class I proteins, and CD8+ T cells. Nature 248:1227–1229

Kremsner PG, Bienzle U (1989) Soluble CD8 antigen in *Plasmodium falciparum* malaria. J Infect Dis 160:357–358

Kurtzhals JA, Adabayeri V, Goka BQ, Akanmori BD, Oliver-Commey JO, Nkrumah FK, Behr C, Hviid L (1998) Low plasma concentrations of interleukin 10 in severe malarial anaemia compared with cerebral and uncomplicated malaria. Lancet 351:1768–1772

Kuziel WA, Morgan SJ, Dawson TC, Griffin S, Smithies O, Ley K, Maeda N (1997) Severe reduction in leukocyte adhesion and monocyte extravasation in mice deficient in CC chemokine receptor 2. Proc Natl Acad Sci USA 94:12053 12058

Kuziel WA, Dawson TC, Quinones M, Garavito E, Chenaux G, Ahuja SS, Reddick RL, Maeda N (2003) CCR5 deficiency is not protective in the early stages of atherogenesis in apoE knockout mice. Atherosclerosis 167:25–32

Kwiatkowski D, Cannon JG, Manogue KR, Cerami A, Dinarello CA, Greenwood BM (1989) Tumour necrosis factor production in Falciparum malaria and its association with schizont rupture. Clin Exp Immunol 77:361–366

Kwiatkowski D, Hill AV, Sambou I, Twumasi P, Castracane J, Manogue KR, Cerami A, Brewster DR, Greenwood BM (1990) TNF concentration in fatal cerebral, non-fatal cerebral, and uncomplicated *Plasmodium falciparum* malaria. Lancet 336:1201–1204

Landau I, Boulard Y (1978) Life cycles and morphology. In: Killick-Kendrick R, Peters W (eds) Rodent malaria. Academic Press, London, pp 53–84

Lisbonne M, Leite de Moraes MC (2003) Invariant Vα14 NKT lymphocytes: a double-edged immuno-regulatory T cell population. Eur Cyt Netw 14:4–14

Lopansri BK, Anstey NM, Weinberg JB, Stoddard GJ, Hobbs MR, Levesque MC, Mwaikambo ED, Granger DL (2003) Low plasma arginine concentrations in children with cerebral malaria and decreased nitric oxide production. Lancet 361:676–678

Lou J, Donati YR, Juillard P, Giroud C, Vesin C, Mili N, Grau GE (1997) Platelets play an important role in TNF-induced microvascular endothelial cell pathology. Am J Pathol 151:1397–405

Lou J, Lucas R, Grau GE (2001) Pathogenesis of cerebral malaria: recent experimental data and possible applications for humans. Clin Microbiol Rev 14:810–820

Lucas R, Juillard P, Decoster E, Redard M, Burger D, Donati Y, Giroud C, Monso-Hinard C, De Kesel T, Buurman WA, Moore MW, Dayer JM, Fiers W, Bluethmann H, Grau GE (1997) Crucial role of tumor necrosis factor (TNF) receptor 2 and membrane-bound TNF in experimental cerebral malaria. Eur J Immunol 27:1719–1725

Mackey LJ, Hochmann A, June CH, Contreras CE, Lambert PH (1980) Immunopathological aspects of *Plasmodium berghei* infection in five strains of mice. II. Immunopathology of cerebral and other tissue lesions during the infection. Clin Exp Immunol 42:412–420

MacMicking J, Xie QW, Nathan C (1997) Nitric oxide and macrophage function. Annu Rev Immunol 15:323–350

MacPherson GG, Warrell MJ, White NJ, Looareesuwan S, Warrell DA (1985) Human cerebral malaria. A quantitative ultrastructural analysis of parasitized erythrocyte sequestration. Am J Pathol 119:385–401

Maegraith BG, Fletcher A (1972) The pathogenesis of mammalian malaria. Adv Parasitol 10:49–72

Maneerat Y, Viriyavejakul P, Punpoowong B, Jones M, Wilairatana P, Pongponratn E, Turner GD, Udomsangpetch R (2000) Inducible nitric oxide synthase expression is increased in the brain in fatal cerebral malaria. Histopathology 37:269–277

Marchiafava E, Bignami A (1900) Malaria. Twentieth century practice of Medicine. Sampson Lowe, London

Margulis MS (1914) Zur frage der pathologish-anatomischen Veränderungen bei bösartige malaria. Neurologishe Zentralblat 33:1019–1024

May J, Lell B, Luty AJ, Meyer CG, Kremsner PG (2000) Plasma interleukin-10:Tumor necrosis factor (TNF)-alpha ratio is associated with TNF promoter variants and predicts malarial complications. J Infect Dis 182:1570–1573

Mercado TI (1965) Paralysis associated with *Plasmodium berghei* malaria in the rat13982. J Infect Dis 115:465–472

Miller LH, Fremount HN (1969) The sites of deep vascular schizogony in chloroquine-resistant *Plasmodium berghei* in mice. Trans R Soc Trop Med Hyg 63:195–197

Monso-Hinard C, Lou JN, Behr C, Juillard P, Grau GE (1997) Expression of major histocompatibility complex antigens on mouse brain microvascular endothelial cells in relation to susceptibility to cerebral malaria. Immunology 92:53–59

Mota MM, Jarra W, Hirst E, Patnaik PK, Holder AA (2000) *Plasmodium chabaudi*-infected erythrocytes adhere to CD36 and bind to microvascular endothelial cells in an organ-specific way. Infect Immun 68:4135–4144

Neill AL, Hunt NH (1992) Pathology of fatal and resolving *Plasmodium berghei* cerebral malaria in mice. Parasitology 105:165–175

Neill AL, Chan-Ling T, Hunt NH (1993) Comparisons between microvascular changes in cerebral and non- cerebral malaria in mice, using the retinal whole-mount technique. Parasitology 107:477–487

Nitcheu J, Bonduelle O, Combadiere C, Tefit M, Seilhean D, Mazier D, Combadiere B (2003) Perforin-dependent brain-infiltrating cytotoxic CD8(+) T lymphocytes mediate experimental cerebral malaria pathogenesis. J Immunol 170:2221–2228

O'Brien SJ, Moore JP (2000) The effect of genetic variation in chemokines and their receptors on HIV transmission and progression to AIDS. Immunol Rev 177:99–111

Pain A, Ferguson DJ, Kai O, Urban BC, Lowe B, Marsh K, Roberts DJ (2001) Platelet-mediated clumping of *Plasmodium falciparum*-infected erythrocytes is a common adhesive phenotype and is associated with severe malaria. Proc Natl Acad Sci USA 98:1805–1810

Patnaik JK, Das BS, Mishra SK, Mohanty S, Satpathy SK, Mohanty D (1994) Vascular clogging, mononuclear cell margination, and enhanced vascular permeability in the pathogenesis of human cerebral malaria. Am J Trop Med Hyg 51:642–647

Perarnau B, Saron MF, San Martin BR, Bervas N, Ong HC, Soloski MJ, Smith AG, Ure JM, Gairin JE, Lemonnier FA (1999) Single H2 K ^{b}, H2D^b and double H2 K^{b}D^b knockout mice: peripheral CD8+ T cell repertoire and anti-lymphocytic chorimeningitis virus cytolytic responses. Eur J Immunol 29:1243–1252

Piguet PF, Da Laperrousaz C, Vesin C, Tacchini-Cottier F, Senaldi G, Grau GE (2000) Delayed mortality and attenuated thrombocytopenia associated with severe malaria in urokinase- and urokinase receptor-deficient mice. Infect Immun 68:3822–3829

Piguet PF, Da Kan C, Vesin C, Rochat A, Donati Y, Barazzone C (2001) Role of CD40-CD40L in mouse severe malaria. Am J Pathol 159:733–742

Pober JS, Cotran RS (1990) Cytokines and endothelial cell biology. Physiol Rev 70:427–451

Pober JS, Cotran RS (1991) Immunologic interactions of T lymphocytes with vascular endothelium. Adv Immunol 50:261–302

Polack B, Delolme F, Peyron F (1998) Protective role of platelets in chronic (BALB/c) and acute (CBA/J) Plasmodium berghei murine malaria. Haemostasis 27:278–285

Polder TW, Jerusalem CR, Eling WMC (1983) Topographical distribution of the cerebral lesions in mice infected with Plasmodium berghei. Trop Med Parasitol 34:235–243

Polder TW, Eling WMC, Curfs JHAJ, Jerusalem CR, Wijers-Rouw M (1992) Ultrastructural changes in the blood-brain barrier of mice infected with Plasmodium berghei. Acta Leidensia 60:31–46

Potter S, Chaudhri G, Hansen A, Hunt NH (1999) Fas and perforin contribute to the pathogenesis of murine cerebral malaria. Redox Rep 4:333–335

Potter SM, Chaudhri G, Hansen AM, Hunt NH (1999) Fas and perforin contribute to the pathogenesis of murine cerebral malaria. Redox Rep 4:333–335

Pouvelle B, Buffet PA, Lepolard C, Scherf A, Gysin J (2000) Cytoadhesion of Plasmodium falciparum ring-stage-infected erythrocytes. Nature Med 6:1264–1268

Rajan AJ, Asensio VC, Campbell IL, Brosnan CF (2000) Experimental autoimmune encephalomyelitis on the SJL mouse: effect of γδ T cell depletion on chemokine and chemokine receptor expression in the central nervous system. J Immunol 164:2120–2130

Rest JR, Wright DH (1979) Electron microscopy of cerebral malaria in golden hamsters (Mesocricetus auratus) infected with Plasmodium berghei. J Pathol 127:115–120

Rest JR (1982) Cerebral malaria in inbred mice. I. A new model and its pathology 2789. Trans R Soc Trop Med Hyg 76:410–415

Rest JR (1983) Pathogenesis of cerebral malaria in golden hamsters and inbred mice4592. Contrib Microbiol Immunol 7:139–146

Rigdon RH, Fletcher DE (1944) Lesions of brain associated with malaria. Pathologic study on man and on experimental animals. Arch Neurol Psych 53:191–198

Ringwald P, Peyron F, Vuillez JP, Touze JE, Le Bras J, Deloron P (1991) Levels of cytokines in plasma during Plasmodium falciparum malaria attacks. J Clin Microbiol 29:2076–2078

Robert C, Peyrol S, Pouvelle B, Gay-Andrieu F, Gysin J (1996) Ultrastructural aspects of *Plasmodium falciparum*-infected erythrocyte adherence to endothelial cells of *Saimiri* brain microvasculature. Am J Trop Med Hyg 54:169–177

Roberts DJ, Craig AG, Berendt AR, Pinches RA, Nash G, Marsh K, Newbold CI (1992) Rapid switching to multiple antigenic and adhesive phenotypes in malaria. Nature 357:689–692

Roberts DJ, Pain A, Kai O, Kortok M, Marsh K (2000) Autoagglutination of malaria-infected red blood cells and malaria severity. Lancet 355:1427–1428

Rowe JA, Moulds JM, Newbold CI, Miller LH (1997) *Plasmodium falciparum* rosetting mediated by a parasite-variant erythrocyte membrane protein and complement-receptor 1. Nature 388:292–295

Rot A, von Andrian UH (2004) Chemokines in Innate and Adaptive Host Defense: Basic Chemokinese Grammar for Immune Cells. Annu Rev Immunol 22:891–928

Rudin W, Eugster HP, Bordmann G, Bonato J, Muller MT, Yamage M, Ryffel B (1997) Resistance to cerebral malaria in tumor necrosis factor-α/β-deficient mice is associated with a reduction of intercellular adhesion molecule-1 up-regulation and T helper type 1 response. Am J Pathol 150:257–266

Rzepczyk CM, Anderson K, Stamatiou S, Townsend E, Allworth A, McCormack J, Whitby M (1997) γδ T cells: their immuno biology and role in malaria infections. Int J Parasitol 27:191–200

Sanni LA, Jarra W, Li C, Langhorne J (2004) Cerebral edema and cerebral hemorrhages in interleukin-10-deficient mice infected with *Plasmodium chabaudi*. Infect Immun 72:3054–3058

Sanni LA, Thomas SR, Tattam BN, Moore DE, Chaudhri G, Stocker R, Hunt NH (1998) Dramatic changes in oxidative tryptophan metabolism along the kynurenine pathway in experimental cerebral and noncerebral malaria. Am J Pathol 152:611–619

Sarfo BY, Singh S, Lillard JW, Quarshie A, Gyasi RK, Armah H, Adjei AA, Jolly P, Stiles JK (2004) The cerebral-malaria-associated expression of RANTES, CCR3 and CCR5 in post-mortem tissue samples. Ann Trop Med Parasitol 98:297–303

Schetters TPM, Curfs JHAJ, van Zon AAJC, Hermsen CC, Eling WMC (1989) Cerebral lesions in mice infected with *Plasmodium berghei* are the result of an immunopathological reaction. Trans R Soc Trop Med Hyg 83:103–104

Schmutzhard E, Gerstenbrand F (1984) Cerebral malaria in Tanzania. Its epidemiology, clinical symptoms and neurological long term sequelae in the light of 66 cases. Trans R Soc Trop Med Hyg 78:351–353

Schofield L, Hackett F (1993) Signal transduction in host cells by a glycosylphosphatidylinositol toxin of malaria parasites. J Exp Med 177:145–53

Schofield L, Hewitt MC, Evans K, Siomos MA, Seeberger PH (2002) Synthetic GPI as a candidate anti-toxic vaccine in a model of malaria. Nature 418:785–789

Scragg IG, Hensmann M, Bate CA, Kwiatkowski D (1999) Early cytokine induction by *Plasmodium falciparum* is not a classical endotoxin-like process. Eur J Immunol 29:2636–2644

Sedgwick JD, Riminton DS, Cyster JG, Korner H (2000) Tumor necrosis factor: a master-regulator of leukocyte movement. Immunol Today 21:110–113

Senaldi G, Vesin C, Chang R, Grau GE, Piguet PF (1994) Role of polymorphonuclear neutrophil leukocytes and their integrin CD11a (LFA-1) in the pathogenesis of severe murine malaria. Infect Immun 62:1144–1149

Senaldi G, Kremsner PG, Grau GE (1992) Nitric oxide and cerebral malaria. Lancet 340:1554

Sexton AC, Good RT, Hansen DS, D'Ombrain MC, Buckingham L, Simpson K, Schofield L (2004) Transcriptional profiling reveals suppressed erythropoiesis, up-regulated glycolysis, and interferon-associated responses in murine malaria. J Infect Dis 189:1245–1256

Sharma MC, Tripathi LM, Rastogi M, Maitra SC, Sagar P, Dutta GP, Pandey VC (1992) Aberrations in cerebral vascular functions due to *Plasmodium yoelii nigeriensis* infection in mice. Exp Mol Pathol 57:62–69

Sharma MR, Sharma MC, Tripathi LM, Pandey VC, Maitra SC (1994) Neuropathological studies on *Plasmodium yoelii nigeriensis*-induced malaria in mice. J Comp Pathol 110:313–317

Silamut K, Phu NH, Whitty C, Turner GDH, Louwrier K, Mai NT, Simpson JA, Hien TT, White NJ (1999) A quantitative analysis of the microvascular sequestration of malaria parasites in the human brain. Am J Pathol 155:395–410

Spitz S (1961) Pathology of tropical diseases. Saunders Co, Philadelphia

Stach JL, Dufrenoy E, Roffi J, Bach MA (1986) T-cell subsets and natural killer activity in *Plasmodium falciparum*-infected children. Clin Immunol Immunopathol 38:129–134

Stager S, Alexander J, Kirby AC, Botto M, Rooijen NV, Smith DF, Brombacher F, Kaye PM (2003) Natural antibodies and complement are endogenous adjuvants for vaccine-induced CD8+ T-cell responses. Nature Med 9:1287–1292

Stevenson MM, Riley EM (2004) Innate immunity to malaria. Nat Rev Immunol 4:169–180

Stoelcker B, Hehlgans T, Weigl K, Bluethmann H, Grau GE, Mannel DN (2002) Requirement for tumor necrosis factor receptor 2 expression on vascular cells to induce experimental cerebral malaria. Infect Immun 70:5857–5859

Sun G, Chang WL, Li J, Berney SM, Kimpel D, van der Heyde HC (2003) Inhibition of platelet adherence to brain microvasculature protects against severe *Plasmodium berghei* malaria. Infect Immun 71:6553–6561

Taniguchi M, Harada M, Kojo S, Nakayama T, Wakao H (2003) The regulatory role of Valpha14NKT cells in innate and acquired immunity. Annu Rev Immunol 21:483–513

Toro G, Roman G (1977) Cerebral malaria. A disseminated vasculomyelinopathy Pathophysiology of atypical malaria. J Assoc Physicians India 25:419–422

Trowell HC, Davies JN, Dean RFA (1954) Kwashiorkor. Edward Arnold, London

Troye-Blomberg M, Romero P, Patarroyo ME, Bjorkman A, Perlmann P (1984) Regulation of the immune response in *Plasmodium falciparum* malaria. III. Proliferative response to antigen in vitro and subset composition of T cells from patients with acute infection or from immune donors. Clin Exp Immunol 58:380–387

Udomsangpetch R, Wahlin B, Carlson J, Berzins K, Torii M, Aikawa M, Perlmann P, Wahlgren M (1987) *Plasmodium falciparum*-infected erythrocytes form spontaneous erythrocytes rosettes. J Exp Med 169:1835–1840

Van den Eertwegh AJ, Boersma WJ, Claassen E (1992) Immunological functions and in vivo cell-cell interactions of T cells in the spleen. Crit Rev Immunol 11:337–380

van der Heyde HC, Bauer PR, Sun G, Chang WL, Yin L, Fuseler J, Granger DN (2001) Assessing vascular permeability during experimental cerebral malaria by a radiolabeled monoclonal antibody technique. Infect Immun 69:3460–3465

van Hensbroek MB, Palmer A, Onyiorah E, Schneider G, Jaffar S, Dolan G, Memming H, Frenkel J, Enwere G, Bennett S, Kwiatkowski D, Greenwood B (1996) The effect of a monoclonal antibody to tumor necrosis factor on survival from childhood cerebral malaria. J Infect Dis 174:1091–1097

Van Kaer L, Ashton-Rickardt PG, Ploegh HL, Tonegawa S (1992) *TAP1* mutant mice are deficient in antigen presentation, surface class I molecules, and CD4-CD8+ T cells 6481. Cell 71:1205–1214

Vincke IH, Lips MAH (1948) Un nouveau *Plasmodium* d'un rongeur sauvage du Congo, *Plasmodium berghei* n. sp. Ann Soc Belge Med Trop 28:97–105

Wallach D, Varfolomeev EE, Malinin NL, Goltsev YV, Kovalenko AV, Boldin MP (1999) Tumor necrosis factor receptor and Fas signaling mechanisms. Annu Rev Immunol 17:331–367

Warrell DA, Molyneux ME, Beales PF (1990) Severe and complicated malaria. World Health Organization, Division of Control of Tropical Diseases. Trans R Soc Trop Med Hyg 84 Suppl 2:1–65

Wassmer SC, Lepolard C, Traore B, Pouvelle B, Gysin J, Grau GE (2004) Platelets reorient *Plasmodium falciparum*-Infected erythrocyte cytoadhesion to activated endothelial cells. J Infect Dis 189:180–189

Weyrich AS, Prescott SM, Zimmerman GA (2002) Platelets, endothelial cells, inflammatory chemokines, and restenosis: complex signaling in the vascular play book. Circulation 106:1433–1435

White NJ, Ho M (1992) The pathophysiology of malaria. Adv Parasitol 31:83–172

World health Organization (1990) Severe and complicated malaria. World Health Organization, Division of Control of Tropical Diseases. Trans R Soc Trop Med Hyg 84:1–65

Wright DH (1968) The effect of neonatal thymectomy on the survival of golden hamsters infected with *Plasmodium berghei*. Br J Exp Pathol 49:379–384

Wright DH, Masembe RM, Bazira ER (1971) The effect of antithymocyte serum on golden hamsters and rats infected with *Plasmodium berghei*. Br J Exp Pathol 52:465–477

Yanez DM, Manning DD, Cooley AJ, Weidanz WP, van der Heyde HC (1996) Participation of lymphocyte subpopulations in the pathogenesis of experimental murine cerebral malaria. J Immunol 157:1620–1624

Yanez DM, Batchelder J, van der Heyde HC, Manning DD, Weidanz WP (1999) γδ T-Cell Function in Pathogenesis of Cerebral Malaria in Mice Infected with *Plasmodium berghei* ANKA. Infect Immun 67:446–448

Yoeli M, Hargreaves BJ (1974) Brain capillary blockage produced by a virulent strain of rodent malaria. Science 184:572–573

CTMI (2005) 297:145–185
© Springer-Verlag Berlin Heidelberg 2005

Glycosylphosphatidylinositols in Malaria Pathogenesis and Immunity: Potential for Therapeutic Inhibition and Vaccination

C. S. Boutlis[1,2] (✉) · E. M. Riley[3] · N. M. Anstey[1,2] · J. B. de Souza[3,4]

[1]International Health Program, Infectious Diseases Division, Menzies School of Health Research, P.O. Box 41096, 0811 Casuarina, NT, Australia
craig.boutlis@menzies.edu.au

[2]Charles Darwin University, 0909 Darwin, NT, Australia

[3]Department of Infectious and Tropical Diseases, London School of Hygiene and Tropical Medicine, Keppel Street, London WC1E 7HT, UK

[4]Department of Immunology and Molecular Pathology, Royal Free and University College London Medical School, Windeyer Institute of Medical Research, 46 Cleveland Street, London WIT 4JF, UK

Abstract Glycosylphosphatidylinositols (GPIs) are found in the outer cell membranes of all eukaryotes. GPIs anchor a diverse range of proteins to the surface of *Plasmodium falciparum*, but may also exist free of protein attachment. In vitro and in vivo studies have established GPIs as likely candidate toxins in malaria, consistent with the prevailing paradigm that attributes induction of inflammatory cytokines, fever and other pathology to parasite toxins released when schizonts rupture. Although evolutionarily conserved, sufficient structural differences appear to exist that impart upon plasmodial GPIs the ability to activate second messengers in mammalian cells and elicit immune responses. In populations exposed to *P. falciparum*, the antibody response to purified GPIs is characterised by a predominance of immunoglobulin (Ig)G over IgM and an increase in the prevalence, level and persistence of responses with increasing age. It remains unclear, however, if these antibodies or other cellular responses to GPIs mediate anti-toxic immunity in humans; anti-toxic immunity may comprise either reduction in the severity of disease or maintenance of the malaria-tolerant state (i.e. persistent asymptomatic parasitaemia). *P. falciparum* GPIs are potentially amenable to specific therapeutic inhibition and vaccination; more needs to be known about their dual roles in malaria pathogenesis and protection for these strategies to succeed.

Abbreviations

GPI	Glycosylphosphatidylinositol
ICAM	Intercellular adhesion molecule
IFN	Interferon
Ig	Immunoglobulin
IL	Interleukin
LPS	Lipopolysaccharide
LT	Lymphotoxin
Man4	Fourth mannose
MHC	Major histocompatibility complex
MSP	Merozoite surface protein
NF	Nuclear factor
NO	Nitric oxide
PKC	Protein kinase C
PTK	Protein tyrosine kinase
TGF	Transforming growth factor
TLR	Toll-like receptor
TNF	Tumour necrosis factor

1
Introduction

Plasmodium falciparum glycosylphosphatidylinositols (GPIs) became the focus of mainstream media attention in 2002 with the publication in *Nature* of a report demonstrating proof of concept for an anti-toxic vaccine that delayed malaria mortality in a rodent model (Schofield et al. 2002). As the best characterised of the putative malaria toxins, interest in GPIs has burgeoned since the early 1990s to the point that strategies for creating fully synthetic GPI analogues are advancing rapidly (Lu et al. 2004; Liu and Seeberger 2004; Seeberger et al. 2004). This should soon enable investigators to clarify the role of GPIs in malaria pathogenesis and immunity. Understanding the potential for anti-GPI therapeutics and vaccination in human malaria requires an understanding of the pathophysiology of toxin-mediated events, as well as the nature of human anti-toxic immune responses. The conceptual framework must account for epidemiological phenomena that have been patiently catalogued by malariologists and withstood years of observation. Thus, the present review comprises three main parts: an outline of the toxic basis of malaria disease, with an emphasis on the proposed role of GPIs; a summary of what is thought clinically to represent anti-toxic immunity to malaria; and a discussion of what is presently known about immune responses to plasmodial GPIs.

2
The Toxic Basis of Malaria

Fever and anaemia are common to all forms of human malaria, whereas severe malaria due to *P. falciparum* is additionally characterised by metabolic acidosis, hypoglycaemia, uraemia, pulmonary oedema and/or coma (referred to as cerebral malaria). These features of malaria pathogenesis are thought to result from a number of mechanisms acting in concert: destruction of red blood cells by the parasite, a cell-mediated inflammatory host response, and in the case of *P. falciparum* only, cytoadherence of parasitised erythrocytes to vascular endothelium. Cytoadherence in particular may lead to sequestration of parasites away from the general circulation and localised organ-based immunopathology. This section will focus on the potential roles played by parasite toxin(s) in initiating and/or exacerbating these key events. Readers seeking more information are referred to comprehensive recent reviews (Clark and Cowden 2003; Clark et al. 2004; Maitland and Marsh 2004).

2.1
The Toxic Paradigm in Malaria

A prevailing view of malaria pathogenesis can be stated as follows: that a parasite toxin (or toxins) induces production of host-derived inflammatory cytokines that are directly responsible for the characteristic febrile paroxysms of malaria, and indirectly contribute to other clinical manifestations. The Italian

Nobel laureate Camillo Golgi first established that paroxysms occurred following malarial shizogony in 1886 (Golgi 1886), but it took another 100 years for the physiological basis of this observation to be elucidated. Parallel lines of research converged in the late 1970s and early 1980s, leading to the recognition that endotoxin-mediated bacterial sepsis and malaria shared striking similarities in their pathophysiological features and cytokine profiles (Clark 1978; Clark et al. 1981). Central to this was the discovery and definition of tumour necrosis factor (TNF)-α, followed by recognition that it mediated pathology in rodent malaria models (Clark et al. 1987) and could be induced by malaria parasites and putative malaria toxins in vitro (Kwiatkowski et al. 1989; Scragg et al. 1999). Subsequently, plasma TNF-α levels were shown to correlate with the severity of human malaria (Grau et al. 1989; Kern et al. 1989), and a causal role was suggested by genetic association studies linking polymorphisms in the TNF-α promoter region to disease outcome (McGuire et al. 1994; Wattavidanage et al. 1999; Aidoo et al. 2001).

With time, it has become clear that TNF-α is but one in a milieu of soluble mediators that together influence the pathophysiology of malaria. Monoclonal anti-TNF-α antibodies given to Gambian children with cerebral malaria reduced fever (Kwiatkowski et al. 1993) but had no effect on mortality in a subsequent randomised placebo-controlled trial (van Hensbroek et al. 1996). Similarly disappointing results were observed using polyclonal anti-TNF-α antibodies in Thai adults with severe malaria (Looareesuwan et al. 1999), and the relevance of TNF-α polymorphisms has since been questioned (Bayley et al. 2004). Recent studies have demonstrated that lymphotoxin (LT)-α (formerly TNF-β), rather than TNF-α, appears to be the principle mediator of murine cerebral malaria in the *P. berghei* (ANKA) model (Engwerda et al. 2002; Rae et al. 2004). Interestingly, this is consistent with research conducted 10 years earlier that showed elevated levels of LT-α in human malaria, and induction of interleukin (IL)-6 and hypoglycaemia in mice injected with the cytokine (Clark et al. 1992). Together, these studies highlight that the pivotal role ascribed to TNF-α in malaria pathogenesis may in part have reflected its study in isolation from the complex interplay of other mediators (Dodoo et al. 2002). Evidence from in vitro, animal and human studies (reviewed by Artavanis-Tsakonas et al. 2003; Clark et al. 2004) suggests that at least the following are also involved in determining the outcome of malaria infection: interferon (IFN)-γ, IL-1, 6, 10, 12 (Dodoo et al. 2002), and 18 (Singh et al. 2002), transforming growth factor (TGF)-β (Omer and Riley 1998), chemokines, nitric oxide (NO) (Anstey et al. 1996; Hobbs et al. 2002) and prostaglandins (Perkins et al. 2001). Moreover, in different settings or at different levels, the same cytokine or mediator may be harmful or protective (reviewed by Hunt and Grau 2003). By way of example, TNF-α itself has been ascribed a protective role in regulating parasite density (Kwiatkowski 1995), which is supported by the demonstration of a parasiticidal effect of TNF-α on *P. falciparum* in vitro (Muniz-Junqueira et al. 2001).

It is generally thought that the soluble mediators induced by malaria toxins contribute not only to fever, but also to the end-organ, metabolic and haematological consequences of disease. TNF-α and LT-α have been shown to increase expression of parasitised erythrocyte receptors such as intercellular adhesion molecule (ICAM)-1 on endothelial cells (Ockenhouse et al. 1992; Engwerda et al. 2002), thus potentially initiating a vicious cycle that may lead to severe malaria by sequestering more parasitised cells and further increasing local cytokine production. Other mediators, such as NO and prostaglandins, decrease cytokine-induced endothelial ICAM-1 and reduce cytoadherence of parasitised erythrocytes (Xiao et al. 1999; Serirom et al. 2003). Other factors are likely to contribute to protection or pathology in CM, including IFN-γ, migration inhibitory factor (Clark et al. 2003b), carbon monoxide (Clark et al. 2003a) and chemokines. The degree of anaemia in malaria is thought to exceed that which can be explained by destruction of parasitised erythrocytes alone, leading to the proposition that erythropoiesis may be depressed by soluble mediators (reviewed by Menendez et al. 2000). Severe metabolic acidosis with hyper-lactataemia is associated with a very high mortality in malaria (English et al. 1996) and probably results from a combination of tissue hypoxia, direct effects of cytokines, lactate production by parasites, and decreased clearance of lactate by the liver (Marsh and Snow 1997). The pathogenesis of other metabolic derangements such as hypoglycaemia may share similar antecedents (Clark et al. 1997).

2.2
Structure of *P. falciparum* GPIs

GPI molecules are evolutionarily conserved glycolipids present in the outer membranes of eukaryotic cells. Their core structure comprises a single membrane-associated phospholipid head, attached linearly to an inositol ring that is followed by a tetrasaccharide containing one glucosamine and three sequentially numbered mannose residues (Fig. 1). A phosphoethanolamine group attached to the terminal mannose affords stable anchorage for a diverse range of proteins. GPIs vary between eukaryotes in a limited number of ways that nonetheless appear to impart a wide range of functional differences. In mammals and yeast, an additional ethanolamine phosphate is invariably present as a side-chain on the first mannose and occasionally on the second mannose. Protozoa such as *Trypanosoma brucei* may carry an additional carbohydrate modification on the first mannose (Ferguson 1999). In contrast,

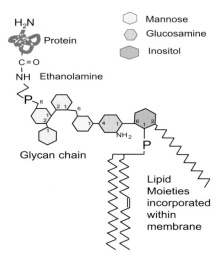

Fig. 1 Schematic representation of *P. falciparum* GPI. The lipid moieties are incorporated into the plasma membrane and joined via glycerol and phosphate (*P*) to an inositol ring. A conserved core glycan chain composed of glucosamine and three mannose residues is attached at the inositol 6 position. The terminal third conserved mannose residue is joined via a P ester to ethanolamine, which facilitates linkage to the C-terminus of a protein via an amide group. *P. falciparum* GPI remains acylated at the inositol 2-position, and a fourth side-chain mannose is typically attached to the ethanolamine-linked mannose

no side-chain modifications of the first two mannose residues have been described in *P. falciparum*. A side-chain fourth mannose (Man$_4$) is typically attached to the terminal mannose in *P. falciparum* and yeast, whereas this was thought to be uncommon until recently in mammals. It has now been demonstrated that *hSMP3* is the human homologue for yeast *SMP3*, and that it encodes the mannosyltransferase responsible for addition of Man$_4$ to GPIs (Taron et al. 2004). Although the gene is only weakly expressed in many cultured mammalian cell lines, it is expressed in most human tissues, challenging the previous paradigm that Man$_4$-GPI formation is relatively unimportant in mammalia.

Mammalian GPI inositol rings may be acylated by palmitate in some cases, although it is common for mammalian inositol to be deacylated following GPI biosynthesis (Chen et al. 1998). In contrast, *P. falciparum* inositol remains acylated, most often with palmitate (90%) but occasionally with myristate (10%) (Naik et al. 2000a). The phosphorylated lipid moiety attached to inositol in *P. falciparum* is invariably diacylglycerol in structure (Naik et al. 2000a), but in mammalian cells is predominantly 1-alkyl, 2-acyl glycerol. Recent examination by gas chromatography-mass spectrometry of protein-anchored "major" GPIs in *P. falciparum* has demonstrated heterogeneity resulting in at least five different structures, which can be fully ascribed to compositional differences in the fatty acyl substituents (Naik et al. 2000a). Importantly, variation in lipid composition did not appear to influence the likelihood of protein anchoring by the GPIs and it is likely that other biologically active "minor" GPIs with unusual fatty acyl substituents remain to be described (Naik et al. 2000a). Plasmodial GPIs from human and rodent malaria species demonstrate a high level of conservation in structure (Gerold et al. 1997; Naik et al. 2000a; Kimmel et al. 2003), which is also seen in widely dispersed geographical isolates of *P. falciparum* (Berhe et al. 1999). To date, GPIs have not been described in other species of plasmodia that cause malaria in humans.

2.3
Biosynthesis of *P. falciparum* GPIs

The general processes involved in GPI biosynthesis have been comprehensively reviewed (Ferguson 1999; Kinoshita and Inoue 2000; Eisenhaber et al. 2003) and will be only briefly summarised here. GPIs are assembled sequentially in the endoplasmic reticulum by a number of proteins/protein complexes that exhibit a variety of catalytic and regulatory roles. These proteins and their genes are well characterised in mammals, and this has enabled matching of sequence homologues in other eukaryotes in a number of instances through database mining. Homologues have been identified in *P. falciparum* for 8 of the approximately 20 known protein components of human GPI biosynthesis, with a 40%–70% similarity in amino acid sequences (Delorenzi et al. 2002; Shams-Eldin et al. 2002). The existence of other homologues may have been concealed by the level of stringency used for database matching or incomplete annotation of the *P. falciparum* genome at the time; also, non-homologous proteins may perform some of the designated functions (Delorenzi et al. 2002). In general, the *P. falciparum* homologues described are for proteins involved in key catalytic roles, rather than in regulating the rate or stability of reactions. Consistent with the proposed structure of *P. falciparum* GPIs, homologues for the mammalian genes that encoded addition of phosphoethanolamine groups to non-terminal mannoses and deacylation of inositol (which appears not to occur in *P. falciparum*) were not found. It has been suggested that this overall economy may have arisen through an adaptation to rapid growth and from lesser requirements for fine tuning compared to higher eukaryotes (Delorenzi et al. 2002).

The transamidation reaction that covalently anchors proteins to GPI inside the endoplasmic reticulum depends on recognition of a signal sequence and proteolytic cleavage of a carboxy-terminal pro-peptide (Eisenhaber et al. 2003). This process appears to be intricately mediated in mammalian cells by the protein PIG-T, which possesses both a hook for the key catalytic subunit (PIG-K) and a hole-like beta propeller structure that regulates access of C terminal oligopeptides to the protease site through a tunnel (Eisenhaber et al. 2003). A similar coding region for the *PIG-T* gene was found in *P. falciparum,* but failed stringency tests (Delorenzi et al. 2002). However, it has been noted that sequence similarity BLAST searching may fail to detect *PIG-T* homologues, unless consideration is given to secondary structural preferences or physical property patterns (Eisenhaber et al. 2003). As cells from mammals and parasitic protozoa appear to differ in their preference for particular amino acid coding regions in the signal sequence (Moran and Caras 1994), the transamidation reaction represents a particularly attractive target for species-specific inhibitors.

2.4
Specific Roles of *P. falciparum* GPIs in Malaria Pathogenesis

A range of in vitro and in vivo animal studies have demonstrated that purified *P. falciparum* GPIs can induce the pathophysiology ascribed to putative malaria toxins and/or that anti-GPI antibodies can neutralise these effects. Mouse macrophages were first shown to produce TNF-α after incubation with erythrocytes parasitised with either *P. yoelii* or *P. berghei in vitro* in 1988 (Bate et al. 1988). Consistent results were soon demonstrated for human monocytes in the presence of *P. falciparum* in vitro (Kwiatkowski et al. 1989). This was followed by partial characterisation of the likely toxin using physical and chemical extraction procedures (Bate et al. 1992b) coupled with monoclonal and polyclonal antibody neutralisation studies (Bate et al. 1992a; Bate and Kwiatkowski 1994a). By 1993, it was clear that the putative toxin was a GPI and that its injection into thioglycollate-primed rodents could reproduce major features of acute clinical malaria, including pyrexia and hypoglycaemia (Schofield and Hackett 1993); similar findings have subsequently been reported in unprimed mice (Elased et al. 2004). Concurrently, it was shown that a monoclonal antibody to *P. falciparum*-derived GPIs could neutralise the TNF-α-inducing activity of whole-parasite extracts in vitro (Schofield et al. 1993), suggesting that GPIs alone may be responsible for TNF-α induction. Polyclonal antibodies raised in T-cell-deficient mice (Bate et al. 1990) and sera from human patients infected with both *P. falciparum* and *P. vivax* (Bate and Kwiatkowski 1994b) were reported to have similar activity. However, we have been unable to confirm this ourselves, with toxin-neutralisation assays showing no clear-cut correlation between anti-GPI antibody titres in serum and the ability of purified immunoglobulin (Ig)G from the same serum to neutralise TNF-α induction by whole-parasite extracts from a macrophage cell line in vitro (J.B. de Souza et al., unpublished data). These data suggest either that GPI is not the only TNF-inducing component of parasite extracts or that not all anti-GPI antibodies are able to neutralise GPI activity.

By the mid-1990s, *P. falciparum* GPIs had been shown capable of inducing macrophage production of IL-1 (Schofield and Hackett 1993) as well as production of NO by macrophages and vascular endothelial cells in a process enhanced by IFN-γ (Tachado et al. 1996). *P. falciparum* GPIs were then shown to increase endothelial cell expression of ICAM-1, vascular cell adhesion molecule-1 and E-selectin (receptors implicated in cytoadherence of parasitised erythrocytes) in a process enhanced by TNF-α and IL-1 (Schofield et al. 1996). This process was also blocked by monoclonal anti-GPI antibodies. Consistent with the ability to induce hypoglycaemia in mice, *P. falciparum* GPIs were shown to possess insulin-mimetic activity through increasing glucose oxidation in murine adipocytes in vitro (Schofield and Hackett 1993). The culmination of these studies was the recent demonstration that murine antibodies raised through vaccination with a *P. falciparum* GPI glycan analogue completely abolished whole schizont extract-induced TNF-α release from mouse macrophages (Schofield et al. 2002). To the extent that the in vitro model matches the clinical situation in humans, this is the most suggestive evidence to date that GPIs are the predominant pro-inflammatory toxins of *P. falciparum*.

It has not yet been determined precisely how *P. falciparum* GPIs initiate the intracellular signalling that results in expression of cytokines, NO and adhesion molecules. Early studies using specific inhibitors supported a two-step model of cellular activation that ultimately ends with activation of the transcription factor nuclear factor (NF)-κB (Schofield et al. 1996; Tachado et al. 1996, 1997; Vijaykumar et al. 2001); the first signal provided by the glycan moiety [activating protein tyrosine kinase (PTK)] and the second by the diacylglycerol [activating protein kinase C (PKC)]. The issue of whether the two signals require insertion and/or endocytosis of whole GPIs or GPI substructures into the plasma membrane (Vijaykumar et al. 2001) or can be provided entirely extracellularly (Vijaykumar et al. 2001) remains unresolved. More recently it has been suggested that *P. falciparum* GPIs can initiate intracellular signalling—without internalisation—through toll-like receptors (TLRs), although the extent to which signalling via the PTK, PKC and TLR pathways may overlap is still unclear. In vitro studies examining TNF-α production by GPI-stimulated macrophages derived from the bone marrow of TLR knockout mice have demonstrated a major role for TLR2, a lesser role for TLR4, and a potential minor role for other pathways not dependent on the TLR2/TLR4 shared adapter protein MyD88 (Krishnegowda et al. 2004). Similar results were apparent in experiments using human monocytes that were pre-treated with monoclonal antibodies to TLR2 and/or TLR4. Subsequent intracellular signalling in both the mouse and human cells involved activation of a number of second messengers, including ERK1/ERK2, JNK and p38, and ultimately the NF-κB pathway. Parallel experiments by the same investigators demonstrated that the pattern of TNF-α, IL-6, IL-12 and NO production by GPI-stimulated mouse macrophages depended on differential activation of these signalling molecules and a variable requirement for co-stimulation with IFN-γ (Zhu et al. 2004). This may have relevance in vivo, as it has previously been shown that CD3$^+$ T cells are required for optimal TNF-α production by human monocytes stimulated by *P. falciparum* ex vivo (Scragg et al. 1999), which may also indicate the involvement of IFN-γ (reviewed by Artavanis-Tsakonas et al. 2003).

The exact structural requirements of *P. falciparum* GPIs for activation of intracellular signalling also require further clarification. The issue of whether glycan-induced signalling is dependent on the third (Tachado et al. 1997) or fourth terminal (Vijaykumar et al. 2001) mannose appears to have been resolved in favour of the former, with Man$_3$ GPIs shown to possess approximately 80% of the TNF-α-inducing activity of Man$_4$ GPIs (Krishnegowda et al. 2004). Insolubility of Man$_3$ GPIs in the solvent (80% ethanol) used for transfer from the stock vial to the culture medium is now thought to explain the previous results (Vijaykumar et al. 2001). More in keeping with their previous findings (Vijaykumar et al. 2001), diacylated *sn*-2 *lyso*-GPIs (resulting from partial deacylation of native GPIs by phospholipase A$_2$) induced levels of TNF-α from mouse macrophages and human monocytes that were similar to those from the intact molecules (Krishnegowda et al. 2004). Interestingly, heterodimerisation of TLR2 (a basic requirement for TLR2-induced signalling) involved TLR1 in the case of triacylated GPIs but TLR6 for the diacylated *sn*-2 *lyso*-GPIs, thus implicating lipid composition as a basis for antigenic discrimination by macrophages—a phenomenon that the authors point out has a precedent in the case of bacterial lipoproteins (Takeda et al. 2002; Akira and Hemmi 2003). Just as intriguing was the finding that GPIs were degraded and inactivated in the presence of mouse macrophages and human monocytes, consistent with cell-surface related activity of phospholipase A$_2$ and phospholipase D (Krishnegowda et al. 2004). To what extent human monocyte phospholipases may be able to regulate the activity of *P. falciparum* GPIs in vivo, and whether this may further be influenced by phospholipases released into serum during human malaria (Vadas et al. 1993), remains to be determined.

In addition to their putative roles as toxins, GPIs may indirectly contribute to malaria pathogenesis both by anchoring protein determinants of parasite virulence and altering their pathological and immune functions. In *P. falciparum*, as in all eukaryotes, the fundamental physiological role of GPIs is to stably anchor a diverse range of proteins on cellular plasma membranes. A number of important proteins appear to be GPI-anchored in *P. falciparum*, including merozoite surface protein (MSP)-1, MSP-2 and MSP-4 (Chatterjee and Mayor 2001; Gowda 2002). In addition, a large pool of *P. falciparum* GPIs exist free of protein attachment (Gerold et al. 1994), which is also common in other parasitic protozoa (Ropert and Gazzinelli 2000). It is possible, although not yet proven, that it is the free GPIs released at the time of schizont rupture that are predominantly responsible for toxin-mediated effects. It has been reported that the presence of GPI anchors on sporozoite protein vaccines impairs the development of antibody (Martinez et al. 2000; Scheiblhofer et al. 2001) and T-cell responses (Bruna-Romero et al. 2004) with consequent attenuation of vaccine-induced immunity; similar observations have been made in other systems (Wood and Elliott 1998). However, following DNA vaccination, antibody responses to a gametocyte-specific antigen are enhanced by the retention of the GPI anchor signal sequence (Fanning et al. 2003). These data suggest that the presence of glycans alters the solubility and membrane interactions of proteins, and thus the pathway of protein trafficking within an antigen-presenting cell. Additionally, GPI attachment may alter the conformation of anchored proteins in a manner that influences the proteins' function and/or immunogenicity. These observations may have important implications for the development of recombinant protein vaccines, many of which are based on GPI-anchored proteins (reviewed by Gowda 2002).

2.5
Putative Malaria Toxins Other than GPI

In addition to GPI, haemozoin (or "malaria pigment"; an insoluble digestion product of trophozoites comprising detoxified haemoglobin, as well as remnants of host and parasite membranes) has been implicated as a malaria toxin (Arese and Schwarzer 1997). Purified and synthetic haemozoin (β-haematin) were linked to inflammatory cytokine production in vitro in a number of studies (Pichyangkul et al. 1994; Prada et al. 1995; Sherry et al. 1995; Mordmuller et al. 1998) conducted in the period preceding identification of *Mycoplasma* contamination of parasite cultures (Turrini et al. 1997; Rowe et al. 1998). Subsequently, de-proteinated haemozoin enriched from *P. falciparum* culture was shown to induce TNF-α and IL-1β production by human peripheral blood mononuclear cells *ex vivo,* which was able to be blocked by naturally occurring IgM antibodies (Biswas et al. 2001). More recently, it was demonstrated that synthetic haemozoin induced inflammatory cytokines (including IL1-α, IL1-β, IL-6, and IL-12), chemokines and their receptors, and migration of neutrophils and monocytes, following injection into mice (Jaramillo et al. 2004). Unlike the case with GPIs, it appears that *P. falciparum* haemozoin is more likely to activate host cells through a hitherto unique TLR9-mediated, MyD88-dependent pathway that is sensitive to inhibition by chloroquine (Pichyangkul et al. 2004; Coban et al. 2005). In addition to induction of soluble mediators, haemozoin-laden macrophages have been shown to produce large quantities of the free fatty acids 12- and 15-hydroxy-arachidonic acid, which may be pathogenic by causing vascular damage and increased cytoadherence (Schwarzer et al. 2003).

Others have shown that *P. falciparum*-derived haemozoin induced NO synthase-2 expression in cultured human blood monocytes ex vivo, which was more pronounced in cells from children with anaemia (Keller et al. 2004). A similar effect has been shown in mouse macrophages with *P. falciparum*-derived and synthetic haemozoin, although a requirement for co-stimulation with IFN-γ was apparent in that study (Jaramillo et al. 2003). In contrast, β-haematin was shown to suppress TNF-α and NO production by lipopolysaccharide (LPS)-stimulated mouse macrophages (Taramelli et al. 1995); an effect later attributed to β-haematin-induced oxidative stress (Taramelli et al. 2000). Another study showed that high levels of haemozoin ingestion by intervillous blood monocytes were associated with suppression of TNF-α, prostaglandin-E_2 and IL-10 in women with placental parasitaemia (Perkins et al. 2003). The source of mononuclear cells in these different studies, and the nature of the interactions between the cells and haemozoin, may be factors to consider in resolving these apparent contradictions (Basilico et al. 2003; Jaramillo et al. 2005).

Other candidates for "malaria toxins" are anti-malarial IgE-antigen complexes and IgE-anti-IgE complexes, which may also induce TNF-α release from peripheral blood mononuclear cells in vitro (Perlmann et al. 1997). These complexes have been proposed to activate NF-κB transcription factors by cross-linking the macrophage low-affinity Fcε receptor for IgE (Perlmann et al. 1997). Using an in vitro toxin-neutralisation assay, which measures TNF-α in supernatants of cultured macrophages incubated with malaria-immune sera and *P. falciparum* schizont lysates, we have shown that some malaria-immune sera themselves induce TNF-α in the absence of exogenous malaria antigen; this activity is absent from purified IgG (J.B. de Souza et al., unpublished data). Although this might be explained by trace amounts of GPI in the serum (as the sera were taken from residents of highly malaria-endemic areas), it is possible that serum IgE complexes induce TNF-α; this notion is further supported by the observation that non-IgG antibodies in other malaria-immune sera synergise with parasite extract to enhance TNF-α production (J.B. de Souza et al., unpublished data). These data are consistent with the likely involvement of an immune complex-mediated TNF-α triggering pathway. Anti-malarial IgE/antigen complexes may exert pathogenic effects by depositing on cerebral microvasculature (Maeno et al. 2000), leading to local induction of pro-inflammatory cytokines, with consequent vascular damage. This would explain the recent finding that West African children with severe malaria had higher anti-*P. falciparum* IgE levels than age-matched children with mild malaria (Calissano et al. 2003).

2.6
Summary

It should be recognised that, at present, the evidence that *P. falciparum* GPIs act as toxins in humans in vivo is circumstantial. Purified or synthetic GPIs have not been injected into humans, and nor have anti-GPI antibodies been shown to inhibit the pathogenesis of *P. falciparum* in vivo; thus, the level of evidence is less than that associating bacterial endotoxin with the clinical manifestations of sepsis. Regardless, in vitro studies and data from animal models of malaria have identified clear avenues of investigation into the role of GPIs in human malaria, as well as other putative toxins such as haemozoin and IgE complexes.

3
The Nature of Anti-toxic Immunity to Malaria

Bewilderment regarding the mechanisms of anti-malarial immunity is reflected by the number of terms used to describe it; among others, natural, clinical, innate, acquired, specific, non-specific, anti-parasitic, anti-disease, anti-toxic, cell-mediated, antibody-mediated, tolerance, premunition and semi-immune. In part, confusion in the use of these terms (sometimes interchangeably) has arisen through a desire to explain observable epidemiological phenomena on the one hand, within the confines of existing immunological paradigms on the other. As the focus of this review is the putative malaria toxin GPI, and immune responses to it, we will generally refer to anti-toxic immune responses, and dispense with the commonly used epithet "anti-disease", as the latter may be considered the sine qua non of all forms of immunity. Hence, this section concerns differences in the clinical condition that can reasonably be expected to infer the existence of anti-toxic immunity, which may in theory act by inhibition of parasite metabolic pathways leading to reduced or defective toxin production (of which little is presently known), neutralisation of toxin at or shortly after the time of release, interference with the cellular mechanisms triggered by toxin activation that lead to production of inflammatory mediators, and/or diminished host responsiveness to one or more of the inflammatory processes that follow.

3.1
Tolerance of Malaria Parasitaemia Without Symptoms

Despite thousands of publications related to anti-malarial immunity, it is probably just as true to say today as it was 100 years ago that the best correlate of immunity to malaria is the presence of malaria parasites in the blood of individuals without symptoms (Sinton 1938; McGregor et al. 1956). It is generally accepted that the likelihood of observing asymptomatic parasitaemia within a population correlates with the intensity of exposure, and that it is unlikely to be observed in previously malaria-naïve individuals. It has been shown by some that asymptomatic infections can become established and persist at reasonably stable densities over time (Sowunmi 1995; Farnert et al. 1997; Smith et al. 1999; Bruce et al. 2000), but others have challenged this notion in longitudinal studies demonstrating an increased future risk of symptoms (Missinou et al. 2003; Njama-Meya et al. 2004). It is evident though, from our own studies in regions of intense malaria transmission, that a high prevalence of asymptomatic infections can be expected in individuals of all ages in whom signs and symptoms are objectively evaluated on multiple occasions over 24 h (Boutlis et al. 2002, 2003b). The levels of parasitaemia observed, especially in children (Rogier et al. 1996; Boutlis et al. 2002), are often much higher than those recorded to cause disease in previously malaria-naïve subjects (Gatton and Cheng 2002; Molineaux et al. 2002). Given that it has long been assumed that malaria parasites release pyrogenic substances (i.e. toxins) during schizogony (Golgi 1886), and there is no evidence to suggest that field strains can become avirulent, it seems reasonable to suppose that host immune responses maintain the healthy phenotype during asymptomatic infection.

Through detailed epidemiological studies conducted in regions of high malaria endemicity, it has been observed that young children will tolerate high levels of malaria parasitaemia; levels that are much more frequently associated with disease in adults (Smith et al. 1994; Rogier et al. 1996). By mathematical modelling, the risk of symptoms has been shown to correlate with the level of parasitaemia in an age-dependent manner, with a peak at approximately 1 year of age that declines steeply through early childhood to a plateau in adolescence (Smith et al. 1994; Rogier et al. 1996). The exponentially decaying curve that describes the relationship between the level of parasitaemia associated with fever and increasing age has been referred to as defining a "pyrogenic threshold" (Rogier et al. 1996). These results were generally in keeping with observations such as those made by Miller in Liberia in 1958: "...while adults were more efficient in suppressing parasite levels and suffered less from clinical attacks of malaria, children could tolerate higher parasite burdens without showing clinical evidence of disease" (Miller 1958). In contrast, the application of mathematical modelling techniques in regions of low or unstable malaria transmission has shown a less discrete relationship between the level of parasitaemia and the risk of symptoms, with generally lower pyrogenic thresholds and less dependence on age (Prybylski et al. 1999; Boisier et al. 2002). This suggests that fully effective anti-toxic immunity may only become manifest in areas of quite high and/or stable malaria transmission. Interestingly, studies of experimental infection in previously malaria-naïve subjects have shown that an individual's pyrogenic threshold may increase following an initial infection, as well as being influenced by host genetics and the "strain" of parasite (Gatton and Cheng 2002; Molineaux et al. 2002).

Considered together, these observations are consistent with a model in which repetitive and ongoing exposure to malaria infection results in relatively short-lived anti-toxic immune responses that abrogate inflammatory pathology. It is evident from studies in hyper-endemic regions that the efficacy of these responses is highest in early childhood and is lowest in adulthood. This creates an apparent paradox in relation to the fact that, in endemic areas, malaria severity is highest in young children and the frequency of malaria attacks reduces with age. This can be resolved, however, by conceptualising disease as resulting from uncontrolled expansion of parasite densities that overcome an individual's pyrogenic threshold. The immune responses that act to limit parasite replication (sometimes referred to as "anti-parasitic" responses) appear to increase with age, in contrast to the anti-toxic responses that maintain tolerance of parasitaemia. The ability to limit the severity of disease in the face of unchecked parasite growth may be expected to result from a number of factors, some of which may be anti-toxic in nature (Sect. 3.2), but in addition may involve prevention of other critical events that are not primarily toxin-mediated, such as cytoadherence and anaemia.

3.2
Limitation of Malaria Severity in the Face of Disease

The model proposed in the previous section is broadly consistent with the concept that anti-malarial immune responses can be categorised as anti-parasitic, anti-fever (i.e. parasite tolerance), and anti-severe disease (Snow

and Marsh 1998). The latter may involve mechanisms that reduce cytoadherence (e.g. antibodies to cytoadherence ligands on infected erythrocytes),
whilst alterations in the balance of inflammatory and anti-inflammatory cytokines may effect both anti-fever and anti-severe disease immunity (Omer
et al. 2000). To better understand the influence of age itself (separated from
exposure) on malaria severity, Baird and colleagues have prospectively studied recently arrived Indonesian transmigrants from very low-endemic Java
into hyper-endemic Papua Province (Baird 1998). Previously malaria-naïve
children appeared to manifest relative resistance to the severity of malaria
compared to adults (Baird et al. 1998). The explanation for these findings is
not entirely clear, and results may have been biased in part by differences in the
use of prophylaxis or in treatment-seeking behaviour in adults and children.
Alternatively, it is plausible that children make lower levels of inflammatory
cytokines in response to a given "dose" of parasites (Riley 1999).

Of the numerous candidate host responses proposed to limit malaria severity, some may be predominantly anti-toxic in nature, whereas others may
act more broadly. For example, a growing body of literature (reviewed by
Anstey et al. 1999a) suggests that genetic (Hobbs et al. 2002) and acquired
influences regulating NO production act to reduce malaria severity through
cross-talk with other soluble mediators, such as TNF-α (Iuvone et al. 1996)
and prostaglandins (N.M. Anstey et al., unpublished data), in addition to
reducing expression of endothelial cytoadherence receptors (Serirom et al.
2003). It had previously been suggested that individuals in malaria-endemic
regions produced NO in an age-dependent manner that was correlated with
the age-dependent pyrogenic threshold (Clark et al. 1996; Anstey et al. 1999b).
However, a recent detailed longitudinal examination of NO production in
malaria-exposed children and adults living in Madang, Papua New Guinea
has shown that NO production differs little across age groups from age 2 to
60 years (Boutlis et al. 2004).

Additionally, the anti-inflammatory cytokines IL-10 and TGF-β have repeatedly been shown to reduce the toxic effects of malaria infections in mice
and in humans. The pathology of *P. chabaudi chabaudi* infection and the mortality in IL-10-deficient mice are ameliorated by anti-TNF-α and exacerbated
by anti-TGF-β antibodies (Omer and Riley 1998; Dodoo et al. 2002; Li et al.
2003), and recent data suggest an important role for regulatory T cells in setting
the pro-inflammatory/anti-inflammatory cytokine balance (Omer et al. 2003;
Hisaeda et al. 2004). Disentangling the influence of a raft of other cell-mediated
and cytokine responses on malaria severity is difficult in isolation, but has
recently been reviewed in the context of an overall model of anti-malarial immunity that also considers factors such as nutrition (Artavanis-Tsakonas et
al. 2003). The subtlety and importance of cross-species interactions between

malaria and other infections, such as intestinal helminths, that may also influence cell-mediated phenomena, are beginning to be appreciated (Nacher 2002; Boutlis et al. 2003b; Le Hesran et al. 2004; Nacher 2005; Hesran 2005), but further discussion is beyond the scope of the present review.

3.3
Summary

It appears that anti-toxic immune responses to malaria may contribute to the maintenance of malarial tolerance on the one hand, while contributing to resistance to severe disease in those unable to limit exponential expansion of parasitaemia on the other. It should be recognised that the potential for multiple anti-toxic effector mechanisms exists, but that they do not necessarily have the same relationship with age. For example, those that mediate tolerance may decrease with age, whereas those underlying resistance to disease severity may increase, with some degree of overlap in the transition from one to another. While an individual's genetic make-up and parasite strain differences may contribute to the overall level of toxicity manifest in the host–parasite relationship, it is likely that the level of exposure to malaria and other infections, and factors related to age per se, are also involved. It seems logical that the sum of an individual's anti-toxic immune responses will act in concert to protect the individual by either neutralising the parasite toxin(s) and/or diminishing the host's response to toxin-triggered events. Furthermore, it is apparent that not all immune responses acting to reduce the severity of malaria need be thought of as being primarily anti-toxic in nature.

4
Immunity to *P. falciparum* GPIs

Assuming that the preparations used were pure and free from contamination (Naik et al. 2000a), it has been consistently demonstrated in a number of studies done in malaria-endemic regions that GPIs purified from *P. falciparum* are recognised by human antibodies (Naik et al. 2000a; de Souza et al. 2002; Boutlis et al. 2002; Hudson Keenihan et al. 2003; Suguitan et al. 2004). This has raised the possibility that these naturally occurring antibodies could neutralise GPIs and influence the outcome of human malaria. The presence of antibodies implies that GPIs are recognised by immune cells; hence, GPIs may also potentially elicit other cellular immune responses that are not antibody-mediated. It is important to understand how GPIs may initiate these immune responses, and how they are effected, if vaccination against GPIs is to be used for protection against malaria.

4.1
GPI Induction of Tolerance-Like Immunity

Obvious parallels exist between the phenomena of malarial tolerance and bacterial endotoxin tolerance, which has led to the proposition that they are mediated by common molecular pathways (Clark et al. 2004). The phenomenon of endotoxin tolerance was initially defined in the 1960s on the basis that rabbits could be effectively immunised with a low dose of bacterial endotoxin (LPS) against death from the subsequent injection of a potentially lethal dose (reviewed by West and Heagy 2002). Similarly, febrile responses in humans decrease with subsequent injections of endotoxin (van der Poll and van Deventer 1999). The tolerant state in animals was later shown to correlate with a reduction in TNF-α production in response to repeated endotoxin injection that persisted for several weeks (Sanchez-Cantu et al. 1989). Subsequently, it was shown that LPS-stimulated production of TNF-α, IL-1β, IL-6, and IL-10 in whole blood taken from human volunteers 3 h after an intravenous injection of *Escherichia coli* LPS was significantly reduced compared to baseline, but restored at 24 h (van der Poll et al. 1996). Further in vitro experiments using human and animal monocytes/macrophages defined the characteristic physiological changes accompanying repeated exposure to endotoxin: inhibition of TNF-α; augmentation of NO and prostaglandin-E_2; and variably altered IL-6, IL-1 and IL-8 secretion (West and Heagy 2002). Given the timescale of the induction of endotoxin tolerance, the simplest interpretation of these data is that cells become temporarily refractory to endotoxin after stimulation.

Optimal responses to LPS derived from *Enterobacteriaceae* depend on cellular recognition by TLR4 complexed with CD-14 and the membrane-associated molecule MD-2 (Latz et al. 2002). Binding of LPS leads to induction of protein kinases, which in turn activate nuclear factors including NF-κB (Ziegler-Heitbrock et al. 1994) that influence transcriptional activation of numerous inflammatory cytokine genes (Dobrovolskaia and Vogel 2002). Desensitised human monocytes rendered tolerant by pre-treatment with LPS accumulate an excess of functionally inactive NF-κB complexes comprising p50 homodimers (Ziegler-Heitbrock et al. 1994; Kastenbauer and Ziegler-Heitbrock 1999) and have elevated concentrations of the NF-κB-inhibitory protein Iκ-Bα (Wahlstrom t al. 1999; Ferlito et al. 2001); the activation of other kinases in the signal transduction cascade is also inhibited in tolerant cells (West and Heagy 2002). Alternatively, although alteration of intracellular signal transduction pathways appears likely to mediate tolerance, down-regulation of LPS receptors on the surface of immune cells or over-production of anti-inflammatory mediators such as IL-10, TGF-β and NO may also be involved (Zingarelli et al. 1995; Fahmi et al. 1995; Dobrovolskaia and Vogel 2002). Indeed, NO had been proposed as a candidate mediator of malarial tolerance in endemic regions on the basis of studies suggesting a role in the mediation of endotoxin tolerance (Zingarelli et al. 1995) and preliminary observations in human studies (Clark et al. 1996; Anstey et al. 1999b). The subsequent demonstration that NO is dispensable to the development of endotoxin tolerance in NO synthase-2-knockout mice (Zingarelli et al. 2002) and recent contradictory data from human studies (Boutlis et al. 2004) casts doubt on these suggestions.

The recent demonstration that *P. falciparum* may initiate intracellular signalling through TLR2 and TLR4 (Krishnegowda et al. 2004) provides insight into the mechanisms that may underlie tolerance to malaria infection. Like *P. falciparum* GPIs, the GPI-mucin of *T. cruzi* appears to be recognised by both TLR2 and TLR4 (Campos et al. 2001; Ropert and Gazzinelli 2004; Oliveira et al. 2004); indeed, detailed studies have demonstrated that *T. cruzi* GPI-mucin and *E. coli* LPS use functionally similar pathways to induce TNF-α and IL-12 production in murine macrophages, with levels of both cytokines reduced in response to secondary stimuli (Ropert et al. 2001). This mirrors other models of cross-tolerance induced by differential induction of TLR2/TLR4 (Lehner et al. 2001; Beutler et al. 2001), consistent with these receptors sharing common intracellular pathways. The practical relevance of these studies to human malaria may have been hinted at as long as 50 years ago when it was shown that even a first malaria infection could induce cross-tolerance to endotoxin in experimentally infected humans (Heyman and Beeson 1949; Rubenstein et al. 1965). It is unclear, however, whether possible LPS contamination of the parasite preparations used in these studies may have confounded this effect. Considering the accumulated evidence, it would appear the most likely candidate model for malarial tolerance is one that parallels bacterial endotoxin tolerance.

4.2
Anti-GPI Antibodies in Human Malaria

The recent purification of GPI in sufficient quantities for analysis has enabled the study of anti-GPI responses in human malaria. The strong theme to emerge from all studies conducted in malaria-endemic regions to date is that both the population prevalence and level of antibody responses increases with age (Naik et al. 2000a; de Souza et al. 2002; Boutlis et al. 2002; Hudson Keenihan et al. 2003; Suguitan et al. 2004). That this was true in a population exposed to perennially intense malaria transmission from birth (Boutlis et al. 2002), as well as Javanese transmigrants experiencing their first malaria attacks in hyper-endemic Indonesian Papua (Hudson Keenihan et al. 2003), would suggest that immunological changes related to ageing are at least as important as those relating to cumulative exposure in determining antibody production. Antibodies to *P. falciparum* GPIs are infrequent in children less than 2 years of age (Naik et al. 2000a), possibly due to the inability of the immune system of small children to respond to carbohydrate antigens, but the age-relationship of anti-GPI antibody production thereafter closely mirrors that of a number of other blood-stage malaria peptide antigens (Al Yaman et al. 1994, 1995a,. 1995b; Johnson et al. 2000). Field studies have shown that the anti-GPI antibody response is boostable by recent infection (de Souza et al. 2002; Hudson Keenihan et al. 2003), predominantly IgG rather than IgM (Naik et al. 2000a; Boutlis et al. 2002), and highly skewed towards the IgG3 subclass, especially in children (Boutlis et al. 2003a). Anti-GPI antibody responses decay rapidly after elimination of parasites by chemotherapy, suggesting that ongoing antigenic stimulation is required to maintain antibody production; the very rapid decline in treated children compared to treated adults (Boutlis et al. 2002) probably reflects the preponderance of IgG3 in children's plasma (Boutlis et al. 2003a), as IgG3 has a shorter half-life in serum than other IgG subclasses.

The relationship between anti-GPI antibodies and clinical malaria has been evaluated in a number of studies. In a study of Kenyan children and their mothers, seropositivity for anti-GPI antibodies was associated with lower body temperature and higher haemoglobin levels after adjusting for age and parasitaemia (Naik et al. 2000a). However, it was unclear from the data presented whether the association with lower body temperatures directly translated to a lower risk of acute febrile illness. In a prospective study in Gambian children aged 3–8 years, antibody levels at the beginning of the transmission season were not significantly predictive of the subsequent risk of mild malaria after controlling for age (de Souza et al. 2002); nor was there any significant difference in anti-GPI response between hospital-admitted Gambian children with severe (mainly cerebral) malaria or mild malaria in an independent case-control study (de Souza et al. 2002). Interestingly, several children with severe malaria had exceedingly high titres of anti-GPI antibodies in this study, which may have been due to rapid boosting of anti-GPI titres by the current infection. A study of Javanese transmigrants appeared to show that children aged 6–12 years (but not adults) with a positive anti-GPI response following infection had reduced subsequent risk of symptomatic disease (Hudson Keenihan et al. 2003). However, the analysis may have been influenced by the use of multiple measurements from the same child and the lack of adjustment for age; a similar finding was initially noted in the Gambian children, but disappeared after adjusting for the confounding effect of age (de

Souza et al. 2002). A cross-sectional study from Cameroon of anti-GPI antibody responses in pregnant women at delivery showed no relationship with acute or chronic placental pathology, TNF-α levels or pregnancy outcomes (Suguitan et al. 2004). Again, boosting of anti-GPI antibody concentration by the current malaria infection may have obscured important differences in GPI levels earlier in pregnancy.

In summary, investigators have consistently shown that the prevalence, persistence and level of anti-GPI antibodies increase with age in malaria-exposed populations. To date, however, there is little evidence to show that the antibody responses measured correlate with protection against clinical malaria or disease severity. However, it should be borne in mind that none of these studies was primarily designed to evaluate the potential clinical roles of anti-GPI antibodies, and that future hypothesis-driven studies will likely provide more robust results. Crucially, more prospective studies are required in which measures of anti-GPI antibodies prior to infection can be tested for association with outcome of subsequent infection; notwithstanding the major logistical problems associated with prospective studies of severe malaria. The use of fully synthetic GPIs (Lu et al. 2004; Liu and Seeberger 2004; Seeberger et al. 2004) will help dispel any doubt that the responses measured are specific, and combining clinical studies with functional assays (such as toxin neutralisation) will provide the clearest outcomes.

4.3
Antigen Recognition and Processing of GPIs

Although several life cycle stages of *Plasmodium* express GPIs, initiation of immune responses likely occurs during asexual schizogony, when the highest concentrations of free GPI are released (Fig. 2). Early studies, conducted in immunocompetent and T-cell-deficient mice, suggested that non-protein antigens derived from the boiled supernatants of in vitro *P. falciparum* cultures induced a predominantly IgM response (Bate et al. 1990; Playfair et al. 1991). Serum from the mice could be used to block toxin-induced TNF-α production in vitro and in vivo (Playfair et al. 1991); this response appeared rapidly after immunisation and did not appear to be enhanced by boosting (Bate et al. 1992a) or common adjuvants (Playfair et al. 1990). This is typical of T-cell-independent antibody responses (Baumgarth 2000), but is at odds with the typical antibody responses to *P. falciparum* GPIs described in humans, which are IgG dominated (Naik et al. 2000a; Boutlis et al. 2002), characterised by skewing toward IgG3 (Boutlis et al. 2003a), and rapidly boosted by reinfection. This contrasts with the IgG2- and IgG1-dominated responses that have been described toward carbohydrate antigens such as bacterial polysaccha-

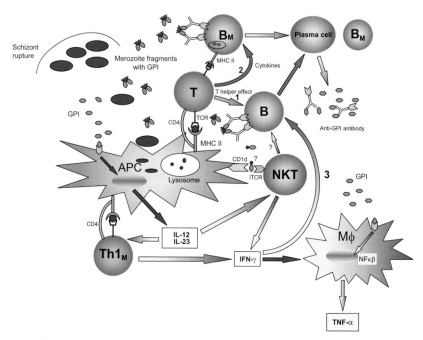

Fig. 2 Proposed cellular interactions in the generation of anti-GPI antibodies. Schizogony is accompanied by the release of merozoites with GPI-linked surface proteins and by free GPI. GPIs provide activation signals for antigen presenting cells (*APC*) and macrophages (*M*ϕ). Parasite material is internalised by APCs and after processing through the endosomal/lysosomal pathway, peptides are presented in association with MHC class II to T cells. Meanwhile B cells may recognise free GPI or GPI bound to merozoites and become activated through cross-linking of the B cell receptor and by helper cytokines released by T cells (*arrows 1* and *2*). B cell activation leads either to plasma cell differentiation and large scale production of anti-GPI antibody or to formation of GPI-specific memory B cells (*B_M*). Alternatively, GPI-specific B cells may internalise GPI-containing parasite material and present processed MHC class II-linked peptides to T cells. GPIs may also trigger APCs to produce IL-12 and IL-23 which regulate the function of other classes of T cell. IL-23-activated memory T cells (*Th1_M*) produce IFN-γ which in turn acts on B cells [(*arrow 3*), contributing to affinity maturation and Ig class switching) or macrophages (inducing anti-parasitic effector activity)]. The role of CD1d in the presentation of GPI-linked peptide to NKT cells remains controversial; however, it is likely that NKT cells respond following activation by IL-12/23 released by GPI-activated APC

rides (reviewed by Ferrante et al. 1990) and may indicate that GPI-anchored proteins act as natural adjuvants in eliciting immunological memory to *P. falciparum* GPIs. The apparent absence of IgG2 and IgG4 and the high ratio of IgG3 to IgG1 subclasses that we have observed (Boutlis et al. 2003a) are remarkably similar to the pattern of responses previously described in Solomon Islanders (Rzepczyk et al. 1997) and Gambians (Taylor et al. 1998) to MSP-2, which is a GPI-linked protein.

Given the absence of peptide epitopes for conventional T cells, antibody responses to free GPIs are likely to be T-cell-independent during a primary malaria infection. During a secondary response, however, activated GPI-specific B-cells may internalise and process GPI-linked proteins, possibly in the form of membrane vesicles (Hoessli et al. 2003), and subsequently present peptides derived from these GPI-linked proteins to CD4[+] T cells in the context of major histocompatibility complex class II (MHC-II). This would allow provision of cognate T-cell help to GPI-specific B-cells, via a classical hapten-carrier interaction, leading to immunoglobulin class switching, somatic mutation and affinity maturation of the BCR and generation of long-lived plasma cells and memory B-cells. As cognate interactions are most likely to take place between GPI-specific B cells and T cells recognising peptide epitopes that are physically linked to GPI, it is probable that T-cell help for GPI-specific B cells is provided by T cells specific for GPI-linked proteins and thus that anti-GPI antibodies may share qualitative features with antibodies to, for example, merozoite surface proteins. It is possible, for example, that the predominantly IgG3 subclass response to GPIs is mediated by T cells specific for MSP-2, which is known to induce IgG3 (Rzepczyk et al. 1997; Taylor et al. 1998). In support of this hypothesis, in the absence of covalently linked proteins, GPIs from the protozoal parasite *T. cruzi* can induce a switch from IgM to IgG production in murine B cells only in the presence of the T-cell-derived cytokines IL-4 and IL-5 (Bento et al. 1996).

Little is known of the primary immune response to *P. falciparum* GPIs, although it is likely to involve interactions with pattern recognition molecules (such as TLRs) expressed by dendritic cells and/or macrophages in the spleen (Stevenson and Riley 2004). Various types of lipid and glycolipid molecules can also be presented to NK T cells by CD1 molecules, which are MHC-like molecules encoded by genes outside the MHC (Sieling et al. 1995). CD1 molecules are expressed on the surface of antigen-presenting cells, e.g. macrophages, dendritic cells and B-cells (Kronenberg et al. 2001). Human CD1b has been shown to bind and present the mycobacterial lipoglycans, lipoarabinomannan and PI mannosides, which have a similar basic lipid anchor to *P. falciparum* GPIs (Sieling et al. 1995). In the presence of lipoarabi-nomannan and CD1[+] antigen-presenting cells, CD1b-restricted T cells taken from the skin of a patient with leprosy have been shown to induce IgG1 and IgG3 subclass antibody production by B cells at the expense of IgG4 and IgE (Fujieda et al. 1998). Mouse CD1d (which is highly homologous to human CD1d) (Porcelli and Modlin 1999) binds GPI with high affinity via the PI moiety (Joyce et al. 1998) and has been shown to strongly stimulate natural killer NK T cells in vitro after binding a variety of purified phospholipids (including PI) (Gumperz et al. 2000).

Whether or not CD1d molecules recognise malarial GPIs is controversial. It has been reported that CD1d-restricted presentation of GPI-anchored *P. falciparum* (sporozoite) surface proteins leads to NK T-cell stimulation and that presentation of *P. berghei* circumsporozoite antigen (thought to be GPI anchored) by CD1d elicits NK T-cell help in regulating IgG production (Schofield et al. 1999). However, two independent laboratories, in attempting to replicate these results using CD1d and MHC-II-deficient mice, have demonstrated that the IgG response to the circumsporozoite protein is solely MHC-II-dependent (Molano et al. 2000; Romero et al. 2001), in line with previous evidence (Romero et al. 1988). Genetic differences between the mice used in the three studies were thought not to explain the discrepant results (Romero et al. 2001). Similarly conflicting results have emerged regarding the role for CD1d-restricted NK T-cell-mediated regulation of antibody responses to *T. cruzi* GPIs (Procopio et al. 2002; Duthie et al. 2002), which share structural similarities with those of *P. falciparum* (Naik et al. 2000a). It may be that differences in the process of antigen presentation (exogenous versus endogenous) (Hansen et al. 2003a) or kinetics of the antibody responses (Hansen et al. 2003b) can explain these apparent contradictions. Most recently it has been demonstrated that CD1d-restricted NK T cells appear to influence the balance of IFN-γ/IL-4 cytokine production, pathogenesis and fatality in the murine *P. berghei* (ANKA) model (Hansen et al. 2003a, 2003b), as well as regulating B-cell-mediated antibody responses, which to MSP-1 at least were shown to arise from both CD1d-dependent and MHC-II-dependent pathways (Hansen et al. 2003b).

5
Potential for Therapeutic Inhibition of *P. falciparum* GPI Biosynthesis

GPIs and their anchored proteins appear to mediate critical events in malaria pathogenesis and immunity (Sects. 2 and 4), and their production appears crucial for the survival of *P. falciparum* (Naik et al. 2000b). Thus, therapeutic targeting of *P. falciparum* GPI biosynthesis has the potential to arrest disease by affecting parasite growth, development and virulence. Although the core structure of GPIs is conserved across eukaryotes, available evidence suggests that sufficient differences exist in the specificity and sequence of GPI synthesis reactions to enable species-specific pharmacological manipulation (reviewed by de Macedo et al. 2003). While an ideal inhibitor of *P.*

falciparum GPI synthesis would have little or no effect on mammalian GPI synthesis, absolute specificity may not be essential, given that normal levels of GPI synthesis are in some instances dispensable for mammalian cell survival (Ferguson 1999).

Proof in the concept of selective enzyme inhibition has been demonstrated for a fungal metabolite that inhibited mammalian, but not protozoal, GPIs (Sutterlin et al. 1997) and has been validated at different stages of GPI assembly in *T. brucei* and *Leishmania mexicana* (Smith et al. 1997, 1999, 2001, 2004; Ferguson 2000). These studies have provided the methodological basis to compare GPI synthesis between *P. falciparum* and man. Consequently, a synthetic glucosamine-*N*-acetyl-PI analogue has been shown to irreversibly inhibit the *P. falciparum* de-*N*-acetylase, and an isomer of glucosamine-*N*-PI appears to competitively inhibit either the inositol-transferase or first mannosyltransferase, with little apparent effect on the human orthologues (Smith et al. 2002). Others have shown that early steps in *P. falciparum* GPI assembly can be aborted by using glucosamine (Naik et al. 2003) or modified sugar residues like mannosamine (2-amino-2-deoxy-*d*-mannose), which inhibits parasite growth (Naik et al. 2000b). However, results have been inconsistent between studies and the precise mechanisms of activity remain unclear (Naik et al. 2000b; Santos de Macedo et al. 2001). Further potential exists for targeting other pathways intricately linked to early GPI biosynthesis, such as the supply of PI, activated sugars and lipid chains (Eisenhaber et al. 2003).

The apparent importance of the side-chain Man_4 of *P. falciparum* GPIs to cell signalling and its likely requirement for protein anchoring (Naik et al. 2000a) makes the process of its addition an attractive therapeutic target. This is particularly so given that the process of cellular activation is currently thought to be novel, as it does not appear to involve membrane insertion or endocytosis (Gowda 2002). The fatty acyl requirements for cellular activation are still somewhat unclear, although it appears that features common to *P. falciparum* but absent in mammalian GPIs are important for activity (Gowda 2002). Although it was recently shown that Man_4-GPIs are much more common in humans than previously realised, it was also demonstrated that protein transfer to human GPIs occurs irrespective of the presence of Man_4 or Man_3-GPI precursors (Taron et al. 2004). Prior addition of Man_4 is mandatory for GPI protein anchoring in *Saccharomyces cerevisiae* (Grimme et al. 2001) and is likely to be a requirement in *P. falciparum*, given that all GPI protein anchors discovered to date possess a fourth mannose (Naik et al. 2000a). Together, these findings suggest that differences in the specificities of human, yeast and *P. falciparum* transamidase complexes for Man_3/Man_4 GPI precursors can be expected and potentially exploited, perhaps even in a tissue-specific manner (Taron et al. 2004). Further definition of the genes and proteins involved in

P. falciparum GPI synthesis, and how their substrate specificities differ from humans, will help to determine whether anti-GPI pharmacological therapy can indeed become a reality.

6
Prospects for Anti-GPI Vaccination

If the primary goal of active malaria vaccination is to protect malaria-exposed children from severe disease, then inhibiting toxin-induced pathophysiological responses is a potentially useful strategy. Immunisation of mice with deacylated synthetic *P. falciparum* GPI glycan conjugated to keyhole limpet haemocyanin reduced the early mortality of *P. berghei* (ANKA) challenge from 100% to 25% (Schofield et al. 2002). The glycan GPI analogue induced IgG antibodies in immunised mice that bound to intact intra-erythrocytic tropho- zoites and schizonts but did not cross-react with uninfected erythrocytes (which express endogenous GPIs on their surface). Serum from immunised mice completely neutralised production of TNF-α by mouse macrophages in response to stimulation by crude *P. falciparum* schizont extracts, suggesting that GPI alone is both sufficient and necessary for the induction of this in- flammatory response. However, the early protection noted was independent of any reduction in parasitaemia, and immunised rodents eventually suc- cumbed to haemolytic anaemia accompanied by massive parasitaemia. Other investigators have thus urged caution with GPI vaccination studies, especially given that *P. falciparum* GPIs are implicated in cell-mediated host-defence responses in addition to pathogenesis (Clark et al. 2004).

Vaccination specifically targeted at GPIs in humans raises concerns that vaccinated individuals with malaria would feel less sick and thus present to hospital later and with extremely high levels of parasitaemia, with the atten- dant risks of severe anaemia and organ failure. Inhibition of GPI-mediated early pro-inflammatory cytokine responses that limit parasite replication may also favour rapid rises in parasitaemia in vaccinated individuals (Kwiatkowski 1995). These concerns may be offset if anti-toxic vaccine antigen(s) were to be combined with epitopes primarily directed at generating an anti-parasitic response that limited exponential expansion in parasitaemia. However, this would require at least partial anti-parasitic efficacy in 100% of subjects receiv- ing a combination vaccine—a target that would be very difficult to achieve. Moreover, the anti-parasitic immune responses induced by such a vaccine combination would need to be of longer duration than that of the anti-GPI immune response— again a difficult target. Active vaccination against GPI antigens may also theoretically interfere with any protective effect of NO against malarial disease severity (Anstey et al. 1996; Hobbs et al. 2002), given that *P. falciparum* GPIs have been shown to induce NO production in vitro (Tachado et al. 1996). Passive immunisation of individuals with severe malaria by administration of monoclonal or polyclonal anti-GPI antibodies is an alternative adjunctive therapeutic strategy that may avoid interfering with early immune responses, and be transient enough to avoid long-term problems. In support of this approach, polyclonal antibody preparations that recognise bacterial super-antigens have been reported to improve clinical outcomes in streptococcal toxic shock syndrome (Kaul et al. 1999), which shares several features of the Th1 cytokine-dominated inflammatory response to severe malaria (Norrby-Teglund et al. 1997).

Field studies highlight the challenges involved in generating a sustained anti-GPI antibody response in children less than 5 years of age, which is the highest priority for vaccination in malaria-endemic areas. Understanding whether the events involved in GPI antigen presentation and processing (Sect. 4.3) can be modified by adjuvants (including other malarial antigens) or immuno-modulators may help to improve vaccine immunogenicity in this age group. Finally, given the conservation in the core structure of GPIs across eukaryotes, it would be important for anti-GPI vaccination to avoid inducing auto-immune responses. The finding that spleen cells primed with parasite-derived or mammalian Thy-1 derived GPI later responded to both homologous and heterologous antigenic challenge (Schofield et al. 1999) highlights these concerns.

7
Conclusion

At present, although data from model systems are encouraging, there is very little firm evidence to suggest that antibody-mediated immune responses to *P. falciparum* GPIs play a significant role in either mediating tolerance or reducing disease severity in human malaria. Concerns over the purity of GPI preparations derived from *P. falciparum,* in relation to the specific induction of both pathological and immune responses, can be effectively dispelled if results can be repeated using fully synthetic preparations. It is exciting to think that the availability of synthetic GPIs may enable detailed and direct examination of the human fever responses in much the same way as human volunteers have contributed to our understanding of the modes of action of bacterial lipopolysaccharides (van der Poll and van Deventer 1999). A theoretical, but real, concern that must be addressed prior to such human studies involves determining the likelihood of cross-reactive, and potentially autoimmune, antibody responses. Should the pathological significance of GPIs be confirmed by further studies of pathophysiology and/or natural immunity, then strategies to address the potential for unchecked parasite replication in the face of vaccination must be considered. Such concerns are less relevant for the development of selective pharmacological inhibitors of *P. falciparum* GPI biosynthesis; although confirmation that GPIs are essential to ongoing parasite replication is a pre-requisite if this approach is to be successful.

References

Aidoo M, McElroy PD, Kolczak MS, Terlouw DJ, ter Kuile FO, Nahlen B, Lal AA, Udhayakumar V (2001) Tumor necrosis factor-alpha promoter variant 2 (TNF2) is associated with pre-term delivery, infant mortality, and malaria morbidity in western Kenya: Asembo Bay Cohort Project IX. Genet Epidemiol 21:201–211

Akira S, Hemmi H (2003) Recognition of pathogen-associated molecular patterns by TLR family. Immunol Lett 85:85–95

Al Yaman F, Genton B, Anders RF, Falk M, Triglia T, Lewis D, Hii J, Beck HP, Alpers MP (1994) Relationship between humoral response to Plasmodium falciparum merozoite surface antigen-2 and malaria morbidity in a highly endemic area of Papua New Guinea. Am J Trop Med Hyg 51:593–602

Al Yaman F, Genton B, Falk M, Anders RF, Lewis D, Hii J, Beck HP, Alpers MP (1995a) Humoral response to Plasmodium falciparum ring-infected erythrocyte surface antigen in a highly endemic area of Papua New Guinea. Am J Trop Med Hyg 52:66–71

Al Yaman F, Genton B, Kramer KJ, Taraika J, Chang SP, Hui GS, Alpers MP (1995b) Acquired antibody levels to Plasmodium falciparum merozoite surface antigen 1 in residents of a highly endemic area of Papua New Guinea. Trans R Soc Trop Med Hyg 89:555–559

Anstey NM, Weinberg JB, Hassanali MY, Mwaikambo ED, Manyenga D, Misukonis MA, Arnelle DR, Hollis D, McDonald MI, Granger DL (1996) Nitric oxide in Tanzanian children with malaria: inverse relationship between malaria severity and nitric oxide production/nitric oxide synthase type 2 expression. J Exp Med 184:557–567

Anstey N, Weinberg J, Granger D (1999a) Nitric oxide and malaria. In: Fang FC (ed) Nitric oxide and infection. Plenum Publishing Corp., New York, pp 311–341

Anstey NM, Weinberg JB, Wang Z, Mwaikambo ED, Duffy PE, Granger DL (1999b) Effects of age and parasitemia on nitric oxide production/leukocyte nitric oxide synthase type 2 expression in asymptomatic, malaria-exposed children. Am J Trop Med Hyg 61:253–258

Arese P, Schwarzer E (1997) Malarial Pigment (Haemozoin) - a Very Active Inert Substance. Annals of Tropical Medicine & Parasitology 91:501–516

Artavanis-Tsakonas K, Tongren JE, Riley EM (2003) The war between the malaria parasite and the immune system: immunity, immunoregulation and immunopathology. Clin Exp Immunol 133:145–152

Baird JK (1998) Age-dependent characteristics of protection v. susceptibility to Plasmodium falciparum. Ann Trop Med Parasitol 92:367–390

Baird JK, Masbar S, Basri H, Tirtokusumo S, Subianto B, Hoffman SL (1998) Age-dependent susceptibility to severe disease with primary exposure to Plasmodium falciparum. J Infect Dis 178:592–595

Basilico N, Tognazioli C, Picot S, Ravagnani F, Taramelli D (2003) Synergistic and antagonistic interactions between haemozoin and bacterial endotoxin on human and mouse macrophages. Parassitologia 45:135–140

Bate CA, Kwiatkowski D (1994a) A monoclonal antibody that recognizes phosphatidylinositol inhibits induction of tumor necrosis factor alpha by different strains of Plasmodium falciparum. Infect Immun 62:5261–5266

Bate CA, Kwiatkowski D (1994b) Inhibitory immunoglobulin M antibodies to tumor necrosis factor-inducing toxins in patients with malaria. Infect Immun 62:3086–3091

Bate CA, Taverne J, Playfair JH (1988) Malarial parasites induce TNF production by macrophages. Immunology 64:227–231

Bate CA, Taverne J, Dave A, Playfair JH (1990) Malaria exoantigens induce T-independent antibody that blocks their ability to induce TNF. Immunology 70:315–320

Bate CA, Taverne J, Bootsma HJ, Mason RC, Skalko N, Gregoriadis G, Playfair JH (1992a) Antibodies against phosphatidylinositol and inositol monophosphate specifically inhibit tumour necrosis factor induction by malaria exoantigens. Immunology 76:35–41

Bate CA, Taverne J, Roman E, Moreno C, Playfair JH (1992b) Tumour necrosis factor induction by malaria exoantigens depends upon phospholipid. Immunology 75:129–135

Baumgarth N (2000) A two-phase model of B-cell activation. Immunol Rev 176:171–180

Bayley JP, Ottenhoff TH, Verweij CL (2004) Is there a future for TNF promoter polymorphisms? Genes Immun 5:315–329

Bento CA, Melo MB, Previato JO, Mendonca-Previato L, Pecanha LM (1996) Glycoinositolphospholipids purified from Trypanosoma cruzi stimulate Ig production in vitro. J Immunol 157:4996–5001

Berhe S, Schofield L, Schwarz RT, Gerold P (1999) Conservation of structure among glycosylphosphatidylinositol toxins from different geographic isolates of Plasmodium falciparum. Mol Biochem Parasitol 103:273–278

Beutler E, Gelbart T, West C (2001) Synergy between TLR2 and TLR4: a safety mechanism. Blood Cells Mol Dis 27:728–730

Biswas S, Karmarkar MG, Sharma YD (2001) Antibodies detected against Plasmodium falciparum haemozoin with inhibitory properties to cytokine production. FEMS Microbiol Lett 194:175–179

Boisier P, Jambou R, Raharimalala L, Roux J (2002) Relationship between parasite density and fever risk in a community exposed to a low level of malaria transmission in Madagascar highlands. Am J Trop Med Hyg 67:137–140

Boutlis CS, Gowda DC, Naik RS, Maguire GP, Mgone CS, Bockarie MJ, Lagog M, Ibam E, Lorry K, Anstey NM (2002) Antibodies to Plasmodium falciparum glycosylphosphatidylinositols: inverse association with tolerance of parasitemia in Papua New Guinean children and adults. Infect Immun 70:5052–5057

Boutlis CS, Fagan PK, Gowda DC, Lagog M, Mgone CS, Bockarie MJ, Anstey NM (2003a) Immunoglobulin G responses to Plasmodium falciparum glycosylphosphatidylinositols are short-lived and predominantly of the IgG3 subclass. J Infect Dis 187:862–865

Boutlis CS, Tjitra E, Maniboey H, Misukonis MA, Saunders JR, Suprianto S, Weinberg JB, Anstey NM (2003b) Nitric oxide production and mononuclear cell nitric oxide synthase activity in malaria-tolerant Papuan adults. Infect Immun 71:3682–3689

Boutlis CS, Weinberg JB, Baker J, Bockarie MJ, Mgone CS, Cheng Q, Anstey NM (2004) Nitric oxide production and nitric oxide synthase activity in malaria-exposed Papua New Guinean children and adults show longitudinal stability and no association with parasitemia. Infect Immun 72:6932–6938

Bruce MC, Donnelly CA, Alpers MP, Galinski MR, Barnwell JW, Walliker D, Day KP (2000) Cross-species interactions between malaria parasites in humans. Science 287:845–848

Bruna-Romero O, Rocha CD, Tsuji M, Gazzinelli RT (2004) Enhanced protective immunity against malaria by vaccination with a recombinant adenovirus encoding the circumsporozoite protein of Plasmodium lacking the GPI-anchoring motif. Vaccine 22:3575–3584

Calissano C, Modiano D, Sirima BS, Konate A, Sanou I, Sawadogo A, Perlmann H, Troye-Blomberg M, Perlmann P (2003) IgE antibodies to Plasmodium falciparum and severity of malaria in children of one ethnic group living in Burkina Faso. Am J Trop Med Hyg 69:31–35

Campos MA, Almeida IC, Takeuchi O, Akira S, Valente EP, Procopio DO, Travassos LR, Smith JA, Golenbock DT, Gazzinelli RT (2001) Activation of Toll-like receptor-2 by glycosylphosphatidylinositol anchors from a protozoan parasite. J Immunol 167:416–423

Chatterjee S, Mayor S (2001) The GPI-anchor and protein sorting. Cell Mol Life Sci 58:1969–1987

Chen R, Walter EI, Parker G, Lapurga JP, Millan JL, Ikehara Y, Udenfriend S, Medof ME (1998) Mammalian glycophosphatidylinositol anchor transfer to proteins and posttransfer deacylation. Proc Natl Acad Sci U S A 95:9512–9517

Clark IA (1978) Does endotoxin cause both the disease and parasite death in acute malaria and babesiosis? Lancet 2:75–77

Clark IA, Cowden WB (2003) The pathophysiology of falciparum malaria. Pharmacol Ther 99:221–260

Clark IA, Virelizier JL, Carswell EA, Wood PR (1981) Possible importance of macrophage-derived mediators in acute malaria. Infect Immun 32:1058–1066

Clark IA, Cowden WB, Butcher GA, Hunt NH (1987) Possible roles of tumor necrosis factor in the pathology of malaria. Am J Pathol 129:192–199

Clark IA, Gray KM, Rockett EJ, Cowden WB, Rockett KA, Ferrante A, Aggarwal BB (1992) Increased lymphotoxin in human malarial serum, and the ability of this cytokine to increase plasma interleukin-6 and cause hypoglycaemia in mice: implications for malarial pathology. Trans R Soc Trop Med Hyg 86:602–607

Clark IA, al Yaman FM, Cowden WB, Rockett KA (1996) Does malarial tolerance, through nitric oxide, explain the low incidence of autoimmune disease in tropical Africa? Lancet 348:1492–1494

Clark IA, al Yaman FM, Jacobson LS (1997) The biological basis of malarial disease. Int J Parasitol 27:1237–1249

Clark IA, Awburn MM, Harper CG, Liomba NG, Molyneux ME (2003a) Induction of HO-1 in tissue macrophages and monocytes in fatal falciparum malaria and sepsis. Malar J 2:41-

Clark IA, Awburn MM, Whitten RO, Harper CG, Liomba NG, Molyneux ME, Taylor TE (2003b) Tissue distribution of migration inhibitory factor and inducible nitric oxide synthase in falciparum malaria and sepsis in African children. Malar J 2:6-

Clark IA, Alleva LM, Mills AC, Cowden WB (2004) Pathogenesis of malaria and clinically similar conditions. Clin Microbiol Rev 17:509–539

Coban C, Ishii KJ, Kawai T, Hemmi H, Sato S, Uematsu S, Yamamoto M, Takeuchi O, Itagaki S, Kumar N, Horii T, Akira S (2005) Toll-like receptor 9 mediates innate immune activation by the malaria pigment hemozoin. J Exp Med 201:19–25

de Macedo CS, Shams-Eldin H, Smith TK, Schwarz RT, Azzouz N (2003) Inhibitors of glycosyl-phosphatidylinositol anchor biosynthesis. Biochimie 85:465–472

de Souza JB, Todd J, Krishegowda G, Gowda DC, Kwiatkowski D, Riley EM (2002) Prevalence and boosting of antibodies to Plasmodium falciparum glycosylphosphatidylinositols and evaluation of their association with protection from mild and severe clinical malaria. Infect Immun 70:5045–5051

Delorenzi M, Sexton A, Shams-Eldin H, Schwarz RT, Speed T, Schofield L (2002) Genes for glycosylphosphatidylinositol toxin biosynthesis in Plasmodium falciparum. Infect Immun 70:4510–4522

Dobrovolskaia MA, Vogel SN (2002) Toll receptors, CD14, and macrophage activation and deactivation by LPS. Microbes Infect 4:903–914

Dodoo D, Omer FM, Todd J, Akanmori BD, Koram KA, Riley EM (2002) Absolute Levels and Ratios of Proinflammatory and Anti-inflammatory Cytokine Production In Vitro Predict Clinical Immunity to Plasmodium falciparum Malaria. J Infect Dis 185:971–979

Duthie MS, Wleklinski-Lee M, Smith S, Nakayama T, Taniguchi M, Kahn SJ (2002) During Trypanosoma cruzi infection CD1d-restricted NK T cells limit parasitemia and augment the antibody response to a glycophosphoinositol- modified surface protein. Infect Immun 70:36–48

Eisenhaber B, Maurer-Stroh S, Novatchkova M, Schneider G, Eisenhaber F (2003) Enzymes and auxiliary factors for GPI lipid anchor biosynthesis and post-translational transfer to proteins. Bioessays 25:367–385

Elased KM, Gumaa KA, de Souza JB, Playfair JH, Rademacher TW (2004) Improvement of glucose homeostasis in obese diabetic db/db mice given Plasmodium yoelii glycosylphosphatidylinositols. Metabolism 53:1048–1053

English M, Waruiru C, Amukoye E, Murphy S, Crawley J, Mwangi I, Peshu N, Marsh K (1996) Deep breathing in children with severe malaria: indicator of metabolic acidosis and poor outcome. Am J Trop Med Hyg 55:521–524

Engwerda CR, Mynott TL, Sawhney S, de Souza JB, Bickle QD, Kaye PM (2002) Locally up-regulated lymphotoxin alpha, not systemic tumor necrosis factor alpha, is the principle mediator of murine cerebral malaria. J Exp Med 195:1371–1377

Fahmi H, Charon D, Mondange M, Chaby R (1995) Endotoxin-induced desensitization of mouse macrophages is mediated in part by nitric oxide production. Infect Immun 63:1863–1869

Fanning SL, Czesny B, Sedegah M, Carucci DJ, van Gemert GJ, Eling W, Williamson KC (2003) A glycosylphosphatidylinositol anchor signal sequence enhances the immunogenicity of a DNA vaccine encoding Plasmodium falciparum sexual-stage antigen, Pfs230. Vaccine 21:3228–3235

Farnert A, Snounou G, Rooth I, Bjorkman A (1997) Daily dynamics of Plasmodium falciparum subpopulations in asymptomatic children in a holoendemic area. Am J Trop Med Hyg 56:538–47

Ferguson MA (1999) The structure, biosynthesis and functions of glycosylphos-phatidylinositol anchors, and the contributions of trypanosome research. J Cell Sci 112 (Pt 17):2799–2809

Ferguson MA (2000) Glycosylphosphatidylinositol biosynthesis validated as a drug target for African sleeping sickness. Proc Natl Acad Sci U S A 97:10673–10675

Ferlito M, Squadrito F, Halushka PV, Cook JA (2001) Signal transduction events in Chinese hamster ovary cells expressing human CD14; effect of endotoxin desensitization. Shock 15:291–296

Ferrante A, Beard LJ, Feldman RG (1990) IgG subclass distribution of antibodies to bacterial and viral antigens. Pediatr Infect Dis J 9:S16-S24

Fujieda S, Sieling PA, Modlin RL, Saxon A (1998) CD1-restricted T-cells influence IgG subclass and IgE production. J Allergy Clin Immunol 101:545–551

Gatton ML, Cheng Q (2002) Evaluation of the pyrogenic threshold for Plasmodium falciparum malaria in naive individuals. Am J Trop Med Hyg 66:467–473

Gerold P, Dieckmann-Schuppert A, Schwarz RT (1994) Glycosylphosphatidylinositols synthesized by asexual erythrocytic stages of the malarial parasite, Plasmodium falciparum. Candidates for plasmodial glycosylphosphatidylinositol membrane anchor precursors and pathogenicity factors. J Biol Chem 269:2597–2606

Gerold P, Vivas L, Ogun SA, Azzouz N, Brown KN, Holder AA, Schwarz RT (1997) Glycosylphosphatidylinositols of Plasmodium chabaudi chabaudi: a basis for the study of malarial glycolipid toxins in a rodent model. Biochem J 328 (Pt 3):905–911

Golgi C (1886) Sull'infezione malarica. Archivio Per Le Scienze Mediche 10:109–135

Gowda DC (2002) Structure and activity of glycosylphosphatidylinositol anchors of Plasmodium falciparum. Microbes Infect 4:983–990

Grau GE, Taylor TE, Molyneux ME, Wirima JJ, Vassalli P, Hommel M, Lambert PH (1989) Tumor necrosis factor and disease severity in children with falciparum malaria. N Engl J Med 320:1586–1591

Grimme SJ, Westfall BA, Wiedman JM, Taron CH, Orlean P (2001) The essential Smp3 protein is required for addition of the side-branching fourth mannose during assembly of yeast glycosylphosphatidylinositols. J Biol Chem 276:27731–27739

Gumperz JE, Roy C, Makowska A, Lum D, Sugita M, Podrebarac T, Koezuka Y, Porcelli SA, Cardell S, Brenner MB, Behar SM (2000) Murine CD1d-restricted T cell recognition of cellular lipids. Immunity 12:211–221

Hansen DS, Siomos MA, Buckingham L, Scalzo AA, Schofield L (2003a) Regulation of murine cerebral malaria pathogenesis by CD1d-restricted NKT cells and the natural killer complex. Immunity 18:391–402

Hansen DS, Siomos MA, Koning-Ward T, Buckingham L, Crabb BS, Schofield L (2003b) CD1d-restricted NKT cells contribute to malarial splenomegaly and enhance parasite-specific antibody responses. Eur J Immunol 33:2588–2598

Heyman A, Beeson PB (1949) Influence of various disease states upon the febrile response to intravenous injection of typhoid bacterial pyrogen: with particular reference to malaria and cirrhosis of the liver. J Lab Clin Med 34:1400–1403

Hisaeda H, Maekawa Y, Iwakawa D, Okada H, Himeno K, Kishihara K, Tsukumo S, Yasutomo K (2004) Escape of malaria parasites from host immunity requires CD4+ CD25+ regulatory T cells. Nat Med 10:29–30

Hobbs MR, Udhayakumar V, Levesque MC, Booth J, Roberts JM, Tkachuk AN, Pole A, Coon H, Kariuki S, Nahlen BL, Mwaikambo ED, Lal AL, Granger DL, Anstey NM, Weinberg JB (2002) A new NOS2 promoter polymorphism associated with increased nitric oxide production and protection from severe malaria in Tanzanian and Kenyan children. Lancet 360:1468–1475

Hoessli DC, Poincelet M, Gupta R, Ilangumaran S, Nasir uD (2003) Plasmodium falciparum merozoite surface protein 1. Eur J Biochem 270:366–375

Hudson Keenihan SN, Ratiwayanto S, Soebianto S, Krisin, Marwoto H, Krishnegowda G, Gowda DC, Bangs MJ, Fryauff DJ, Richie TL, Kumar S, Baird JK (2003) Age-dependent impairment of IgG responses to glycosylphosphatidylinositol with equal exposure to Plasmodium falciparum among Javanese migrants to Papua, Indonesia. Am J Trop Med Hyg 69:36–41

Hunt NH, Grau GE (2003) Cytokines: accelerators and brakes in the pathogenesis of cerebral malaria. Trends Immunol 24:491–499

Iuvone T, D'Acquisto F, Carnuccio R, Di Rosa M (1996) Nitric oxide inhibits LPS-induced tumor necrosis factor synthesis in vitro and in vivo. Life Sci 59:L207-L211

Jaramillo M, Gowda DC, Radzioch D, Olivier M (2003) Hemozoin increases IFN-gamma-inducible macrophage nitric oxide generation through extracellular signal-regulated kinase- and NF-kappa B-dependent pathways. J Immunol 171:4243–4253

Jaramillo M, Plante I, Ouellet N, Vandal K, Tessier PA, Olivier M (2004) Hemozoin-inducible proinflammatory events in vivo: potential role in malaria infection. J Immunol 172:3101–3110

Jaramillo M, Godbout M, Olivier M (2005) Hemozoin induces macrophage chemokine expression through oxidative stress-dependent and -independent mechanisms. J Immunol 174:475–484

Johnson A, Leke R, Harun L, Ginsberg C, Ngogang J, Stowers A, Saul A, Quakyi IA (2000) Interaction of HLA and age on levels of antibody to Plasmodium falciparum rhoptry-associated proteins 1 and 2. Infect Immun 68:2231–2236

Joyce S, Woods AS, Yewdell JW, Bennink JR, De S, Boesteanu A, Balk SP, Cotter RJ, Brutkiewicz RR (1998) Natural ligand of mouse CD1d1: cellular glycosylphos-phatidylinositol. Science 279:1541–1544

Kastenbauer S, Ziegler-Heitbrock HW (1999) NF-kappaB1 (p50) is upregulated in lipopolysaccharide tolerance and can block tumor necrosis factor gene expression. Infect Immun 67:1553–1559

Kaul R, McGeer A, Norrby-Teglund A, Kotb M, Schwartz B, O'Rourke K, Talbot J, Low DE (1999) Intravenous immunoglobulin therapy for streptococcal toxic shock syndrome–a comparative observational study. The Canadian Streptococcal Study Group. Clin Infect Dis 28:800–807

Keller CC, Kremsner PG, Hittner JB, Misukonis MA, Weinberg JB, Perkins DJ (2004) Elevated nitric oxide production in children with malarial anemia: hemozoin-induced nitric oxide synthase type 2 transcripts and nitric oxide in blood mononuclear cells. Infect Immun 72:4868–4873

Kern P, Hemmer CJ, Van Damme J, Gruss HJ, Dietrich M (1989) Elevated tumor necrosis factor alpha and interleukin-6 serum levels as markers for complicated Plasmodium falciparum malaria. Am J Med 87:139–143

Kimmel J, Ogun SA, de Macedo CS, Gerold P, Vivas L, Holder AA, Schwarz RT, Azzouz N (2003) Glycosylphosphatidyl-inositols in murine malaria: Plasmodium yoelii yoelii. Biochimie 85:473–481

Kinoshita T, Inoue N (2000) Dissecting and manipulating the pathway for glycosylphosphatidylinositol-anchor biosynthesis. Curr Opin Chem Biol 4:632–638

Krishnegowda G, Hajjar AM, Zhu J, Douglass EJ, Uematsu S, Akira S, Woods AS, Gowda DC (2004) Induction of proinflammatory responses in macrophages by the glycosylphosphatidylinositols (GPIs) of Plasmodium falciparum: Cell signaling receptors, GPI structural requirement, and regulation of GPI activity. J Biol Chem Dec 28: Epub ahead of print

Kronenberg M, Naidenko O, Koning F (2001) Right on target: novel approaches for the direct visualization of CD1-specific T cell responses. Proc Natl Acad Sci U S A 98:2950–2952

Kwiatkowski D (1995) Malarial toxins and the regulation of parasite density. Parasitology Today 11:206–212

Kwiatkowski D, Cannon JG, Manogue KR, Cerami A, Dinarello CA, Greenwood BM (1989) Tumour necrosis factor production in Falciparum malaria and its association with schizont rupture. Clin Exp Immunol 77:361–366

Kwiatkowski D, Molyneux ME, Stephens S, Curtis N, Klein N, Pointaire P, Smit M, Allan R, Brewster DR, Grau GE (1993) Anti-TNF therapy inhibits fever in cerebral malaria. Q J Med 86:91–98

Latz E, Visintin A, Lien E, Fitzgerald K, Monks BG, Kurt-Jones E, Golenbock DT, Espevik T (2002) LPS rapidly traffics to and from the Golgi apparatus with the TLR4/MD-2/CD14 complex in a process that is distinct from the initiation of signal transduction. J Biol Chem 277:47834–47843

Le Hesran JY, Akiana J, Ndiaye eH, Dia M, Senghor P, Konate L (2004) Severe malaria attack is associated with high prevalence of Ascaris lumbricoides infection among children in rural Senegal. Trans R Soc Trop Med Hyg 98:397–399

Le Hesran JY (2005) Reply to comment on: Severe malaria attack is associated with high prevalence of Ascaris lumbricoides infection among children in rural Senegal. Trans R Soc Trop Med Hyg 99:164–165

Lehner MD, Morath S, Michelsen KS, Schumann RR, Hartung T (2001) Induction of cross-tolerance by lipopolysaccharide and highly purified lipoteichoic acid via different Toll-like receptors independent of paracrine mediators. J Immunol 166:5161–5167

Li C, Sanni LA, Omer F, Riley E, Langhorne J (2003) Pathology of Plasmodium chabaudi chabaudi infection and mortality in interleukin-10-deficient mice are ameliorated by anti-tumor necrosis factor alpha and exacerbated by anti-transforming growth factor beta antibodies. Infect Immun 71:4850–4856

Liu X, Seeberger PH (2004) A Suzuki-Miyaura coupling mediated deprotection as key to the synthesis of a fully lipidated malarial GPI disaccharide. Chem Commun (Camb) 1708–1709

Looareesuwan S, Sjostrom L, Krudsood S, Wilairatana P, Porter RS, Hills F, Warrell DA (1999) Polyclonal anti-tumor necrosis factor-alpha Fab used as an ancillary treatment for severe malaria. Am J Trop Med Hyg 61:26–33

Lu J, Jayaprakash KN, Schlueter U, Fraser-Reid B (2004) Synthesis of a malaria candidate glycosylphosphatidylinositol (GPI) structure: a strategy for fully inositol acylated and phosphorylated GPIs. J Am Chem Soc 126:7540–7547

Maeno Y, Perlmann P, PerlmannH, Kusuhara Y, Taniguchi K, Nakabayashi T, Win K, Looareesuwan S, Aikawa M (2000) IgE deposition in brain microvessels and on parasitized erythrocytes from cerebral malaria patients. Am J Trop Med Hyg 63:128–132

Maitland K, Marsh K (2004) Pathophysiology of severe malaria in children. Acta Trop 90:131–140

Marsh K, Snow RW (1997) Host-parasite interaction and morbidity in malaria endemic areas. Philos Trans R Soc Lond B Biol Sci 352:1385–94

Martinez AP, Margos G, Barker G, Sinden RE (2000) The roles of the glycosylphosphatidylinositol anchor on the production and immunogenicity of recombinant ookinete surface antigen Pbs21 of Plasmodium berghei when prepared in a baculovirus expression system. Parasite Immunol 22:493–500

McGregor IA, Gilles HM, Walters JH, Davies AH, Pearson FA (1956) Effects of heavy and repeated malarial infections on Gambian infants and children: effects of erythrocytic parasitization. Br Med J 4994:686–692

McGuire W, Hill AV, Allsopp CE, Greenwood BM, Kwiatkowski D (1994) Variation in the TNF-alpha promoter region associated with susceptibility to cerebral malaria. Nature 371:508–510

Menendez C, Fleming AF, Alonso PL (2000) Malaria-related anaemia. Parasitol Today 16:469–476

Miller MJ (1958) Observations of the natural history of malaria in the semi-resistant west African. Trans R Soc Trop Med Hyg 52:152–168

Missinou MA, Lell B, Kremsner PG (2003) Uncommon asymptomatic Plasmodium falciparum infections in Gabonese children. Clin Infect Dis 36:1198–1202

Molano A, Park SH, Chiu YH, Nosseir S, Bendelac A, Tsuji M (2000) Cutting edge: the IgG response to the circumsporozoite protein is MHC class II-dependent and CD1d-independent: exploring the role of GPIs in NK T cell activation and antimalarial responses. J Immunol 164:5005–5009

Molineaux L, Trauble M, Collins WE, Jeffery GM, Dietz K (2002) Malaria therapy reinoculation data suggest individual variation of an innate immune response and independent acquisition of antiparasitic and antitoxic immunities. Trans R Soc Trop Med Hyg 96:205–209

Moran P, Caras IW (1994) Requirements for glycosylphosphatidylinositol attachment are similar but not identical in mammalian cells and parasitic protozoa. J Cell Biol 125:333–343

Mordmuller B, Turrini F, Long H, Kremsner PG, Arese P (1998) Neutrophils and monocytes from subjects with the Mediterranean G6PD variant: effect of Plasmodium
falciparum hemozoin on G6PD activity, oxidative burst and cytokine production.
Eur Cytokine Netw 9:239–245

Muniz-Junqueira MI, dos Santos-Neto LL, Tosta CE (2001) Influence of tumor necrosis
factor-alpha on the ability of monocytes and lymphocytes to destroy intraerythrocytic Plasmodium falciparum in vitro. Cell Immunol 208:73–79

Nacher M (2002) Worms and malaria: noisy nuisances and silent benefits. Parasite
Immunol 24:391–393

Nacher M (2005) Comment on: Severe malaria attack is associated with high prevalence
of Ascaris lumbricoides infection among children in rural Senegal. Trans R Soc
Trop Med Hyg 99:161–163

Naik RS, Branch OH, Woods AS, Vijaykumar M, Perkins DJ, Nahlen BL, Lal AA, Cotter
RJ, Costello CE, Ockenhouse CF, Davidson EA, Gowda DC (2000a) Glycosylphosphatidylinositol anchors of Plasmodium falciparum: molecular characterization
and naturally elicited antibody response that may provide immunity to malaria
pathogenesis. J Exp Med 192:1563–1576

Naik RS, Davidson EA, Gowda DC (2000b) Developmental stage-specific biosynthesis
of glycosylphosphatidylinositol anchors in intraerythrocytic Plasmodium falciparum and its inhibition in a novel manner by mannosamine. J Biol Chem
275:24506–24511

Naik RS, Krishnegowda G, Gowda CD (2003) Glucosamine inhibits inositol acylation
of the glycosylphosphatidylinositol anchors in intraerythrocytic plasmodium
falciparum. J Biol Chem 278:2036–2042

Njama-Meya D, Kamya MR, Dorsey G (2004) Asymptomatic parasitaemia as a risk
factor for symptomatic malaria in a cohort of Ugandan children. Trop Med Int
Health 9:862–868

Norrby-Teglund A, Lustig R, Kotb M (1997) Differential induction of Th1 versus Th2
cytokines by group A streptococcal toxic shock syndrome isolates. Infect Immun
65:5209–5215

Ockenhouse CF, Tegoshi T, Maeno Y, Benjamin C, Ho M, Kan KE, Thway Y, Win K,
Aikawa M, Lobb RR (1992) Human vascular endothelial cell adhesion receptors
for Plasmodium falciparum-infected erythrocytes: roles for endothelial leukocyte
adhesion molecule 1 and vascular cell adhesion molecule 1. J Exp Med 176:1183–
1189

Oliveira AC, Peixoto JR, de Arruda LB, Campos MA, Gazzinelli RT, Golenbock DT,
Akira S, Previato JO, Mendonca-Previato L, Nobrega A, Bellio M (2004) Expression
of functional TLR4 confers proinflammatory responsiveness to Trypanosoma
cruzi glycoinositolphospholipids and higher resistance to infection with T. cruzi.
J Immunol 173:5688–5696

Omer FM, Riley EM (1998) Transforming growth factor beta production is inversely
correlated with severity of murine malaria infection. J Exp Med 188:39–48

Omer FM, Kurtzhals JA, Riley EM (2000) Maintaining the immunological balance in
parasitic infections: a role for TGF-beta? Parasitol Today 16:18–23

Omer FM, de Souza JB, Riley EM (2003) Differential induction of TGF-beta regulates
proinflammatory cytokine production and determines the outcome of lethal and
nonlethal Plasmodium yoelii infections. J Immunol 171:5430–5436

Perkins DJ, Kremsner PG, Weinberg JB (2001) Inverse relationship of plasma prostaglandin E2 and blood mononuclear cell cyclooxygenase-2 with disease severity in children with Plasmodium falciparum malaria. J Infect Dis 183:113–118

Perkins DJ, Moore JM, Otieno J, Shi YP, Nahlen BL, Udhayakumar V, Lal AA (2003) In vivo acquisition of hemozoin by placental blood mononuclear cells suppresses PGE2, TNF-alpha, and IL-10. Biochem Biophys Res Commun 311:839–846

Perlmann P, Perlmann H, Flyg BW, Hagstedt M, Elghazali G, Worku S, Fernandez V, Rutta AS, Troye-Blomberg M (1997) Immunoglobulin E, a pathogenic factor in Plasmodium falciparum malaria. Infect Immun 65:116–121

Pichyangkul S, Saengkrai P, Webster HK (1994) Plasmodium falciparum pigment induces monocytes to release high levels of tumor necrosis factor-alpha and interleukin-1 beta. Am J Trop Med Hyg 51:430–435

Pichyangkul S, Yongvanitchit K, Kum-arb U, Hemmi H, Akira S, Krieg AM, Heppner DG, Stewart VA, Hasegawa H, Looareesuwan S, Shanks GD, Miller RS (2004) Malaria blood stage parasites activate human plasmacytoid dendritic cells and murine dendritic cells through a Toll-like receptor 9-dependent pathway. J Immunol 172:4926–4933

Playfair JH, Taverne J, Bate CA, de Souza JB (1990) The malaria vaccine: anti-parasite or anti-disease? Immunol Today 11:25–27

Playfair JH, Taverne J, Bate CA (1991) Don't kill the parasite: control the disease. Acta Leiden 60:157–165

Porcelli SA, Modlin RL (1999) The CD1 system: antigen-presenting molecules for T cell recognition of lipids and glycolipids. Annu Rev Immunol 17:297–329

Prada J, Malinowski J, Muller S, Bienzle U, Kremsner PG (1995) Hemozoin differentially modulates the production of interleukin 6 and tumor necrosis factor in murine malaria. Eur Cytokine Netw 6:109–112

Procopio DO, Almeida IC, Torrecilhas AC, Cardoso JE, Teyton L, Travassos LR, Bendelac A, Gazzinelli RT (2002) Glycosylphosphatidylinositol-anchored mucin-like glycoproteins from Trypanosoma cruzi bind to CD1d but do not elicit dominant innate or adaptive immune responses via the CD1d/NKT cell pathway. J Immunol 169:3926–3933

Prybylski D, Khaliq A, Fox E, Sarwari AR, Strickland GT (1999) Parasite density and malaria morbidity in the Pakistani Punjab. Am J Trop Med Hyg 61:791–801

Rae C, McQuillan JA, Parekh SB, Bubb WA, Weiser S, Balcar VJ, Hansen AM, Ball HJ, Hunt NH (2004) Brain gene expression, metabolism, and bioenergetics: interrelationships in murine models of cerebral and noncerebral malaria. FASEB J 18:499–510

Riley EM (1999) Is T-cell priming required for initiation of pathology in malaria infections? Immunol Today 20:228–233

Rogier C, Commenges D, Trape JF (1996) Evidence for an age-dependent pyrogenic threshold of Plasmodium falciparum parasitemia in highly endemic populations. Am J Trop Med Hyg 54:613–619

Romero PJ, Tam JP, Schlesinger D, Clavijo P, Gibson H, Barr PJ, Nussenzweig RS, Nussenzweig V, Zavala F (1988) Multiple T helper cell epitopes of the circumsporozoite protein of Plasmodium berghei. Eur J Immunol 18:1951–1957

Romero JF, Eberl G, MacDonald HR, Corradin G (2001) CD1d-restricted NK T cells are dispensable for specific antibody responses and protective immunity against liver stage malaria infection in mice. Parasite Immunol 23:267–269

Ropert C, Gazzinelli RT (2000) Signaling of immune system cells by glycosylphosphatidylinositol (GPI) anchor and related structures derived from parasitic protozoa. Curr Opin Microbiol 3:395–403

Ropert C, Gazzinelli RT (2004) Regulatory role of Toll-like receptor 2 during infection with Trypanosoma cruzi. J Endotoxin Res 10:425–430

Ropert C, Almeida IC, Closel M, Travassos LR, Ferguson MA, Cohen P, Gazzinelli RT (2001) Requirement of mitogen-activated protein kinases and I kappa B phosphorylation for induction of proinflammatory cytokines synthesis by macrophages indicates functional similarity of receptors triggered by glycosylphosphatidylinositol anchors from parasitic protozoa and bacterial lipopolysaccharide. J Immunol 166:3423–3431

Rowe JA, Scragg IG, Kwiatkowski D, Ferguson DJ, Carucci DJ, Newbold CI (1998) Implications of mycoplasma contamination in Plasmodium falciparum cultures and methods for its detection and eradication. Mol Biochem Parasitol 92:177–180

Rubenstein M, Mulholland J, Jeffery G, Wolff S (1965) Malaria induced endotoxin tolerance. Proc Soc Exp Biol Med 118:283–287

Rzepczyk CM, Hale K, Woodroffe N, Bobogare A, Csurhes P, Ishii A, Ferrante A (1997) Humoral immune responses of Solomon Islanders to the merozoite surface antigen 2 of Plasmodium falciparum show pronounced skewing towards antibodies of the immunoglobulin G3 subclass. Infect Immun 65:1098–1100

Sanchez-Cantu L, Rode HN, Christou NV (1989) Endotoxin tolerance is associated with reduced secretion of tumor necrosis factor. Arch Surg 124:1432–1435

Santos de Macedo C, Gerold P, Jung N, Azzouz N, Kimmel J, Schwarz RT (2001) Inhibition of glycosyl-phosphatidylinositol biosynthesis in Plasmodium falciparum by C-2 substituted mannose analogues. Eur J Biochem 268:6221–6228

Scheiblhofer S, Chen D, Weiss R, Khan F, Mostbock S, Fegeding K, Leitner WW, Thalhamer J, Lyon JA (2001) Removal of the circumsporozoite protein (CSP) glycosylphosphatidylinositol signal sequence from a CSP DNA vaccine enhances induction of CSP-specific Th2 type immune responses and improves protection against malaria infection. Eur J Immunol 31:692–698

Schofield L, Hackett F (1993) Signal transduction in host cells by a glycosylphosphatidylinositol toxin of malaria parasites. J Exp Med 177:145–153

Schofield L, Vivas L, Hackett F, Gerold P, Schwarz RT, Tachado S (1993) Neutralizing monoclonal antibodies to glycosylphosphatidylinositol, the dominant TNF-alpha-inducing toxin of Plasmodium falciparum: prospects for the immunotherapy of severe malaria. Ann Trop Med Parasitol 87:617–626

Schofield L, Novakovic S, Gerold P, Schwarz RT, McConville MJ, Tachado SD (1996) Glycosylphosphatidylinositol toxin of Plasmodium up-regulates intercellular adhesion molecule-1, vascular cell adhesion molecule-1, and E-selectin expression in vascular endothelial cells and increases leukocyte and parasite cytoadherence via tyrosine kinase-dependent signal transduction. J Immunol 156:1886–1896

Schofield L, McConville MJ, Hansen D, Campbell AS, Fraser-Reid B, Grusby MJ, Tachado SD (1999) CD1d-restricted immunoglobulin G formation to GPI-anchored antigens mediated by NKT cells. Science 283:225–229

Schofield L, Hewitt MC, Evans K, Siomos MA, Seeberger PH (2002) Synthetic GPI as a candidate anti-toxic vaccine in a model of malaria. Nature 418:785–789

Schwarzer E, Kuhn H, Valente E, Arese P (2003) Malaria-parasitized erythrocytes and hemozoin nonenzymatically generate large amounts of hydroxy fatty acids that inhibit monocyte functions. Blood 101:722–728

Scragg IG, Hensmann M, Bate CA, Kwiatkowski D (1999) Early cytokine induction by Plasmodium falciparum is not a classical endotoxin-like process. Eur J Immunol 29:2636–2644

Seeberger PH, Soucy RL, Kwon YU, Snyder DA, Kanemitsu T (2004) A convergent, versatile route to two synthetic conjugate anti-toxin malaria vaccines. Chem Commun (Camb) 1706–1707

Serirom S, Raharjo WH, Chotivanich K, Loareesuwan S, Kubes P, Ho M (2003) Anti-adhesive effect of nitric oxide on Plasmodium falciparum cytoadherence under flow. Am J Pathol 162:1651–1660

Shams-Eldin H, Azzouz N, Kedees MH, Orlean P, Kinoshita T, Schwarz RT (2002) The GPI1 homologue from Plasmodium falciparum complements a Saccharomyces cerevisiae GPI1 anchoring mutant. Mol Biochem Parasitol 120:73–81

Sherry BA, Alava G, Tracey KJ, Martiney J, Cerami A, Slater AF (1995) Malaria-specific metabolite hemozoin mediates the release of several potent endogenous pyrogens (TNF, MIP-1 alpha, and MIP-1 beta) in vitro, and altered thermoregulation in vivo. J Inflamm 45:85–96

Sieling PA, Chatterjee D, Porcelli SA, Prigozy TI, Mazzaccaro RJ, Soriano T, Bloom BR, Brenner MB, Kronenberg M, Brennan PJ, . (1995) CD1-restricted T cell recognition of microbial lipoglycan antigens. Science 269:227–230

Singh RP, Kashiwamura S, Rao P, Okamura H, Mukherjee A, Chauhan VS (2002) The role of IL-18 in blood-stage immunity against murine malaria Plasmodium yoelii 265 and Plasmodium berghei ANKA. J Immunol 168:4674–4681

Sinton JA (1938) Immunity or tolerance in malarial infections. Proc R Soc Med 31:1298–1302

Smith T, Genton B, Baea K, Gibson N, Taime J, Narara A, Al Yaman F, Beck HP, Hii J, Alpers M (1994) Relationships between Plasmodium falciparum infection and morbidity in a highly endemic area. Parasitology 109:539–549

Smith T, Felger I, Tanner M, Beck HP (1999) Premunition in Plasmodium falciparum infection: insights from the epidemiology of multiple infections. Trans R Soc Trop Med Hyg 93:S59-S64

Smith TK, Sharma DK, Crossman A, Dix A, Brimacombe JS, Ferguson MA (1997) Parasite and mammalian GPI biosynthetic pathways can be distinguished using synthetic substrate analogues. EMBO J 16:6667–6675

Smith TK, Sharma DK, Crossman A, Brimacombe JS, Ferguson MA (1999) Selective inhibitors of the glycosylphosphatidylinositol biosynthetic pathway of Trypanosoma brucei. EMBO J 18:5922–5930

Smith TK, Crossman A, Borissow CN, Paterson MJ, Dix A, Brimacombe JS, Ferguson MA (2001) Specificity of GlcNAc-PI de-N-acetylase of GPI biosynthesis and synthesis of parasite-specific suicide substrate inhibitors. EMBO J 20:3322–3332

Smith TK, Gerold P, Crossman A, Paterson MJ, Borissow CN, Brimacombe JS, Ferguson MA, Schwarz RT (2002) Substrate specificity of the Plasmodium falciparum glyco-sylphosphatidylinositol biosynthetic pathway and inhibition by species-specific suicide substrates. Biochemistry 41:12395–12406

Smith TK, Crossman A, Brimacombe JS, Ferguson MA (2004) Chemical validation of GPI biosynthesis as a drug target against African sleeping sickness. EMBO J 23:4701–4708

Snow RW, Marsh K (1998) New insights into the epidemiology of malaria relevant for disease control. Br Med Bull 54:293–309

Sowunmi A (1995) Body temperature and malaria parasitaemia in rural African children. East Afr Med J 72:427–430

Stevenson MM, Riley EM (2004) Innate immunity to malaria. Nat Rev Immunol 4:169–180

Suguitan AL, Jr., Gowda DC, Fouda G, Thuita L, Zhou A, Djokam R, Metenou S, Leke RG, Taylor DW (2004) Lack of an association between antibodies to Plasmodium falciparum glycosylphosphatidylinositols and malaria-associated placental changes in Cameroonian women with preterm and full-term deliveries. Infect Immun 72:5267–5273

Sutterlin C, Horvath A, Gerold P, Schwarz RT, Wang Y, Dreyfuss M, Riezman H (1997) Identification of a species-specific inhibitor of glycosylphosphatidylinositol synthesis. EMBO J 16:6374–6383

Tachado SD, Gerold P, McConville MJ, Baldwin T, Quilici D, Schwarz RT, Schofield L (1996) Glycosylphosphatidylinositol toxin of Plasmodium induces nitric oxide synthase expression in macrophages and vascular endothelial cells by a protein tyrosine kinase-dependent and protein kinase C-dependent signaling pathway. J Immunol 156:1897–1907

Tachado SD, Gerold P, Schwarz R, Novakovic S, McConville M, Schofield L (1997) Signal transduction in macrophages by glycosylphosphatidylinositols of Plasmodium, Trypanosoma, and Leishmania: activation of protein tyrosine kinases and protein kinase C by inositolglycan and diacylglycerol moieties. Proc Natl Acad Sci U S A 94:4022–4027

Takeda K, Takeuchi O, Akira S (2002) Recognition of lipopeptides by Toll-like receptors. J Endotoxin Res 8:459–463

Taramelli D, Basilico N, Pagani E, Grande R, Monti D, Ghione M, Olliaro P (1995) The heme moiety of malaria pigment (beta-hematin) mediates the inhibition of nitric oxide and tumor necrosis factor-alpha production by lipopolysaccharide-stimulated macrophages. Exp Parasitol 81:501–511

Taramelli D, Recalcati S, Basilico N, Olliaro P, Cairo G (2000) Macrophage preconditioning with synthetic malaria pigment reduces cytokine production via heme iron-dependent oxidative stress. Lab Invest 80:1781–1788

Taron BW, Colussi PA, Wiedman JM, Orlean P, Taron CH (2004) Human Smp3p adds a fourth mannose to yeast and human glycosylphosphatidylinositol precursors in vivo. J Biol Chem 279:36083–36092

Taylor RR, Allen SJ, Greenwood BM, Riley EM (1998) IgG3 antibodies to Plasmodium falciparum merozoite surface protein 2 (MSP2): increasing prevalence with age and association with clinical immunity to malaria. Am J Trop Med Hyg 58:406–413

Turrini F, Giribaldi G, Valente E, Arese P (1997) *Mycoplasma* contamination of *Plasmodium* cultures—a case of parasite parasitism. Parasitol Today 13:367–368

Vadas P, Taylor TE, Chimsuku L, Goldring D, Stefanski E, Pruzanski W, Molyneux ME (1993) Increased serum phospholipase A2 activity in Malawian children with falciparum malaria. Am J Trop Med Hyg 49:455–9

van der Poll T., Coyle SM, Moldawer LL, Lowry SF (1996) Changes in endotoxin-induced cytokine production by whole blood after in vivo exposure of normal humans to endotoxin. J Infect Dis 174:1356–1360

van der Poll T, van Deventer SJH (1999) Endotoxemia in healthy subjects as a human model of inflammation. 1st:335–357

van Hensbroek MB, Palmer A, Onyiorah E, Schneider G, Jaffar S, Dolan G, Memming H, Frenkel J, Enwere G, Bennett S, Kwiatkowski D, Greenwood B (1996) The effect of a monoclonal antibody to tumor necrosis factor on survival from childhood cerebral malaria. J Infect Dis 174:1091–1097

Vijaykumar M, Naik RS, Gowda DC (2001) Plasmodium falciparum Glycosylphosphatidylinositol-induced TNF-alpha Secretion by Macrophages Is Mediated without Membrane Insertion or Endocytosis. J Biol Chem 276:6909–6912

Wahlstrom K, Bellingham J, Rodriguez JL, West MA (1999) Inhibitory kappaBalpha control of nuclear factor-kappaB is dysregulated in endotoxin tolerant macrophages. Shock 11:242–247

Wattavidanage J, Carter R, Perera KL, Munasingha A, Bandara S, McGuinness D, Wickramasinghe AR, Alles HK, Mendis KN, Premawansa S (1999) TNFalpha*2 marks high risk of severe disease during Plasmodium falciparum malaria and other infections in Sri Lankans. Clin Exp Immunol 115:350–355

West MA, Heagy W (2002) Endotoxin tolerance: A review. Crit Care Med 30:S64-S73

Wood P, Elliott T (1998) Glycan-regulated antigen processing of a protein in the endoplasmic reticulum can uncover cryptic cytotoxic T cell epitopes. J Exp Med 188:773–778

Xiao L, Patterson PS, Yang C, Lal AA (1999) Role of eicosanoids in the pathogenesis of murine cerebral malaria. Am J Trop Med Hyg 60:668–673

Zhu J, Krishnegowda G, Gowda DC (2004) Induction of proinflammatory responses in macrophages by the glycosylphosphatidylinositols (GPIs) of Plasmodium falciparum: The requirement of ERK, p38, JNK and NF-kappa B pathways for the expression of proinflammatory cytokines and nitric oxide. J Biol Chem Dec 15: Epub ahead of print

Ziegler-Heitbrock HW, Wedel A, Schraut W, Strobel M, Wendelgass P, Sternsdorf T, Bauerle PA, Haas JG, Riethmuller G (1994) Tolerance to lipopolysaccharide involves mobilization of nuclear factor kappa B with predominance of p50 homodimers. J Biol Chem 269:17001–17004

Zingarelli B, Halushka PV, Caputi AP, Cook JA (1995) Increased nitric oxide synthesis during the development of endotoxin tolerance. Shock 3:102–108

Zingarelli B, Hake PW, Cook JA (2002) Inducible nitric oxide synthase is not required in the development of endotoxin tolerance in mice. Shock 17:478–484

CTMI (2005) 297:187–227
© Springer-Verlag Berlin Heidelberg 2005

The Immunology and Pathogenesis of Malaria During Pregnancy

J. G. Beeson[1] (✉) · P. E. Duffy[2,3]

[1]The Walter and Eliza Hall Institute of Medical Research,
Parkville, Victoria, Australia
beeson@wehi.edu.au

[2]Seattle Biomedical Research Institute, Seattle, WA, USA

[3]Walter Reed Army Institute of Research, Silver Spring, MD, USA

Abstract   Women in endemic areas become highly susceptible to malaria during first and second pregnancies, despite immunity acquired after years of exposure. Recent insights have advanced our understanding of pregnancy malaria caused by *Plasmodium falciparum*, which is responsible for the bulk of severe disease and death. Accumulation of parasitized erythrocytes in the blood spaces of the placenta is a key feature of maternal infection with *P. falciparum*. Placental parasites express surface ligands and antigens that differ from those of other *P. falciparum* variants, facilitating evasion of existing immunity, and mediate adhesion to specific molecules, such as chondroitin sulfate A, in the placenta. The polymorphic and clonally variant *P. falciparum* erythrocyte membrane protein 1, encoded by *var* genes, binds to placental receptors in vitro and may be the target of protective antibodies. An intense infiltration of immune cells, including macrophages, into the placental intervillous spaces, and the production of pro-inflammatory cytokines often occur in response to infection, and are associated with low birth weight and maternal anemia. Expression of α and β chemokines may initiate or facilitate this cellular infiltration during placental malaria. Specific immunity against placental-binding parasites may prevent infection or facilitate clearance of parasites prior to the influx of inflammatory cells, thereby avoiding a cascade of events leading to disease and death. Much less is known about pathogenic processes in *P. vivax* infections, and corresponding immune responses. Emerging knowledge of the pathogenesis and immunology of malaria in pregnancy will increasingly lead to new opportunities for the development of therapeutic and preventive interventions and new tools for diagnosis and monitoring.

1
Introduction

Malaria during pregnancy is a major global health problem that kills both mothers and infants. In non-immune women, malaria during pregnancy frequently causes severe disease and maternal and fetal death. However, the greater loss of life occurs among semi-immune women living in areas of stable malaria transmission, owing to the huge population at risk. Annually, an estimated 50 million women living in areas of malaria transmission become pregnant [177]. Each year, many thousands of pregnant women die due to malaria, up to 93 per 100,000 live births in a recent study from The Gambia [7], and 62,000–363,000 African infants die due to pregnancy malaria-related low birth weight (LBW) [127].

Of the four malaria species infecting humans, *Plasmodium falciparum* causes the bulk of severe disease and complications, both among pregnant and non-pregnant individuals, partly because of its ability to adhere to endothelium and sequester in deep vascular beds during its intraerythrocytic developmental stage [10, 122]. *P. falciparum* is the predominant species in tropical Africa, eastern Asia, Oceania and the Amazon basin of South America [199]. *P. vivax* is also widely distributed geographically and causes a sub-stantial amount of clinical malaria, including pregnancy malaria [119].

The earliest medical records indicated that malaria was more likely to cause severe syndromes in pregnant women [59]. Many studies over the last half-century have further demonstrated that parasitemias due to *P. falciparum* or *P. vivax* (but not *P. malariae* or *P. ovale*) are more frequent and more dense in pregnant women than in their non-pregnant counterparts. Among women living in endemic areas, susceptibility is greatest during first pregnancy and diminishes over successive pregnancies, a parity-specific susceptibility that is unique to malaria (reviewed in [25]) [26, 115]. Histologically, the hallmark of pregnancy malaria due to *P. falciparum* is the accumulation of mature-stage parasites and macrophages in the placenta (reviewed in [26]) [42, 83].

Until recently, the underlying basis for the susceptibility of pregnant women to malaria remained elusive. Although pregnancy-related im-munomodulation (required to prevent rejection of the fetal allograft) was commonly invoked as an explanation [115], this did not explain parity-specific susceptibility, or the higher susceptibility of pregnant women to malaria but not to all infectious agents. New insights have greatly advanced our understanding of pregnancy malaria caused by *P. falciparum*. Parasitized erythrocytes that sequester in the placenta are now known to express surface adhesins and antigens that differ from those of other *P. falciparum* variants, allowing evasion of immune responses acquired before first pregnancy, and mediating adhesion to specific molecules in the placenta. These new insights have focused studies of antimalarial immunity acquired during pregnancy, leading to a deeper understanding of protective and pathogenic host responses to maternal malaria.

2
Clinical Features and Complications of Malaria in Pregnancy

Maternal malaria can lead to a range of complications, and the impact of malaria during pregnancy appears to depend on the intensity and stability of transmission, the level of pre-existing immunity, and parity (reviewed in [115, 132]). In areas of high malaria transmission, maternal anemia, LBW, and infant anemia are common, whereas in areas of low endemicity or where malaria occurs in epidemics, spontaneous abortions, stillbirths, prematurity, and severe maternal disease occur more frequently [115, 132]. Parity has a significant influence on the susceptibility to parasitemia and disease. Prim-igravid women typically experience a higher prevalence of parasitemia than multigravid women and the sequelae are more severe [25, 117, 132], suggesting that effective immunity to maternal malaria develops over successive pregnancies. With increasing malaria transmission, the effect of parity becomes more marked [132]. In areas of stable malaria transmission, the prevalence of malaria increases at the end of the first trimester, then remains constant or declines after mid-gestation [25, 26, 28, 115, 117]. Infection with HIV-1, which is highly prevalent in many malaria-endemic areas, increases susceptibility to *P. falciparum* malaria in pregnancy, manifest by higher prevalence and density of infection and complications [178, 190, 193].

2.1
Consequences of Malaria for Mothers

The accumulation of parasitized erythrocytes in the blood spaces of the placenta is a key feature of maternal infection with *P. falciparum*. The density of infection in the placenta can be striking, with over 50% of erythrocytes infected by parasites in some cases [9, 35], and in areas of stable transmission, high-density infections are more prevalent in primigravid women [115, 132]. Placental parasitemia is typically higher than that seen in the peripheral blood, and may be observed in the absence of a detectable peripheral blood parasitemia [42, 158, 167, 196]. Although placental sequestration of *P. falciparum* is a prominent feature of maternal infection, peripheral parasitemia has been observed in the absence of placental infection [114, 158, 167]. This presentation occurs infrequently, and the factors that lead to maternal infection without placental involvement are unknown.

In non-immune women, such as travelers or victims of malaria epidemics, pregnancy increases malaria morbidity and mortality. Severe syndromes, such as cerebral malaria, severe anemia and respiratory distress, are common and life-threatening [132, 197]. In immune women living in areas of stable malaria transmission, malaria is an important contributing factor in the prevalence and severity of anemia during pregnancy [67, 115]. Anemia consequently increases the incidence of maternal death during pregnancy or post-partum [85], and is associated with increased fetal and infant mortality, prematurity, and LBW [67]. Although other factors contribute to the development of maternal anemia, malaria is a significant treatable cause and several studies have demonstrated that malaria chemoprophylaxis during pregnancy reduces the prevalence and degree of maternal anemia (reviewed in [82]).

2.2
Consequences of Maternal Malaria for Infants

LBW is the major complication of maternal malaria, being the single greatest risk factor for infant mortality and morbidity [22, 112]. Both fetal growth restriction and prematurity contribute to reduced birth weight in newborns delivered from malaria-exposed pregnancies [25, 90, 121]. In areas with stable and high levels of malaria transmission, LBW probably results mainly from growth restriction rather than prematurity, whereas in settings of unstable endemicity prematurity is a significant effect of maternal malaria [120, 132, 133]. Convincing evidence supporting the contribution of *P. falciparum* infection to LBW comes from randomized placebo-controlled trials that demonstrate increases in mean birth weight, up to 500 g higher in some studies [196], following the use of effective antimalarial chemoprophylaxis during pregnancy (reviewed in [82]).

Malaria during pregnancy has been associated with anemia in newborns [67, 192], a paradoxical finding because maternal anemia can elicit an increase in fetal hemoglobin [24]. Newborns are rarely born with patent parasitemia, making it unlikely that fetal anemia is directly due to malaria. Other factors must be involved, and more research is needed to determine whether factors such as reduced placental weight, altered placental function or fetal growth restriction contribute to the development of fetal anemia.

Numerous reports of congenital malaria cases have established that this syndrome occurs, although the frequency with which it occurs remains controversial. While some reports contend that cord blood parasitemia is a common complication of maternal infection [145], most reports have found that congenital malaria is uncommon among deliveries to immune women in areas of stable malaria transmission. An important consideration in such studies is the possibility that cord blood may be contaminated by highly infected placental blood, leading to a false diagnosis of congenital malaria. True congenital malaria can result in severe malaria and death, but infection is often self-limited [117, 120]. Infection and disease during the neonatal period may be limited due to placentally transferred maternal antibodies [61, 88], activation of the fetal immune system by maternal malaria during gestation [53, 94], a predominance of hemoglobin F in newborns [140], limiting amounts of *para*-amino-benzoic acid in breastfed infants [44], or other reasons.

3
Parasite Adhesion and Sequestration in the Placenta

3.1
Sequestration of *P. falciparum*-Infected Erythrocytes

P. falciparum infected erythrocytes adhere to vascular and other host cells, mediating organ-specific accumulation or sequestration of parasites that is thought to contribute to the pathogenesis of severe disease [10, 122]. Parasite-derived proteins are inserted into the membrane of the infected erythrocyte, enabling adhesion to a range of host molecules (reviewed in [10, 47]). Generally speaking, studies that have sought to link specific receptors to severe malaria syndromes have not reported consistent associations [10, 102]. Such studies are challenging, due to the inability to recover live parasites from specific organs and the difficulty of working with and limited availability of post-mortem tissue.

By contrast, studies of placental malaria have provided a unique opportunity to study sequestration. Viable parasites can be isolated relatively easily from infected placentas following delivery rather than relying on examination of tissue post-mortem. Studies of placental parasite adhesion have therefore contributed more broadly to our understanding of organ-specific sequestration and disease resulting from *P. falciparum*.

In *P. falciparum* infections, parasitized erythrocytes accumulate throughout the intervillous space [195, 200], and cell adhesion appears to play a significant role in this process. The great majority of placentally sequestered parasites consist of the mature pigmented stages of parasitized erythrocytes [9, 42, 195] that adhere to candidate placental receptors in vitro [11, 19, 71], whereas young ring-stage parasites are uncommon in the placenta [9] and generally do not adhere at high levels in vitro [11, 81, 141, 188]. Infected individuals, pregnant or non-pregnant, rarely display mature-stage parasitized erythrocytes in their peripheral blood [9, 103, 168, 195]. Whereas ring-stage parasitized erythrocytes predominate in the peripheral blood, mature *P. falciparum* parasites sequester in deep vascular beds presumably to avoid clearance by the spleen [49, 153]. Sequestration in the placenta or other organs has not been reported for *P vivax*; *P. vivax*-parasitized erythrocytes have been detected in placental tissue, although this appears to be uncommon [114]. Placental parasite sequestration does occur in rodent malarias [185].

3.2
Receptors for Adhesion of *P. falciparum*-Infected Erythrocytes in the Placenta

3.2.1
Chondroitin Sulfate A

Substantial evidence supports an important role for chondroitin sulfate A (CSA) as a receptor for adhesion of *P. falciparum* in the placenta [71, 139]. CSA immobilized on solid matrices or expressed on cell surfaces can support high levels of adhesion of laboratory isolates [151, 157] or patient isolates [70, 157] of *P. falciparum*, including under conditions of physiologically relevant flow [45]. Studies among pregnant women in western Kenya demonstrated that parasitized erythrocytes infecting the placenta bind to placental tissue in a CSA-dependent manner [71]. All placental parasite isolates tested bound immobilized CSA, whereas there was little or no binding to CD36, a common receptor for adhesion of parasite isolates from non-pregnant donors [135], clearly distinguishing placental parasites from other parasite phenotypes [71]. Subsequently, studies in Malawi found the majority of placental isolates bound immobilized CSA, although there was substantial variability in the extent to which different isolates adhere [12]. Among women in Cameroon, placental parasite isolates were shown to bind cultured endothelial cells [86] and syncytiotrophoblast [110] in a CSA-dependent manner. By contrast, adhesion to CSA is generally uncommon among peripheral blood isolates from non-pregnant persons [12, 40, 71, 161]; instead these isolates usually adhere to CD36, often bind to intercellular adhesion molecule (ICAM)-1 and other receptors, and frequently form erythrocyte rosettes.

Placental parasites do not typically adhere to other receptors such as CD36 and ICAM-1 [12, 71, 86] or form erythrocyte rosettes [109, 155]. Selection of parasitized erythrocytes for adhesion to CSA in vitro, or to hyaluronic acid (discussed in the next section), leads to a loss of CD36 and ICAM-1 binding and rosette-forming capacity [11, 19, 80, 157], suggesting that these contrasting phenotypes are largely mutually exclusive. However, some cloned CSA-binding parasitized erythrocytes yield parasite lines that bind both CD36 and CSA [134]. Peripheral blood isolates from pregnant women may bind to CSA, CD36, or both [12, 71], and may form erythrocyte rosettes [109, 155], but they do not adhere to ICAM-1, suggesting that the circulating ring-stage parasites may have arisen from CSA-binding parasites sequestered in the placenta or from endothelial cell-binding parasites sequestered elsewhere in the microvasculature [71].

Parasite adhesion to CSA involves interactions with specific structural motifs dependent on sulfation pattern and chain length. Parasitized erythrocytes do not adhere to chondroitin sulfate B or C, nor do these inhibit adhesion [71, 157]. Oligosaccharides from CSA were shown to inhibit adhesion to immobilized CSA and thrombomodulin, but not CD36 or ICAM-1, in a size-dependent manner, with dodecasaccharides being the minimum length for activity [13]; by contrast, CSC oligosaccharides differing only in sulfation pattern and content were non-inhibitory. Removal of 4-O-sulfation abrogates the binding and inhibitory activity of CSA [5, 74]. Detailed studies with clonal parasite lines using highly defined and structurally characterized oligosaccharides revealed that the optimal motif for interaction with parasitized erythrocytes comprises dodecasaccharide sequences formed by mixed non-sulfated and 4-O-sulfated N-acetyl-galactosamine alternating with glucuronic acid, with 6- or 2-O-sulfation inhibiting the interaction [5, 37]. Others have reported that smaller oligosaccharides can inhibit adhesion of placental parasitized erythrocytes to endothelial cells expressing CSA [142].

Chondroitin sulfates are expressed as proteoglycans (CSPGs) on cell surfaces and the identity of their core proteins in the placenta is not currently known. Low sulfated forms of chondroitin sulfate predominate in placental blood and appear optimal for adhesion of parasitized erythrocytes compared to fully sulfated forms of CSA [3]. These placental CSPGs comprise two major forms in which 2%–3% and 9%–14% of disaccharides are sulfated but sulfate groups cluster within sequences of 6–14 repeating disaccharide units; these contain 20%–28% 4-O-sulfated disaccharides, whereas other regions have little or no sulfation [4]. These 4-sulfated disaccharide clusters are required for efficient adhesion of parasitized erythrocytes [4]. Thrombomodulin, which may have CSA chains attached [84], is a potential receptor as it supports parasite adhesion in vitro [87, 159] and is detected by specific antibody on the surface of human syncytiotrophoblast [106], but it was not detected as the core protein for CSPGs in extracts from placental blood and tissue [3]. Further studies of the structural requirements for *P. falciparum* adhesion in the placenta will be aided by the identification of CSA-binding sites of *P. falciparum* ligands.

3.2.2
Hyaluronic Acid (Hyaluronan)

The non-sulfated glycosaminoglycan hyaluronic acid (HA) has been identified as a receptor for parasitized erythrocyte adhesion in vitro [11, 18, 19, 36], and implicated in mediating placental sequestration of *P. falciparum* in one study to date. In Malawi 80% of placental isolates bound to immobilized HA, whereas adhesion of isolates from the peripheral blood of pregnant women or children was less prevalent and occurred at lower levels [19]. Many isolates bound both HA and CSA, but some bound only one of the receptors. Subsequent studies with clonal isolates have demonstrated that some *P. falciparum* isolates may co-express separate, but overlapping, binding sites for adhesion to CSA and HA [11]. In contrast, a study in Kenya concluded that none of seven placental isolates tested bound to HA in a specific manner [74] and further studies examining the role of adhesion to HA are needed.

Factors that may influence adhesion to HA in vitro include chain length and/or conformation of HA and different HA preparations vary in their binding or inhibitory activity in parasite assays [11, 18]. The presence of co-purified chondroitin sulfates in many formulations of HA, or inadequate immobilization of HA on solid surfaces, are important considerations in studies of parasite adhesion to HA [18, 74 189]. These issues have been addressed through the use of specific enzymatic degradation of HA or proteins on the surface of parasitized erythrocytes, the use of defined oligosaccharide inhibitors, and other approaches [11, 18, 19, 36, 172]. In studies using laboratory isolates of *P. falciparum*, HA differed from CSA by its ability to mediate clumping or aggregation of parasitized erythrocytes [11], which may be relevant to sequestration in vivo. The minimum chain length for interactions between parasitized erythrocytes appears to be 10–12 monosaccharide units [19, 36].

HA appears to be expressed on the syncytiotrophoblast surface [108, 183], and constitutes approximately 1%–2% of glycosaminoglycans in extracts of placental blood from uninfected placentas [3]. One study suggested that the expression of HA is low in normal placentas, but markedly increased in inflammatory conditions such as pre-eclamptic toxemia [108]. This may suggest that HA is not a major receptor for initiating parasite sequestration, but could augment adhesion of HA-binding parasites as inflammation develops. There are presently no published studies of expression of HA in malaria-exposed placentas, and further studies are needed to evaluate binding of parasitized erythrocytes to HA expressed in placental tissue.

3.2.3
Immunoglobulins

Non-immune immunoglobulin (Ig) has also been proposed to be involved in mediating or enhancing parasite sequestration in the placenta by acting as a bridge between parasitized erythrocytes and Fc receptors on the surface of syncytiotrophoblast [68]. IgG and IgM can be detected on placental parasites in situ by immunohistochemistry, and a laboratory-adapted parasite clone was found to adhere in an Ig-dependent manner to placental sections in vitro. Four placental isolates tested demonstrated some IgG binding, in addition to adhesion to CSA [68]. The extent to which the CSA-binding and IgG-binding phenotypes overlap is unclear; however, the Ig-binding laboratory line did not adhere to CSA indicating that these binding properties can arise independently. Others have shown that CSA-binding parasitized erythrocytes adsorb IgM, but not IgG, to the parasitized erythrocyte surface [48]. Additional studies are required to formally demonstrate that placental parasite isolates adhere to syncytiotrophoblast through Ig bridging to Fc receptors, and to localize Fc receptors to the external surface of syncytiotrophoblast.

3.2.4
Binding of Ring-Stage *P. falciparum*

Some investigators have proposed that parasites may replicate locally within the placenta [195], and recent studies have further promoted this hypothesis by demonstrating that early developmental stages, or ring forms, can adhere to placental tissue in vitro [141]. The receptor for binding of ring-stage parasites has not yet been identified, but it is neither CSA nor HA. Rhoptry-associated protein 2 has been proposed as the parasite ligand [55]. Further studies are needed to more clearly elucidate the role of these adhesive events in placental sequestration, since numerous studies have documented mature-stage but not ring-stage parasites sequestered in the placenta. A quantitative study of parasite stages and density in peripheral and placental blood strongly supported specific sequestration of mature-stage parasites that are known to express adhesion ligands and adhere in vitro, but did not support a major role for sequestration of ring-stage parasites [9].

3.2.5
Relative Roles of Different Parasite–Receptor Interactions

Determining the diversity of adhesion phenomena involved in placental sequestration of parasites will be important for understanding the acquisition of specific immunity and for guiding the development of preventive interventions such as vaccines. Most placental isolates bind CSA at significant levels, and CSA appears to be expressed in infected and uninfected placentas, suggesting that it plays a major role in placental infection. In Kenya, all placental parasite isolates with measurable adhesion bound to CSA, and binding to placental cryosections was inhibited by more than 95% by soluble CSA [71]. In Malawi, not all placental isolates bound to CSA in vitro, some bound only at low levels, and some isolates did not bind CSA but did bind HA [12, 19]. The lack of binding did not appear to be explained by poor parasite viability or differences in parasite extraction methods, and serologic assays suggested that the lack of adhesiveness was not due to the absence of parasite antigens on the infected red cell surface [12]. Existing in vitro assays may not be sufficiently sensitive to detect the binding properties of all isolates. Further studies are particularly needed to evaluate the roles of binding to HA, Ig and ring-stage parasites in the pathogenesis of placental malaria.

Most parasitized erythrocytes in the intervillous space are not directly adherent to the syncytiotrophoblast layer, suggesting that other processes may also contribute to placental sequestration [29, 195, 200]. Parasites in the intervillous spaces are often observed to be enmeshed in fibrinoid strands or masses that appear to progressively enlarge [29, 195]. Fibrinoid deposits in the placenta are composed of numerous molecules, including several extra-cellular matrix molecules [130]. Specifically, a recent immunohistochemical study suggested that low-sulfated CS proteoglycans are dispersed throughout the intervillous space and co-localize with parasitized erythrocytes [128]. These results support the notion that CSA is a major receptor for parasitized erythrocyte adhesion in the placenta, including throughout the intervillous spaces.

4
Humoral Immunity to Malaria in Pregnancy

4.1
Emergence of Antigenically Distinct Parasite Populations in Pregnancy

Antigenic variation of *P. falciparum* [20, 104], and other *Plasmodium* species [30, 118], enables evasion of immune responses resulting in repeat and chronic infections and this property appears important for infection during pregnancy. Non-pregnant adults and older children in endemic areas, who typically demonstrate substantial immunity to malaria, possess a large repertoire of variant-specific agglutinating antibodies against different *P. falciparum* isolates indicative of past exposures [104, 148]. These antibodies are associated with protection from infection and clinical disease in children [33, 105]. This aspect of naturally acquired immunity appears to be intact in pregnancy as pregnant women have antibodies to isolates from non-pregnant donors [12].

In pregnancy, novel antigenic variants of *P. falciparum* emerge that are poorly recognized by antibodies acquired prior to first pregnancy [12, 76]. A striking finding is that antibodies able to inhibit adhesion to CSA or bind to the surface of placental isolates or CSA-binding parasite lines are rare in those not exposed to placental malaria, observed in different populations [12, 76, 149]. The emergence of new parasite variants or serotypes in pregnancy would enable evasion of an important aspect of the acquired immune response [17, 72].

P. vivax in pregnancy has not been extensively studied, but prevalence and density decrease with increasing gravidity, as with *P. falciparum* [131, 166, 170]. Unlike *P. falciparum*, *P. vivax* appears more likely to cause disease in multigravid than primigravid women [131, 169]. The basis for this interest-ing epidemiology is unknown. One possibility is that the reticulocytosis of pregnancy increases susceptibility to *P. vivax*, a parasite that exclusively in-fects reticulocytes. Susceptibility to infection might decrease over successive pregnancies due to worsening micronutrient deficiency, which would simultaneously exacerbate anemia and other sequelae when *P. vivax* did occur [58]. More research is needed to understand the pathogenesis and immunology of *P. vivax* during pregnancy.

4.2
Acquired Antibodies and Protective Immunity

Passive transfer of antimalarial IgG antibodies purified from immune adults can reduce parasitemia and illness in susceptible humans [43, 116]. Presumably, these antibodies act against surface proteins expressed by merozoites or parasitized erythrocytes, although few target antigens have been identified. At the population level, susceptibility to *P. falciparum* malaria diminishes over successive pregnancies [25, 115], suggesting an acquired immune response to parasite variants that specifically infect pregnant women [71, 76].

4.2.1
Antibodies to Infected Erythrocytes

Antibodies against *P. falciparum* parasitized erythrocyte surface proteins can be measured in several formats (Table 1), using either fresh clinical isolates or laboratory-adapted isolates and clonal parasite lines, and the different formats most likely measure different and overlapping repertoires of antibody [16]. These assays include those that measure the degree to which sera inhibit parasite adhesion to specific receptors or cells [76, 187], the ability and extent to which sera agglutinate parasitized erythrocytes [12, 104], and total surface antibody reactivity detected by indirect immunofluorescence using microscopy or flow cytometry [174].

Following exposure to malaria during pregnancy, women acquire antibodies to surface antigens and CSA-binding ligands expressed by placental or CSA-binding *P. falciparum* [12, 76, 111, 149]. Antibodies acquired from exposure in one pregnancy appear to be carried through into subsequent pregnancies where they may reduce the risk of infection or complications [16, 175].

Over successive pregnancies, women resident in malaria-endemic areas of Africa, Thailand and Papua New Guinea acquire antibodies that can inhibit parasite adhesion to CSA and/or react with the surface of placental or CSA-binding parasites (summarized in Table 1) [12, 15, 16, 76, 86, 111, 136, 149, 175]. In assays with fresh placental parasites, anti-adhesion antibodies were uniformly absent in sera collected from infected or uninfected primigravid women in Kenya [76], and were uncommon, but not absent, among primigravid women in Malawi [16]. In assays with parasites selected for adhesion

Table 1 Summary of studies examining associations between antibodies to the surface of placental and/or CSA-binding *P. falciparum*-infected erythrocytes and parity, parasitemia, and/or pregnancy outcomes

Study[a]	Population	Source of *P. falciparum*[b]	Antibody measure[c]	Antibody associations
Fried et al. 1998	Kenya, Malawi, Thailand	Placenta (Kenya)	Adhesion inhibition	Parity[d]; Negatively associated with placental parasitemia in Kenyan SGs
Beeson et al. 1999	Malawi	Placenta; Peripheral blood	Agglutination	Parity (with placental isolates, but not isolates from children)
Maubert et al. 1999	Cameroon	Peripheral blood; CSA-binding line (RP5/FCR3)	Agglutination	Parity (with CSA-binding isolate, but not isolates from non-pregnant donors; among women in 2nd trimester and at delivery)
Ricke et al. 2000	Ghana	CSA-binding line (PA/FCR3)	IgG binding	Parity (with CSA-binding line but not CD36-binding line)
Staalsoe et al. 2001	Cameroon	CSA-binding line (FCR3) and isolate (2H3)	IgG binding	Parity; Inverse association with placental parasitemia among MGs (but not PGs)
O'Neill-Dunne et al. 2002	Cameroon	CSA-binding line (3D7/NF54)	Adhesion inhibition	Parity (among women in 2nd trimester, but not at delivery); Not associated with presence of placental infection, inverse correlation with placental parasitemia[e]

Table 1 (continued)

Study[a]	Population	Source of P. falciparum[b]	Antibody measure[c]	Antibody associations
Duffy and Fried 2003	Kenya	Placental isolates	Adhesion inhibition	Positively associated with birth weight. Inversely correlated with placental parasitemia. Not associated with anemia
Staalsoe et al. 2004a	Kenya	CSA-binding lines	IgG binding	Positively associated with birth weight. Inversely associated with anemia
Beeson et al. 2004	Malawi	CSA-binding line (CS2). Placental isolates	IgG binding. Agglutination. Adhesion inhibition	Parity (2nd trimester and at delivery). Placental infection among PGs for all antibody measures; Not associated with placental parasite density or outcomes
Taylor et al. 2004	Cameroon	CSA-binding line (3D7/NF54)	Adhesion inhibition	Inversely correlated with placental parasite density[e]
Mount et al. 2004	Malawi	CSA-binding line (CS2)	IgG binding. Agglutination	Antibodies lower in HIV-1-infected women; Inversely correlated with immunosuppression and HIV viral load; Not correlated with parasite density or associated with pregnancy outcomes
Khattab et al. 2004	Gabon	CSA-selected placental isolates	IgG binding	Parity. Placental infection in PGs

Table 1 (continued)

Study[a]	Population	Source of P. falciparum[b]	Antibody measure[c]	Antibody associations
Staalsoe et al. 2004b	Kenya	CSA-binding lines (FCR3 and Busua)	IgG binding	Lower among women receiving intermittent presumptive treatment/prophylaxis

[a] Studies listed by date of publication. Not all findings from the studies listed have been included in the table (see text for details)

[b] CSA-binding lines are laboratory adapted isolates (usually clonal) that have been selected for high levels of adhesion to CSA in vitro

[c] All antibody assays used intact parasitized erythrocytes—adhesion inhibition measures the ability of serum to inhibit adhesion of PRBCs to CSA in vitro; agglutination measures antibodies to the surface of parasitized erythrocytes by the ability of serum to agglutinate; IgG binding is a measure of antibodies to the parasitized erythrocytes surface by indirect immunofluorescence using flow cytometry (see text for details)

[d] An association between parity and antibodies is defined by a higher level or prevalence of antibodies among women of two or more pregnancies compared to primigravidae, or a correlation between antibody levels and number of pregnancies

[e] Analysis did not control for parity

Abbreviations: PGs, primigravidae; SGs, secundigravidae; MGs, multigravidae; CSA, chondroitin sulfate A; IgG, immunoglobulin G to CSA and maintained in prolonged culture in vitro, primigravid women demonstrated higher levels of antibody, measured by flow cytometry, agglutination, and adhesion inhibition, during placental malaria episodes [16, 14, 93]. Studies of women over the course of pregnancy found that the antibody responses to CSA-binding parasitized erythrocytes detected in primigravid women were delayed compared with multigravid women [136]. Malaria in non-pregnant individuals appears to induce broadly reactive antibody responses against parasitized erythrocyte surface proteins, some of which are short-lived [32, 95].

Antibodies acquired against placental parasites have been related to protection from pregnancy malaria (Table 1). Serum inhibition of parasite adhesion to CSA has been related to reduced prevalence [76] and reduced density [60, 175] of placental parasitemia among women in Kenya and Cameroon. In western Kenya, anti-adhesion antibodies in secundigravid women were associated with increased birth weight and gestational age of the newborn, but were not associated with increased maternal hemoglobin level [60]. Among women residing in coastal Kenya, IgG to the surface of CSA-binding isolates measured by flow cytometry was associated with increased birth weight and maternal hemoglobin level, but these associations were only observed among women with placental histologic changes defined as 'chronic infection' (the presence of parasites and fibrinoid deposits) [176].

Among women in Blantyre, Malawi, similar antibodies were not associated with reduced placental parasitemia or prevalence, or with birth weight or hemoglobin level after controlling for parity, malaria infection status and HIV-1 infection [16, 126]. Co-infection with HIV-1 in these studies was shown to be associated with reduced antibodies to the surface of CSA and HA-binding parasitized erythrocytes [16, 126], which may account for the greater susceptibility to pregnancy malaria seen with HIV-1 [178]. Both the prevalence and levels of antibodies were lower in HIV-1 infected women, being most marked in primigravidae and women with immunosuppression. Specific IgG levels correlated with $CD4^+$ cell counts and inversely with viral load [126].

Prospective studies are needed to further evaluate the role and specificities of antibodies in protective immunity and to examine the relative contribution of adhesion-inhibitory antibodies versus total antibodies to surface antigens (measured by flow cytometry or agglutination assays). The targets of these different antibody types appear to overlap, as expected, but not all samples with antibodies to the parasitized erythrocyte surface inhibit adhesion [16]. The different specificities of antibodies measured in these assays may have different associations with protective immunity and exposure, and the use of different assays may account for some of the differences observed between separate studies. The idea that anti-adhesion antibodies will limit parasitemia by blocking adhesion and sequestration is of course appealing. Agglutinating antibodies may also interfere with parasite adhesion, although placental parasites agglutinate poorly in comparison to isolates collected from non-pregnant individuals [12, 76]. Antibodies that react with the parasitized erythrocyte surface without inhibiting adhesion could still limit parasitemia by opsonizing parasites to promote phagocytosis and lysis. Possibly, a combination of antibody types could be most effective in limiting placental malaria, but studies to test this idea await the identification of surface proteins of placental parasites.

4.2.2
Antibodies to Other Antigens

Studies of antibodies to other blood-stage antigens have generally not found the strong associations with gravidity or placental malaria as have been observed for antibodies to placental parasites (reviewed in [58]). In pregnancy, there is no evidence to support a general reduction in antibody levels and the titer of total antimalarial antibodies does not appear to be reduced or influenced by parity [115, 120]. Antibodies to surface antigens expressed by CD36 and ICAM-1 binding isolates [76], or isolates from children [12], have not been found to differ between pregnant women and nulliparous adults. Some associations have been found between pregnancy and the level of antibodies to the ring-infected erythrocyte surface antigen (RESA), measured by erythrocyte membrane immunofluorescence assays against ring-stage parasites. Titers of RESA-specific antibodies were lower in pregnant than non-pregnant women in some studies [129], but not others [52, 64], or were lower in primigravid than multigravid women in some studies [52, 129], but not others [2, 51]. Anti-RESA antibody levels by immunofluorescence or ELISA were inversely associated with parasitemia in some studies [8, 129], but not others [52, 184]. Higher levels of antibodies to merozoite surface protein 1 have also been associated with reduced risk of placental malaria in some studies [27, 184] but not in others [76, 126]. No protective association has been found for antibodies against circumsporozoite protein [8, 76, 129], liver stage antigen-1 [184], or to a glycosylphosphatidylinositol extract from *P. falciparum* [180].

4.3
Surface Antigens of Placental *P. falciparum*

Despite the highly polymorphic nature of variant surface antigens of *P. falciparum* parasitized erythrocytes, serologic studies suggest that the surface antigens of placental parasites, including the parasite ligand for adhesion to

CSA, have conserved features or epitopes, making these antigens appealing vaccine targets [76]. Sera from women in Africa inhibit the adhesion of parasites collected from pregnant women in Asia, and vice versa [76]. Laboratory parasite isolates selected to bind to CSA in vitro acquire surface reactivity with sera collected from gravid women in geographically distant locations [16, 93, 149, 175]. Furthermore, serum antibody reactivity to different CSA-binding *P. falciparum* isolates was significantly correlated [76, 93]. Such findings have raised expectations that the antigens required for a pregnancy malaria vaccine may be conserved or finite in number.

Presently, the extent of conservation or diversity of placental parasite surface antigens, or whether women acquire cross-reactive antibodies to conserved epitopes or a repertoire of antibodies with different specificities, is unknown. Testing serum from pregnant women in Malawi against different placental isolates found that agglutinating antibodies, which target *P. falciparum* erythrocyte membrane protein 1 (PfEMP1) [20, 171], were largely isolate-specific, rather than pan-reactive, suggesting they target diverse epitopes [12]. However, these antibodies do not necessarily target receptor-binding domains [16], which probably have a greater degree of conservation [76]. The presence of cross-reactive or conserved epitopes on CSA-binding and placental parasitized erythrocytes has been suggested by vaccination with whole parasitized erythrocytes or recombinant PfEMP1 domains [46, 62, 100], although such studies can be confounded by non-specific binding of IgM or IgG [48, 68].

Nearly all studies that have sought to identify CSA or placental-binding ligands have focused on PfEMP1, as it is one of the few known parasitized erythrocyte surface antigens and has been implicated in several adhesive phenomena of *P. falciparum* (reviewed in [10, 47]). Other antigens have been suggested to be surface antigens of parasitized erythrocytes, including the variant antigens called rifins (encoded by *rif* genes) [63, 98], as well as numerous proteins encoded by single-copy genes that have been identified by tandem mass spectrometry [69, 77]. However, it is presently unclear how the expression of any of these proteins influences antigenic and adhesive phenotypes of placental parasites.

4.3.1
PfEMP1 and *var* Genes

PfEMP1 molecules are predicted to be multi-domain proteins of 200–400 kDa formed by highly polymorphic cysteine-rich Duffy-binding-like domains (DBL) and cysteine-rich interdomain regions (CIDR). Typically, PfEMP1s contain several DBL domains and one or two CIDR domains [173]. These domains have been clustered into α, β, γ, δ, ε and unclassified X types for DBL domains, and α, β, and γ types for CIDR domains, based on the presence of key sequence motifs [173]. The complexity and diversity of PfEMP1 (and its encoding *var* gene) have made this molecule exceedingly difficult to study. Studies of *var* gene transcription in CSA-binding parasites have yielded similarly complex results.

In initial studies, fragments of *var* transcripts were amplified by reverse transcription-PCR with degenerate primers from laboratory isolates selected to bind CSA, and the entire *var* gene subsequently sequenced. Two *var* genes were identified by this approach—*varCS2* [146] and *FCR3varCSA* [31]. Both *varCS2* and *FCR3varCSA* contain DBLγ domains that bound CSA in vitro [31, 80, 147] and elicited antibodies that inhibited parasite adhesion to CSA and cross-reacted with placental parasites [100, 146]. *varCS2* does not appear to be well conserved and sequences with homology to it have only rarely been detected among clinical isolates [73, 92]. Genes with substantial homology to *FCR3varCSA* have been identified in many isolates of different geographic origin, demonstrating that it has a relatively conserved sequence [73, 163, 164]. Despite these promising initial results, subsequent studies suggest that these PfEMP1 forms are not associated with CSA-binding or with placental parasites [56, 73, 77, 97, 134, 165, 198]. Recent studies suggest *FCR3varCSA* is expressed at similar levels in CSA-binding and non-binding isolates, and the timing of its expression is atypical [97]. Furthermore, *FCR3varCSA* disruption mutants are able to recover the ability to bind CSA, suggesting other genes can encode the phenotype [6]. Although *varCS2* is differentially expressed in the CSA-binding line from which it was sequenced, compared to the non-binding parent line [146], subsequent studies have shown it is not quantitatively dominant and is expressed at low levels [56, 57].

Although binding to CSA has been largely attributed to DBLγ domains, many expressed DBLγ domains do not bind to CSA [79], and glycosaminoglycan binding activity has also been reported for CIDR1α domains [50, 147]. Among DBLγ domains, there are varying amounts of homology in primary sequence and substantial diversity, without any clearly conserved sequence among DBLγ types that bind to CSA [79]. An analysis of five different DBLγ sequences from placental isolates in one population revealed 39%–55% homology [92]. There was also substantial homology between DBLγ sequences collected from different populations [91], although the number of sequences examined was small.

Quantitative studies of *var* gene transcription are technically challenging [56, 162]. Post-transcriptional events may also regulate the expression of PfEMP1 on the cell surface. An advancing knowledge of *var* gene expression together with a greater body of data from *P. falciparum* sequencing is continuing to facilitate quantitative and more detailed studies. Using quantitative analysis, recent studies have identified the *var2csa* as the dominant transcript in several parasite isolates selected for adhesion to CSA in vitro as well as placental isolates [57, 165]. *var2csa* is highly conserved across genetically different isolates [96, 165], and may fulfill the criteria of a conserved ligand that was suggested from serologic studies [76]. *Var2csa* has an atypical structure that lacks DBLγ or CIDR domains. There is substantial homology between the third DBL domain of *var2csa* and the minimum binding region of the *FCR3varCSA* DBLγ domain [79]. An analysis of PRBC membrane proteins by mass spectrometry did not find that *var2csa* or *FCR3varCSA* were preferentially expressed by CSA-binding or placental isolates, although other PfEMP1 sequences were found to be so expressed [77]. Further validation of these results is needed[1].

As discussed earlier, other adhesive interactions may contribute to the pathogenesis of placental malaria, and therefore the role of antibodies targeting these parasite phenotypes requires investigation. Antibodies that inhibit parasite adhesion to CSA may not be fully protective against placental malaria if alternative mechanisms of sequestration exist. In studies of parasite adhesion to HA, substantial overlap between adhesion of isolates to CSA and HA was identified, suggesting that ligands for adhesion to the two receptors may be co-expressed, although there appear to be separate, possibly overlapping, receptor binding sites [11, 18, 19, 36]. Domain(s) that mediate adhesion to HA have not yet been identified, but the isolate-specific adhesion to HA and sensitivity to trypsin suggest PfEMP1 is involved [11, 19]. Recombinant DBLβ and CIDR1α domains of PfEMP1 have been found to bind IgG [41, 68]. Separate antibody responses would presumably also be required for protection against placental sequestration of ring-stage parasites, if this phenomenon contributes to the pathogenesis of placental malaria [55].

---

[1] Since preparing this review, it has been reported that antibodies against *var2csa* recombinant proteins labeled the surface of CSA-binding IEs, recombinant *var2csa* proteins were recognized in a gravidity-associated manner by plasma antibodies among pregnant women, and these antibodies were associated with improved infant birth weight (Salanti et al. 2004, J Exp Med 200:1197–1203). Recombinant DBL2, DBL3, and DBL6 domains of *var2csa* expressed on CHO cells were shown to bind CSA, although the CSA-binding properties of some domains varied between the two parasite isolates tested (Gamain et al. 2005, J Infect Dis 191:1010–1013).

5
Cellular Immune Responses and Immunopathology

5.1
Inflammatory Responses and Pathology in the Placenta

The mechanisms that lead to disease and death during pregnancy malaria are incompletely understood, but the inflammatory response in the placenta has been related to both severe anemia in the mother and LBW in the newborn (summarized in Table 2). An intense and sometimes massive infiltrate of immune cells is often observed in placental malaria, and may appear in the intervillous spaces several days after *P. falciparum* parasites begin to accumulate in the placenta [83]. In clinicopathologic studies, the accumulation of macrophages in the placenta may be more strongly associated with poor pregnancy outcomes than placental parasitemia per se [58] [101, 121, 137, 160]. *P. vivax* infection has not been associated with placental pathologic changes [114], suggesting that the detrimental effects of infection on pregnancy are mediated through mechanisms other than obstruction to blood flow. *P. berghei* infection in rodents is associated with monocyte infiltrates and many of the placental histologic changes observed with *P. falciparum* in humans [185].

Monocytes and macrophages are the most distinctive cellular component of the inflammatory infiltrate that accompanies placental malaria, and often appear grossly enlarged and engorged with parasite pigment (reviewed in [26, 58, 154]) [35, 89, 137, 195]. Occasionally, macrophages can be seen to have ingested intact parasitized erythrocytes. Monocytes/macrophages can phagocytose parasitized erythrocytes though both opsonic and non-opsonic mechanisms [113], but the mechanisms occurring in the placenta have not been sufficiently studied. The placental infiltrate also commonly includes lymphocytes and less commonly polymorphonuclear cells, but natural killer (NK) cells appear to be absent [101, 138, 144]. The presence of placental monocytes and macrophages has been associated with severe maternal anemia and LBW across many populations (Table 2) [90, 101, 121, 137, 160]. Although many studies have demonstrated an association between placental malaria and LBW [26, 82], placental parasitemia in the absence of inflammation was not related to LBW in Zanzibar [101], suggesting that inflammation plays a key role in the genesis of fetal growth restriction. In Tanzania, monocytes were associated with LBW probably due to fetal growth restriction, whereas parasites were associated with premature delivery [121].

Current evidence suggests that in the absence of specific immunity, parasites accumulate in large numbers in the placenta, inducing an infiltrate of inflammatory cells, accelerated by expression of chemokines. Inflammatory

Table 2 Summary of studies since 1996 examining associations between maternal malaria and cellular immune responses (placental inflammatory cells, cytokines, and chemokines)

Measure	Study[a]	Population	Association with malaria[b]	Association with pregnancy outcome	Other
Intervillous inflammatory cells	Leopardi et al. 1996	Tanzania (Zanzibar)	Increased	Low birth weight	
	Ordi et al. 1998	Tanzania	Increased Massive intervillositis, particularly in PGs	Low birth weight Prematurity	
	Menendez et al. 2000	Tanzania	Increased mononuclear cells	Low birth weight (associated with monocytes)	Placental parasites associated with prematurity
	Ismail et al. 2000	Tanzania	Increased, particularly in PGs		
	Ordi et al. 2001	Tanzania	Increased monocytes, macrophages, CTLs	Reduced birth weight (for CD68[+] cells)	
	Rogerson et al. 2003	Malawi	Increased	Low birth weight Maternal anemia	
	McGready et al. 2004	Thai-Burma border	Increased in *P. falciparum*, but not *P. vivax*, infection; greater in PGs		Inflammatory cell numbers higher when infected close to delivery

Table 2 (continued)

Measure	Study[a]	Population	Association with malaria[b]	Association with pregnancy outcome	Other
Cytokines	Fried et al. 1998	Kenya[c]	↑ TNF-α	Low birth weight (for TNF-α and IFNγ)	
			↑ IFNγ, TGF-β1 among MGs ↔ IL-4, IL-6, IL-10, IL-2	Maternal anemia (for TNF-α)	
	Moore et al. 1999, 2000	Kenya[d]	↑ IFNγ in uninfected MGs ↑ TNF-α among infected PGs	Low birth weight (for TNF-α and IL-8)	↓ IFNγ, IL4, IL10 in HIV-1-infection
	Moorman et al. 1999	Malawi[e]	↑ TNF-α, IL-1β, TGF-β1 ↔ TNF-β, IL-10, IL-1α IFNγ not detected		
	Fievet et al. 2001	Cameroon	↑ TNF-α[c], IFNγ[d] ↔ IL-1, IL-4, IL-6, IL-10, TGF-β, GM-CSF		
	Rogerson et al. 2003	Malawi[f]	↑ TNF-α IFNγ levels generally low or undetectable	Low birth weight (for TNF-α)[g]	Levels not associated with HIV-1 infection

Table 2 (continued)

Measure	Study[a]	Population	Association with malaria[b]	Association with pregnancy outcome	Other
Chemokines	Abrams et al. 2002	Malawi	↑ MIP1α,β, MCP-1, IL-8, I-309 ↔ RANTES	Reduced birth weight (IL-8 and MIP-1β only)	Correlation between chemokines and monocyte density
	Suguitan et al. 2003	Cameroon	↑ MIP1α,β, MCP-1, IP-10 ↔ RANTES, IP-10, IL-8		
	Chaisavanee-yakorn et al. 2003	Kenya	↑ MIP1β ↔ MIP1α		

[a] Studies listed by date of publication. Not all findings from the studies listed have been included in the table (see text for details). Only recent papers have been listed. For comprehensive reviews, see Duffy 2001, Brabin et al. 2004

[b] Infection defined by presence of malaria parasites and/or parasite pigment

[c] Cytokines measured in placental serum/plasma

[d] Cytokines measured in cultures of stimulated placental intervillous mononuclear cells; results varied with different cell stimulants used

[e] Measured cytokine mRNA levels

[f] Cytokines measured in placental and peripheral blood; infection defined as placental or peripheral blood parasitemia

[g] Association did not remain significant in multivariate analysis

PGs, primigravidae; SGs, secundigravidae; MGs, multigravidae; ↔ no change/association; ↑ increased/raised; ↓ reduced/lower; CTL, cytotoxic lymphocyte; TNF, tumor necrosis factor; IFN, interferon; IL, interleukin; TGF, transforming growth factor; MIP, macrophage inflammatory protein; MCP, macrophage chemoattractant protein; IP, IFNγ-inducible protein cells may reduce parasite multiplication, but are inefficient for clearing parasitemia, allowing a prolonged inflammatory response associated with poor pregnancy outcomes including LBW and maternal anemia. The acquisition of specific antibody against placental-binding parasites may facilitate the clearance of parasites prior to the influx of inflammatory cells, thereby avoiding the cascade of events leading to disease and death.

Not long after the discovery of the malaria parasite, early observers described the heavy accumulation of pigment-containing phagocytic cells that can accompany malaria parasites in the placenta [21]. Pigment, or hemozoin, is the heme crystal generated by parasitized erythrocytes as they digest hemoglobin. Hemozoin indicates a current or recent episode of malaria, and can persist for an unknown and variable period of time after clearance of parasites, but perhaps as long as weeks [114, 196]. In Malawi, the presence or amount of hemozoin in the placenta was not specifically associated with pregnancy outcomes [182], but the presence of pigment has been associated with LBW in other studies [196].

The pathologic changes in a malarious placentae are most marked in the intervillous spaces, whereas pathology of the villous tissue during placental malaria is usually subtle [34, 35, 78, 137, 195]. In the syncytiotrophoblast layer, common findings include segmental loss of microvilli, pigment deposits, and focal necrosis adjacent to fibrinoid and pigment deposits (reviewed in [26, 58]). Below the syncytiotrophoblast layer, changes include cytotrophoblast proliferation, thickening of the cytotrophoblast basement membrane, and occasional pigment deposits in Hofbauer cells, cytotrophoblast, or stroma. Specifically, the inflammatory infiltrate does not involve the villi [34, 137, 195], and parasitemia is rarely patent in the fetal circulation.

5.2
Cytokines and Chemokines in Placental Malaria

Cytokines and chemokines most likely play key roles in the genesis of both the inflammatory response and the clinical sequelae (see Table 2). Placental levels of β and α chemokines increase during malaria and could promote the influx of immune cells into the placenta. Macrophage inflammatory protein (MIP)-1α and β, monocyte chemoattractant protein-1, I-309, and IL-8 (but not RANTES) are increased in placental infection [1, 38, 181] and levels correlate with monocyte density [1]. The expression of chemokine receptor CCR5 on the infiltrating macrophages [186] further supports a role for chemokine-induced ingress of the inflammatory infiltrate.

Healthy pregnancy appears to be generally biased toward anti-inflammatory or type 2 cytokines [75, 99, 107]. In an area of Kenya with heavy *P. falci-*

parum transmission, inflammatory cytokines including tumor necrosis factor (TNF)-α, interferon (IFN)γ, and interleukin (IL)-2 were elevated in the placentas of women, including women without parasitemia at delivery, compared to women in an area without malaria [75]. Raised levels of TNF-α, measured in plasma, mRNA, and leukocyte cultures, have been consistently associated with placental malaria in different populations [65, 75, 125, 156, 179]. During episodes of placental malaria, TNF-α and IL-8 are produced by the infiltrating macrophages [125], while IFNγ may derive in part from the chorionic villi of the placental tissue [179]. Severe maternal anemia and/or LBW have been related to TNF-α [75, 125, 156], IFNγ [75], and IL-8 [125]. In one study, IFNγ production by intervillous leukocytes was highest among uninfected multigravid women, perhaps suggesting a protective role for IFNγ [123].

In areas of stable transmission, the relationship between inflammatory cytokines and poor pregnancy outcomes appears to be strongest among primigravid women, who suffer disproportionately from malaria and malaria-related complications. This may be due to the chronicity of infection and the prolonged cytokine responses observed in this parity group [75]. The mass of placental parasites and macrophages that accumulate in the placenta could theoretically impair the transplacental exchange of oxygen and nutrients, but studies to test this hypothesis have failed to yield confirmatory evidence [58].

5.3
Changes in Cellular Immune Function During Pregnancy and Susceptibility

A number of changes in cell-mediated immune function have been reported in pregnant women that could substantially influence susceptibility to malaria. Lymphoproliferative responses of peripheral and placental blood lymphocytes to malaria and other antigens are reduced in pregnant women compared to their non-pregnant counterparts [64, 150]. Additionally, reflecting the accumulation of parasites seen in the placenta during infection, lymphoproliferative responses were found to be lower in placental than peripheral blood [143], although placental samples are also more likely to be contaminated with fetal cells known to suppress maternal responses. Recent studies have reported that lymphoproliferative responses to CSA-binding parasitized erythrocytes [66] and NK cell cytolytic activity in peripheral blood [23] were lower in primigravidae compared to multigravidae. HIV-1 infection can have profound effects on immune function and has been associated with altered cytokine responses to placental malaria. IFNγ and IL-12, which stimulates IFNγ production, were reduced among HIV-1-infected Kenyan women, and may contribute to a reduced capacity to clear placental infection [39, 124].

Hormone-mediated immunosuppression may contribute to the susceptibility of pregnant women to infection with *P. falciparum*. In particular,
increased serum cortisol levels are observed in pregnancy, being highest in
primigravid women in areas of malaria transmission [23, 143, 194], but these
differences are not marked and the progressive increase in cortisol during
pregnancy does not correspond to the prevalence of malaria which peaks
or plateaus in the second trimester. Increased cortisol levels were associated
with malaria during pregnancy in a Kenyan study [194], and because primigravidae are infected most frequently this may confound studies that compare
cortisol levels between parity groups. Similar associations were found in *P.
berghei*-infected pregnant mice [191]. Estrogens, progesterone, and other sex
hormones that are increased in pregnancy can influence the function and
development of T cells and production of cytokines that could contribute to
an increased susceptibility to *P. falciparum* [152]. Epidemiologic studies have
shown that women retain a higher susceptibility to malaria for several weeks
post-partum [54], suggesting that systemic changes induced by pregnancy
play a role in susceptibility to malaria, although trauma and surgery may also
increase malaria susceptibility for unknown reasons that may pertain to the
post-partum period.

6
Conclusion

Malaria during pregnancy is a major cause of maternal and fetal disease and
death. Pregnant women are infected with distinct variants of *P. falciparum*
that accumulate in the placenta through adhesion to specific receptors, such
as CSA. Over successive pregnancies, women acquire antibodies against placental and CSA-binding parasites, and these antibody responses have been
associated with protection from infection and disease. Recent research advances, reviewed here, have shed light on specific mechanisms of placental
infection, humoral and cellular immune responses, and the pathogenic processes of placental injury and maternal and fetal complications. This emerging
body of knowledge will increasingly lead to opportunities for the development
of therapeutic and preventative interventions, as well as new tools for diagnosis, monitoring, and identification of those at greatest risk. More broadly,
studies of malaria in pregnancy have provided unique insights into maternal
immune responses to infection, particularly in the placenta, and the complex
nature of host–parasite interactions in malaria. Such insights can only lead to
improvements in maternal and child health in the future.

Acknowledgements J. Beeson is supported by funding from the National Health and Medical Research Council of Australia (Career Development Award) and the Miller Fellowship of the Walter and Eliza Hall Institute of Medical Research. P. Duffy is supported by funding from the US National Institutes of Health (R01 AI52059), Bill & Melinda Gates Foundation, and the US Department of Defense. The views expressed in this article may not necessarily reflect those of the US Department of Defense.

References

1. Abrams ET, Brown H, Chensue SW, Turner GD, Tadesse E, Lema VM, Molyneux ME, Rochford R, Meshnick SR, Rogerson SJ (2003) Host Response to Malaria During Pregnancy: Placental Monocyte Recruitment Is Associated with Elevated beta Chemokine Expression. J Immunol 170:2759–2764

2. Achidi EA, Perlmann H, Salimonu LS, Asuzu MC, Perlmann P, Berzins K (1995) Antibodies to Pf155/RESA and circumsporozoite protein of *Plasmodium falciparum* in paired maternal-cord sera from Nigeria. Parasite Immunol 17:535–540

3. Achur RN, Valiyaveettil M, Alkhalil A, Ockenhouse CF, Gowda DC (2000) Characterization of proteoglycans of human placenta and identification of unique chondroitin sulfate proteoglycans of the intervillous spaces that mediate the adherence of *Plasmodium falciparum*-infected erythrocytes to the placenta. J Biol Chem 275:40344–56

4. Achur RN, Valiyaveettil M, Gowda DC (2003) The low sulfated chondroitin sulfate proteoglycans of human placenta have sulfate group-clustered domains that can efficiently bind *Plasmodium falciparum*-infected erythrocytes. J Biol Chem 278:11705–13

5. Alkhalil A, Achur RN, Valiyaveettil M, Ockenhouse CF, Gowda DC (2000) Structural requirements for the adherence of *Plasmodium falciparum*-infected erythrocytes to chondroitin sulfate proteoglycans of human placenta. J Biol Chem 275:40357–64

6. Andrews KT, Pirrit LA, Przyborski JM, Sanchez CP, Sterkers Y, Ricken S, Wickert H, Lepolard C, Avril M, Scherf A, Gysin J, Lanzer M (2003) Recovery of adhesion to chondroitin-4-sulphate in *Plasmodium falciparum* varCSA disruption mutants by antigenically similar PfEMP1 variants. Mol Microbiol 49:655–69

7. Anya SE (2004) Seasonal variation in the risk and causes of maternal death in the Gambia: malaria appears to be an important factor. Am J Trop Med Hyg 70:510–3

8. Astagneau P, Steketee RW, Wirima JJ, Khoromana CO, Millet P (1994) Antibodies to ring-infected erythrocyte surface antigen (Pf155/RESA) protect against *P.falciparum* parasitemia in highly exposed multigravid women in Malawi. Acta Trop 57:317–325

9. Beeson JG, Amin N, Kanjala M, Rogerson SJ (2002) Selective accumulation of mature asexual stages of *Plasmodium falciparum*-infected erythrocytes in the placenta. Infect Immun 70:5412–5415

10. Beeson JG, Brown GV (2002) Pathogenesis of *Plasmodium falciparum* malaria: the roles of parasite adhesion and antigenic variation. Cell Molec Life Sci 59:258–271

11. Beeson JG, Brown GV (2004) *Plasmodium falciparum*-infected erythrocytes demonstrate dual specificity for adhesion to hyaluronic acid and chondroitin sulfate A and have distinct adhesive properties. J Infect Dis 189:169–179

12. Beeson JG, Brown GV, Molyneux ME, Mhango C, Dzinjalamala F, Rogerson SJ (1999) *Plasmodium falciparum* isolates from infected pregnant women and children are associated with distinct adhesive and antigenic properties. J Infect Dis 180:464–472

13. Beeson JG, Chai W, Rogerson SJ, Lawson AM, Brown GV (1998) Inhibition of binding of malaria-infected erythrocytes by a tetradecasaccharide fraction from chondroitin sulfate A. Infect Immun 66:3397–3402

14. Beeson JG, Cooke BM, Rowe JA, Rogerson SJ (2002) Expanding the paradigms of placental malaria. Trends Parasitol 18:145–7

15. Beeson JG, Hallamore SL, Kelly G, Mann EJ, Elliott SR, Shulman CE, Cortes A, Reeder JC, Molyneux ME, Marsh K, Rogerson SJ, Brown GV (2003) Distinct antigenic determinants of placental-type *P. falciparum*-infected erythrocytes are frequently recognised by antibodies from pregnant women across diverse populations [abstract]. Exp Parasitol 105:30

16. Beeson JG, Mann EM, Elliott SR, Lema VM, Tadesse E, Molyneux ME, Brown GV, Rogerson SJ (2004) Antibodies to variant surface antigens of *Plasmodium falciparum*-infected erythrocytes and adhesion inhibitory antibodies are associated with placental malaria and have overlapping and distinct targets. J Infect Dis 189:540–551

17. Beeson JG, Reeder JC, Rogerson SJ, Brown GV (2001) Parasite adhesion and immune evasion in placental malaria. Trends Parasitol 17:331–337

18. Beeson JG, Rogerson SJ, Brown GV (2002) Evaluating specific adhesion of *Plasmodium falciparum*-infected erythrocytes to immobilised hyaluronic acid with comparison to binding of mammalian cells. Intl J Parasitol 32:1245–1252

19. Beeson JG, Rogerson SJ, Cooke BM, Reeder JC, Chai W, Lawson AM, Molyneux ME, Brown GV (2000) Adhesion of *Plasmodium falciparum*-infected erythrocytes to hyaluronic acid in placental malaria. Nature Med 6:86–90

20. Biggs BA, Goozé L, Wycherley K, Wollish W, Southwell B, Leech JH, Brown GV (1991) Antigenic variation in *Plasmodium falciparum*. Proc Natl Acad Sci USA 88:9171–9174

21. Bignami A (1898) Sulla questione della malaria congenita. Al Policlinico (Supplemento) 4:763–767

22. Bloland P, Slutsker L, Steketee RW, Wirima JJ, Heymann DL, Breman JG (1996) Rates and risk factors for mortality during the first two years of life in rural Malawi. Am J Trop Med Hyg 55:82–86

23. Bouyou-Akotet MK, Issifou S, Meye JF, Kombila M, Ngou-Milama E, Luty AJ, Kremsner PG, Mavoungou E (2004) Depressed natural killer cell cytotoxicity against *Plasmodium falciparum*-infected erythrocytes during first pregnancies. Clin Infect Dis 38:342–7

24. Brabin B (1992) Fetal anaemia in malarious areas: its causes and significance. Ann Trop Paediatr 12:303–10

25. Brabin BJ (1983) An analysis of malaria in pregnancy in Africa. Bull World Health Organ 61:1005–16

26. Brabin BJ, Romagosa C, Abdelgalil S, Menendez C, Verhoeff FH, McGready R, Fletcher KA, Owens S, D'Alessandro U, Nosten F, Fischer PR, Ordi J (2004) The sick placenta-the role of malaria. Placenta 25:359–78

27. Branch O, Udhayakumar V, Hightower A, Oloo A, Hawley W, Nahlen B, Bloland P, Kaslow D, Lal A (1998) A longitudinal investigation of IgG and IgM antibody responses to the merozoite surface protein-119-kiloDalton domain of *Plasmodium falciparum* in pregnant women and infants: associations with febrileillness, parasitemia, and anemia. Am J Trop Med Hyg 58:211–9

28. Bray RS, Anderson MJ (1979) Falciparum malaria and pregnancy. Trans R Soc Trop Med Hyg 73:427–431

29. Bray RS, Sinden RE (1979) The sequestration of *Plasmodium falciparum* infected erythrocytes in the placenta. Trans R Soc Trop Med Hyg 73:716–719

30. Brown KN, Brown IN (1965) Immunity to malaria: Antigenic variation in chronic infection of *Plasmodium knowlesi*. Nature 208:1286–1288

31. Buffet PA, Gamain B, Scheidig C, Baruch D, Smith JD, Hernandez-Rivas R, Pouvelle B, Oishi S, Fujii N, Fusai T, Parzy D, Miller LH, Gysin J, Scherf A (1999) *Plasmodium falciparum* domain mediating adhesion to chondroitin sulfate A: a receptor for human placental infection. Proc Natl Acad Sci U S A 96:12743–8

32. Bull PC, Lowe BS, Kaleli N, Njuga F, Kortok M, Ross A, Ndungu F, Snow RW, Marsh K (2002) *Plasmodium falciparum* infections are associated with agglutinating antibodies to parasite-infected erythrocyte surface antigens among healthy Kenyan children. J Infect Dis 185:1688–91

33. Bull PC, Lowe BS, Kortok M, Molyneux CS, Newbold CI, Marsh K (1998) Parasite antigens on the infected red cell surface are targets for naturally acquired immunity to malaria. Nature Med 4:358–360

34. Bulmer JN, Rasheed FN, Francis N, Morrison L, Greenwood BM (1993) Placental malaria II: a semi quantitative investigation of the pathological features. Histopathology 22:219–225

35. Bulmer JN, Rasheed FN, Francis N, Morrison L, Greenwood BM (1993) Placental malaria. I. Pathological classification. Histopathology 22:211–218

36. Chai W, Beeson JG, Kogelberg H, Brown GV, Lawson AM (2001) Inhibition of adhesion of *Plasmodium falciparum*-infected erythrocytes by structurally defined hyaluronic acid dodecasaccharides. Infect Immun 69:420–5

37. Chai W, Beeson JG, Lawson AM (2002) The structural motif in chondroitin sulfate for adhesion of *Plasmodium falciparum*-infected erythrocytes comprises disaccharide units of 4-*O*-sulfated and non-sulfated *N*-acetylgalactosamine linked to glucuronic acid. J Biol Chem 277:22438–22446

38. Chaisavaneeyakorn S, Moore JM, Mirel L, Othoro C, Otieno J, Chaiyaroj SC, Shi YP, Nahlen BL, Lal AA, Udhayakumar V (2003) Levels of macrophage inflammatory protein 1 alpha (MIP-1 alpha) and MIP-1 beta in intervillous blood plasma samples from women with placental malaria and human immunodeficiency virus infection. Clin Diagn Lab Immunol 10:631–6

39. Chaisavaneeyakorn S, Moore JM, Otieno J, Chaiyaroj SC, Perkins DJ, Shi YP, Nahlen BL, Lal AA, Udhayakumar V (2002) Immunity to placental malaria. III. Impairment of interleukin (IL)-12, not IL-18, and interferon-inducible protein-10 responses in the placental intervillous blood of human immunodeficiency virus/malaria-coinfected women. J Infect Dis 185:127–131

40. Chaiyaroj SC, Angkasekwinai P, Buranakiti A, Looareesuwan S, Rogerson SJ, Brown GV (1996) Cytoadherence characteristics of *Plasmodium falciparum* isolates from Thailand: Evidence for chondroitin sulfate A as a cytoadherence receptor. Am J Trop Med Hyg 55:76–80

41. Chen Q, Heddini A, Barragan A, Fernandez V, Pearce S, Wahlgren M (2000) The semiconserved head structure of *Plasmodium falciparum* erythrocyte membrane protein 1 mediates binding to multiple independent host receptors. J Exp Med 192:1–10

42. Clark HC (1915) The diagnostic value of the placental film in aestivo-autumnal malaria. J Exp Med 22:427–444

43. Cohen S, McGregor IA, Carrington SC (1961) Gamma-globulin and acquired immunity to human malaria. Nature 192:733–737

44. Colbourne MJ, Sowah EM (1956) Does milk protect infants against malaria? Trans R Soc Trop Med Hyg 50:82–90

45. Cooke BM, Rogerson SJ, Brown GV, Coppel RL (1996) Adhesion of malaria-infected red blood cells to chondroitin sulfate A under flow conditions. Blood 88:4040–4044

46. Costa FT, Fusai T, Parzy D, Sterkers Y, Torrentino M, Douki JB, Traore B, Petres S, Scherf A, Gysin J (2003) Immunization with recombinant duffy binding-like-gamma3 induces pan-reactive and adhesion-blocking antibodies against placental chondroitin sulfate A-binding *Plasmodium falciparum* parasites. J Infect Dis 188:153–64

47. Craig A, Scherf A (2001) Molecules on the surface of the *Plasmodium falciparum* infected erythrocyte and their role in malaria pathogenesis and immune evasion. Mol Biochem Parasitol 115:129–43

48. Creasey AM, Staalsoe T, Raza A, Arnot DE, Rowe JA (2003) Nonspecific immunoglobulin M binding and chondroitin sulfate A binding are linked phenotypes of *Plasmodium falciparum* isolates implicated in malaria during pregnancy. Infect Immun 71:4767–71

49. David PH, Hommel M, Miller LH, Udeinya IJ, Oligino LD (1983) Parasite sequestration in *Plasmodium falciparum* malaria: spleen and antibody modulation of cytoadherence of infected erythrocytes. Proc Natl Acad Sci USA 80:5075–5079

50. Degen R, Weiss N, Beck HP (2000) *Plasmodium falciparum*: cloned and expressed CIDR domains of PfEMP1 bind to chondroitin sulfate A. Exp Parasitol 95:113–121

51. Deloron P, Dubois B, Le Hesran JY, Riche D, Fievet N, Cornet M, Ringwald P, Cot M (1997) Isotypic analysis of maternally transmitted *Plasmodium falciparum*-specific antibodies in Cameroon, and relationship with risk of *P.falciparum* infection. Clin Exp Immunol 110:212–218

52. Deloron P, Steketee RW, Campbell GH, Peyron F, Kaseje DCO (1989) Serological reactivity to the ring-infected erythrocyte surface antigen and circumsporozoite protein in gravid and nulligravid women infected with *Plasmodium falciparum*. Trans R Soc Trop Med Hyg 83:58–62

53. Desowitz RS (1988) Prenatal immune priming in malaria: antigen-specific blastogenesis of cord blood lymphocytes from neonates born in a setting of holoendemic malaria. Ann Trop Med Parasitol 82:121–125

54. Diagne N, Rogier C, Sokhna CS, Tall A, Fontenille D, Roussilhon C, Spiegel A, Trape JF (2000) Increased susceptibility to malaria during the early postpartum period. New England Journal of Medicine 343:598–603

55. Douki JB, Sterkers Y, Lepolard C, Traore B, Costa FT, Scherf A, Gysin J (2003) Adhesion of normal and *Plasmodium falciparum* ring-infected erythrocytes to endothelial cells and the placenta involves the rhoptry-derived ring surface protein-2. Blood 101:5025–32

56. Duffy MF, Brown GV, Basuki W, Krejany EO, Noviyanti R, Cowman AF, Reeder JC (2002) Transcription of multiple var genes by individual, trophozoite-stage *Plasmodium falciparum* cells expressing a chondroitin sulphate A binding phenotype. Mol Microbiol 43:1285–93

57. Duffy MF, Byrne TJ, Elliott SR, Wilson DW, Rogerson SJ, Beeson JG, Noviyanti R, Brown GV (2005) Broad analysis reveals a consistent pattern of var gene transcription in Plasmodium falciparum repeatedly selected for a defined adhesion phenotype. Molec Microbiol 56:774–788

58. Duffy PE (2001) Immunity to malaria during pregnancy: different host, different parasite. In Duffy PE, Fried M (eds): Malaria in pregnancy Deadly parasite, susceptible host, Taylor and Francis, London, pp 71–126

59. Duffy PE, Desowitz RS (2001) Pregnancy malaria throughout history: dangerous labors. In Duffy PE, Fried M (eds): Malaria in pregnancy: deadly parasite, susceptible host, Taylor and Francis, London, pp 1–26

60. Duffy PE, Fried M (2003) Antibodies that inhibit *Plasmodium falciparum* adhesion to chondroitin sulfate A are associated with increased birth weight and the gestational age of newborns. Infect Immun 71:6620–3

61. Edozien JC, Gilles HM, Udeozo IQK (1962) Adult and cord blood gamma globulin and immunity to malaria in Nigerians. Lancet 2:951–955

62. Elliott SR, Duffy MF, Byrne TJ, Beeson JG, Mann EJ, Wilson DW, Rogerson SJ, Brown GV (2005) Cross-reactive surface epitopes on chondroitin sulfate A-adherent *Plasmodium falciparum* infected erythrocytes are associated with transcription of var2csa. Infect Immun 73:2848–2856

63. Fernandez V, Hommel M, Chen Q, Hagblom P, Wahlgren M (1999) Small, clonally variant antigens expressed on the surface of *Plasmodium falciparum*-infected erythrocytes are encoded by the *rif* gene family and are targets of human immune responses. J Exp Med 190:1393–1403

64. Fievet N, Cot M, Chougnet C, Maubert B, Bickii J, Dubois B, Le Hesran JY, Frobert Y, Migot F, Romain F, Verhave JP, Louis F, Deloron P (1995) Malaria and pregnancy in Cameroonian primigravidae: Humoral and cellular immune responses to *Plasmodium falciparum* blood-stage antigens. Am J Trop Med Hyg 53:612–617

65. Fievet N, Moussa M, Tami G, Maubert B, Cot M, Deloron P, Chaouat G (2001) *Plasmodium falciparum* induces a Th1/Th2 disequilibrium, favoring the Th1-type pathway, in the human placenta. J Infect Dis 183:1530–1534

66. Fievet N, Tami G, Maubert B, Moussa M, Shaw IK, Cot M, Holder AA, Chaouat G, Deloron P (2002) Cellular immune response to *Plasmodium falciparum* after pregnancy is related to previous placental infection and parity. Malar J 1:16

67. Fleming AF (1989) Tropical obstetrics and gynaecology. 1. Anaemia in pregnancy in tropical Africa. Trans Roy Soc Trop Med Hyg 83:441–448

68. Flick K, Scholander C, Chen Q, Fernandez V, Pouvelle B, Gysin J, Wahlgren M (2001) Role of nonimmune IgG bound to PfEMP1 in placental malaria. Science 293:2098–100
69. Florens L, Liu X, Wang Y, Yang S, Schwartz O, Peglar M, Carucci DJ, Yates JR, 3rd, Wub Y (2004) Proteomics approach reveals novel proteins on the surface of malaria-infected erythrocytes. Mol Biochem Parasitol 135:1–11
70. Fried M, Duffy PE (1995) Chondroitin sulfate A is the adhesion receptor for *Plasmodium falciparum*-infected erythrocytes in the human placenta [Abstract]. Mol Biol Cell 6:47
71. Fried M, Duffy PE (1996) Adherence of *Plasmodium falciparum* to chondroitin sulfate A in the human placenta. Science 272:1502–1504
72. Fried M, Duffy PE (1998) Maternal malaria and parasite adhesion. J Mol Med 76:162–171
73. Fried M, Duffy PE (2002) Two DBLgamma subtypes are commonly expressed by placental isolates of *Plasmodium falciparum*. Mol Biochem Parasitol 122:201–10
74. Fried M, Lauder RM, Duffy PE (2000) *Plasmodium falciparum*: adhesion of placental isolates modulated by the sulfation characteristics of the glycosaminoglycan receptor. Exp Parasitol 95:75–8
75. Fried M, Muga RO, Misore AO, Duffy PE (1998) Malaria elicits type 1 cytokines in the human placenta: IFN-γ and TNF-α associated with pregnancy outcomes. J Immunol 160:2523–2530
76. Fried M, Nosten F, Brockman A, Brabin BJ, Duffy PE (1998) Maternal antibodies block malaria. Nature 395:851–852
77. Fried M, Wendler JP, Mutabingwa TK, Duffy PE (2004) Mass spectrometric analysis of *Plasmodium falciparum* erythrocyte membrane protein-1 variants expressed by placental malaria parasites. Proteomics 4:1086–93
78. Galbraith RM, Fox H, Hsi B, Galbraith GM, Bray RS, Faulk WP (1980) The human materno-foetal relationship in malaria. II. Histological, ultrastructural and immunopathological studies of the placenta. Trans R Soc Trop Med Hyg 74:61–72
79. Gamain B, Smith JD, Avril M, Baruch DI, Scherf A, Gysin J, Miller LH (2004) Identification of a 67-amino-acid region of the *Plasmodium falciparum* variant surface antigen that binds chondroitin sulphate A and elicits antibodies reactive with the surface of placental isolates. Mol Microbiol 53:445–55
80. Gamain B, Smith JD, Miller LH, Baruch DI (2001) Modifications in the CD36 binding domain of the *Plasmodium falciparum* variant antigen are responsible for the inability of chondroitin sulfate A adherent parasites to bind CD36. Blood 97:3268–74
81. Gardner JP, Pinches RA, Roberts DJ, Newbold CI (1996) Variant antigens and endothelial receptor adhesion in *Plasmodium falciparum*. Proc Natl Acad Sci USA 93:3503–3508
82. Garner P, Brabin B (1994) A review of randomized controlled trials of routine antimalarial drug prophylaxis during pregnancy in endemic malarious areas. Bull WHO 72:89–99
83. Garnham PCC (1938) The placenta in malaria with special reference to reticuloendothelial immunity. Trans R Soc Hyg Trop Med 32:13–48

84. Gerlitz B, Hassell T, Vlahos CJ, Parkinson JF, Bang NU, Grinnell BW (1993) Identification of the predominant glycosaminoglycan-attachment site in soluble recombinant human thrombomodulin: potential regulation of functionality by glycosyltransferase competition for serine[474]. Biochem J 295:131–140

85. Granja AC, Machungo F, Gomes A, Bergstrom S, Brabin B (1998) Malaria-related maternal mortality in urban Mozambique. Ann Trop Med Parasitol 92:257–263

86. Gysin J, Pouvelle B, Fievet N, Scherf A, Lepolard C (1999) Ex vivo desequestration of *Plasmodium falciparum*-infected erythrocytes from human placenta by chondroitin sulfate A. Infect Immun 67:6596–6602

87. Gysin J, Pouvelle B, Le Tonqueze M, Edelman L, Boffa M-C (1997) Chondroitin sulfate of thrombomodulin is an adhesion receptor for *Plasmodium falciparum*-infected erythrocytes. Mol Biochem Parasitol 88:267–271

88. Hogh B, Marbiah NT, Burghaus PA, Andersen PK (1995) Relationship between maternally derived anti-*Plasmodium falciparum* antibodies and risk of infection and disease in infants living in an area of Liberia, West Africa, in which malaria is highly endemic. Infect Immun 63:4034–4038

89. Ismail MR, Ordi J, Menendez C, Ventura PJ, Aponte JJ, Kahigwa E, Hirt R, Cardesa A, Alonso PL (2000) Placental pathology in malaria: a histological, immunohistochemical, and quantitative study. Hum Pathol 31:85–93

90. Jilly P (1969) Anaemia in parturient women, with special reference to malaria infection of the placenta. Ann Trop Med Parasitol 63:109–16

91. Khattab A, Kremsner PG, Klinkert MQ (2003) Common surface-antigen var genes of limited diversity expressed by *Plasmodium falciparum* placental isolates separated by time and space. J Infect Dis 187:477–83

92. Khattab A, Kun J, Deloron P, Kremsner PG, Klinkert MQ (2001) Variants of *Plasmodium falciparum* erythrocyte membrane protein 1 expressed by different placental parasites are closely related and adhere to chondroitin sulfate A. J Infect Dis 183:1165–9

93. Khattab A, Reinhardt C, Staalsoe T, Fievet N, Kremsner PG, Deloron P, Hviid L, Klinkert MQ (2004) Analysis of IgG with specificity for variant surface antigens expressed by placental *Plasmodium falciparum* isolates. Malar J 3:21

94. King CL, Malhotra I, Wamachi A, Kioko J, Mungai P, Wahab SA, Koech D, Zimmerman P, Ouma J, Kazura JW (2002) Acquired immune responses to *Plasmodium falciparum* merozoite surface protein-1 in the human fetus. J Immunol 168:356–64

95. Kinyanjui SM, Bull P, Newbold CI, Marsh K (2003) Kinetics of antibody responses to *Plasmodium falciparum*-infected erythrocyte variant surface antigens. J Infect Dis 187:667–674

96. Kraemer SM, Smith JD (2003) Evidence for the importance of genetic structuring to the structural and functional specialization of the *Plasmodium falciparum* var gene family. Mol Microbiol 50:1527–38

97. Kyes SA, Christodoulou Z, Raza A, Horrocks P, Pinches R, Rowe JA, Newbold CI (2003) A well-conserved *Plasmodium falciparum* var gene shows an unusual stage-specific transcript pattern. Mol Microbiol 48:1339–48

98. Kyes SA, Rowe JA, Kriek N, Newbold CI (1999) Rifins: A second family of clonally variant proteins expressed on the surface of red cells infected with *Plasmodium falciparum*. Proc Natl Acad Sci USA 96:9333–9338

99. Lea RG, Calder AA (1997) The immunology of pregnancy. Curr Opin Infect Dis 10:171–176

100. Lekana Douki J-B, Traore B, Costa FTM, Fusai T, Pouvelle B, Sterkers Y, Scherf A, Gysin J (2002) Sequestration of *Plasmodium falciparum*-infected erythrocytes to chondroitin sulfate A, a receptor for maternal malaria: monoclonal antibodies against the native parasite ligand reveal pan-reactive epitopes in placental isolates. Blood 100:1478–1483

101. Leopardi O, Naughten W, Salvia L, Colecchia M, Matteelli A, Zucchi A, Shein A, Muchi JA, Carosi G, Ghione M (1996) Malaric placentas. A quantitative study and clinico-pathological correlations. Path Res Pract 192:892–898

102. Mackintosh CL, Beeson JG, Marsh K (2004) Clinical features and pathogenesis of severe malaria. Trends Parasitol in press

103. MacPherson GG, Warrell MJ, White NJ, Looareesuwan S, Warrell DA (1985) Human cerebral malaria. A quantitative ultrastructural analysis of parasitized erythrocyte sequestration. Am J Pathol 119:385–401

104. Marsh K, Howard RJ (1986) Antigens induced on erythrocytes by *P. falciparum*: expression of diverse and conserved determinants. Science 231:150–153

105. Marsh K, Otoo L, Hayes RJ, Carson DC, Greenwood BM (1989) Antibodies to blood stage antigens of *Plasmodium falciparum* in rural Gambians and their relation to protection against infection. Trans R Soc Trop Med Hyg 83:293–303

106. Maruyama I, Bell CE, Majerus PW (1985) Thrombomodulin is found on endothelium of arteries, veins, capillaries, and lymphatics, and on syncytiotrophoblast of human placenta. J Cell Biol 101:363–371

107. Marzi M, Vigano A, Trabattoni D, Villa ML, Salvaggio A, Clerici E, Clerici M (1996) Characterization of type 1 and type 2 cytokine production profile in physiologic and pathologic human pregnancy. Clin Exp Immunol 106:127–33

108. Matejevic D, Neudeck H, Graf R, Muller T, Dietl J (2001) Localization of hyaluronan with a hyaluronan-specific hyaluronic acid binding protein in the placenta in preeclampsia. Gynecol Obstet Invest 52:257–9

109. Maubert B, Fievet N, Tami G, Boudin C, Deloron P (1998) *Plasmodium falciparum*-isolates from Cameroonian pregnant women do not rosette. Parasite 5:281–3

110. Maubert B, Fievet N, Tami G, Boudin C, Deloron P (2000) Cytoadherence of *Plasmodium falciparum*-infected erythrocytes in the human placenta. Parasite Immunol 22:191–9

111. Maubert B, Fievet N, Tami G, Cot M, Boudin C, Deloron P (1999) Development of antibodies against chondroitin sulfate A-adherent *Plasmodium falciparum* in pregnant women. Infect Immun 67:5367–5371

112. McCormick MC (1985) The contribution of low birth weight to infant mortality and child morbidity. N Engl J Med 312:82–90

113. McGilvray ID, Serghides L, Kapus A, Rotstein OD, Kain KC (2000) Nonopsonic monocyte/macrophage phagocytosis of *Plasmodium falciparum*-parasitized erythrocytes: a role for CD36 in malarial clearance. Blood 96:3231–40

114. McGready R, Davison BB, Stepniewska K, Cho T, Shee H, Brockman A, Udomsangpetch R, Looareesuwan S, White NJ, Meshnick SR, Nosten F (2004) The effects of *Plasmodium falciparum* and P. vivax infections on placental histopathology in an area of low malaria transmission. Am J Trop Med Hyg 70:398–407

115. McGregor I (1984) Epidemiology, malaria and pregnancy. American Journal of Tropical Medicine and Hygiene 33:517–525
116. McGregor IA, Carrington S (1961) Gamma-globulin and acquired immunity to human malaria. Nature 192:733–737
117. McGregor IA, Wilson ME, Billewicz WZ (1983) Malaria infection of the placenta in The Gambia, West Africa; its incidence and relationship to stillbirth, birthweight and placental weight. Trans R Soc Trop Med Hyg 77:232–244
118. McLean SA, Pearson CD, Phillips RS (1982) *Plasmodium chabaudi*: antigenic variation during recrudescent parasitaemias in mice. Exp Parasitol 54:296–302
119. Mendis K, Sina BJ, Marchesini P, Carter R (2001) The neglected burden of Plasmodium vivax malaria. Am J Trop Med Hyg 64:97–106
120. Menendez C (1995) Malaria during pregnancy: a priority area of malaria research and control. Parasitol Today 11:178–183
121. Menendez C, Ordi J, Ismail MR, Ventura PJ, Aponte JJ, Kahigwa E, Font F, Alonso PL (2000) The impact of placental malaria on gestational age and birth weight. J Infect Dis 181:1740–5
122. Miller LH, Baruch DI, Marsh K, Doumbo OK (2002) The pathogenic basis of malaria. Nature 415:673–9
123. Moore J, Nahlen B, Misore A, Lal A, Udhayakumar V (1999) Immunity to placental malaria. I. Elevated production of interferon-gamma by placental blood mononuclear cells is associated with protection in an area with hightransmission of malaria. J Infect Dis 179:1218–25
124. Moore JM, Ayisi J, Nahlen BL, Misore A, Lal AA, Udhayakumar V (2000) Immunity to placental malaria. II. Placental antigen-specific cytokine responses are impaired in human immunodeficiency virus-infected women. J Infect Dis 182:960–964
125. Moormann AM, Sullivan AD, Rochford RA, Chensue SW, Bock PJ, Nyirenda T, Meshnick SR (1999) Malaria and pregnancy: placental cytokine expression and its relationship to intrauterine growth retardation. J Infect Dis 180:1987–93
126. Mount AM, Mwapasa V, Elliott SR, Beeson JG, Tadesse E, Lema VM, Molyneux ME, Meshnick SR, Rogerson SJ (2004) Impairment of humoral immunity to *Plasmodium falciparum* malaria in pregnancy by HIV infection. Lancet 363:1860–7
127. Murphy SC, Breman JG (2001) Gaps in the childhood malaria burden in Africa: cerebral malaria, neurological sequelae, anemia, respiratory distress, hypoglycemia, and complications of pregnancy. Am J Trop Med Hyg 64 (Suppl):57–67
128. Muthusamy A, Achur RN, Bhavanandan VP, Fouda GG, Taylor DW, Gowda DC (2004) *Plasmodium falciparum*-infected erythrocytes adhere both in the intervillous space and on the villous surface of human placenta by binding to the low-sulfated chondroitin sulfate proteoglycan receptor. Am J Pathol 164:2013–25
129. Mvondo JL, James MA, Sulzer AJ, Campbell CC (1992) Malaria and pregnancy in Cameroonian women. Naturally acquired antibody responses to asexual blood-stage antigens and the circumsporozoite protein of *Plasmodium falciparum*. Trans R Soc Trop Med Hyg 86:486–490
130. Nanaev AK, Milovanov AP, Domogatsky SP (1993) Immunohistochemical localization of extracellular matrix in perivillous fibrinoid of normal human term placenta. Histochemistry 100:341–6

131. Nosten F, McGready R, Simpson JA, Thwai KL, Balkan S, Cho T, Hkirijaroen L, Looareesuwan S, White NJ (1999) Effects of *Plasmodium vivax* malaria in pregnancy. Lancet 354:546–9

132. Nosten F, Rogerson SJ, Beeson JG, McGready R, Mutabingwa TK, Brabin B (2004) Malaria in pregnancy and the endemicity spectrum: what can we learn? Trends Parasitol 20:425–32

133. Nosten F, ter Kuile F, Maelankirri L, Decludt B, White NJ (1991) Malaria during pregnancy in an area of unstable endemicity. Trans R Soc Trop Med Hyg 85:424–9

134. Noviyanti R, Brown GV, Wickham ME, Duffy MF, Cowman AF, Reeder JC (2001) Multiple var gene transcripts are expressed in *Plasmodium falciparum* infected erythrocytes selected for adhesion. Mol Biochem Parasitol 114:227–37

135. Ockenhouse CF, Ho M, Tandon NN, Van-Seventer GA, Shaw S, White NJ, Jamieson GA, Chulay JD, Webster HK (1991) Molecular basis of sequestration in severe and uncomplicated *Plasmodium falciparum* malaria: Differential adhesion of infected erythrocytes to CD36 and ICAM-1. J Infect Dis 164:163–169

136. O'Neil-Dunne I, Achur RN, Agbor-Enoh ST, Valiyaveettil M, Naik RS, Ockenhouse CF, Zhou A, Megnekou R, Leke R, Taylor DW, Gowda DC (2001) Gravidity-dependent production of antibodies that inhibit binding of *Plasmodium falciparum*-infected erythrocytes to placental chondroitin sulfate proteoglycan during pregnancy. Infect Immun 69:7487–92

137. Ordi J, Ismail MR, Ventura P, Kahigwa E, Hirt R, Cardesa A, Alonso P, Menendez C (1998) Massive chronic intervillositis of the placenta associated with malarial infection. Am J Surg Path 22:1006–1011

138. Ordi J, Menendez C, Ismail MR, Ventura PJ, Palacin A, Kahigwa E, Ferrer B, Cardesa A, Alonso PL (2001) Placental malaria is associated with cell-mediated inflammatory responses with selective absence of natural killer cells. J Infect Dis 183:1100–7

139. Parmley RT, Takagi M, Denys FR (1984) Ultrastructural localization of glycosaminoglycans in human term placenta. Anat Rec 210:477–484

140. Pasvol G, Weatherall DJ, Wilson RJ, Smith DH, Gilles HM (1976) Fetal haemoglobin and malaria. Lancet 1:1269–72

141. Pouvelle B, Buffet PA, Lepolard C, Scherf A, Gysin J (2000) Cytoadhesion of *Plasmodium falciparum* ring-stage-infected erythrocytes. Nature Med 6:1264–1268

142. Pouvelle B, Fusai T, Lepolard C, Gysin J (1998) Biological and biochemical characteristics of cytoadhesion of *Plasmodium falciparum*-infected erythrocytes to chondroitin-4-sulfate. Infect Immun 66:4950–6

143. Rasheed FN, Bulmer JN, Dunn DT, Mendendez C, Jawla MFB, Jepson A, Jakobsen PH, Greenwood BM (1993) Suppressed peripheral and placental blood lymphoproliferative responses in first pregnancies: relevance to malaria. Am J Trop Med Hyg 48:154–160

144. Rasheed FN, Bulmer JN, Morrison L, Jawla MFB, Greenwood BM (1992) Isolation of maternal mononuclear cells from placenta for use in in vitro functional assays. J Immunol Methods 146:185–193

145. Redd SC, Wirima JJ, Steketee RW, Breman JG, Heymann DL (1996) Transplancental transmission of *Plasmodium falciparum* in rural Malawi. Am J Trop Med Hyg 55:57–60

146. Reeder JC, Cowman AF, Davern KM, Beeson JG, Thompson JK, Rogerson SJ, Brown GV (1999) The adhesion of *Plasmodium falciparum*-infected erythrocytes to chondroitin sulfate A is mediated by PfEMP1. Proc Natl Acad Sci USA 96:5198–5202

147. Reeder JC, Hodder AN, Beeson JG, Brown GV (2000) Identification of glycosaminoglycan binding domains in *Plasmodium falciparum* erythrocyte membrane protein 1 of a chondroitin sulfate A-adherent parasite. Infect Immun 68:3923–6

148. Reeder JC, Rogerson SJ, Al-Yaman F, Anders RF, Coppel RL, Novakovic S, Alpers MP, Brown GV (1994) Diversity of agglutinating phenotype, cytoadherence, and rosette-forming characteristics of *Plasmodium falciparum* isolates from Papua New Guinean children. Am J Trop Med Hyg 51:45–55

149. Ricke CH, Staalsoe T, Koram K, Akanmori BD, Riley EM, Theander TG, Hviid L (2000) Plasma antibodies from malaria-exposed pregnant women recognize variant surface antigens on *Plasmodium falciparum*-infected erythrocytes in a parity-dependent manner and block parasite adhesion to chondroitin sulfate A. J Immunol 165:3309–16

150. Riley EM, Schneider G, Sambou I, Greenwood BM (1989) Suppression of cell-mediated immune responses to malaria antigens in pregnant Gambian women. Am J Trop Med Hyg 40:141–144

151. Robert C, Pouvelle B, Meyer P, Muanza K, Fukioka H, Aikawa M, Scherf A, Gysin J (1995) Chondroitin-4-sulphate (proteoglycan), a receptor for *Plasmodium falciparum*-infected erythrocyte adherence on brain microvascular endothelial cells. Res Immunol 146:383–393

152. Roberts C, Satoskar A, Alexander J (1996) Sex steroids, pregnancy-associated hormones and immunity to parasitic infections. Parasitol Today 12:382–8

153. Roberts DJ, Biggs B-A, Brown G, Newbold CI (1994) Protection, pathogenesis and phenotypic plasticity in *Plasmodium falciparum* malaria. Parasitol Today 9:281–286

154. Rogerson SJ, Beeson JG (1999) The placenta in malaria: mechanisms of infection, disease and fetal morbidity. Ann Trop Med Parasitol 93 Suppl. 1:S35–42

155. Rogerson SJ, Beeson JG, Mhango C, Dzinjalamala F, Molyneux ME (2000) *Plasmodium falciparum* rosette formation is uncommon in isolates from pregnant women. Infect Immun 68:391–3

156. Rogerson SJ, Brown HC, Pollina E, Abrams ET, Tadesse E, Lema VM, Molyneux ME (2003) Placental tumor necrosis factor alpha but not gamma interferon is associated with placental malaria and low birth weight in Malawian women. Infect Immun 71:267–70

157. Rogerson SJ, Chaiyaroj SC, Ng K, Reeder JC, Brown GV (1995) Chondroitin sulfate A is a cell surface receptor for *Plasmodium falciparum*-infected erythrocytes. J Exp Med 182:15–20

158. Rogerson SJ, Mkundika P, Kanjala MK (2003) Diagnosis of *Plasmodium falciparum* malaria at delivery: a comparison of blood film preparation methods, and of blood films with histology. J Clin Microbiol 41:1370–1374

159. Rogerson SJ, Novakovic S, Cooke BM, Brown GV (1997) *Plasmodium falciparum*-infected erythrocytes adhere to the proteoglycan thrombomodulin in static and flow-based systems. Exp Parasitol 86:8–18

160. Rogerson SJ, Pollina E, Getachew A, Tadesse E, Lema VM, Molyneux ME (2003) Placental monocyte infiltrates in response to *Plasmodium falciparum* malaria infection and their association with adverse pregnancy outcomes. Am J Trop Med Hyg 68:115–119

161. Rogerson SJ, Tembenu R, Dobano C, Plitt S, Taylor TE, Molyneux ME (1999) Cytoadherence characteristics of *Plasmodium falciparum*-infected erythrocytes from Malawian children with severe and uncomplicated malaria. Am J Trop Med Hyg 61:467–72

162. Rowe JA, Kyes SA (2004) The role of *Plasmodium falciparum* var genes in malaria in pregnancy. Mol Microbiol 53:1011–9

163. Rowe JA, Kyes SA, Rogerson SJ, Babiker HA, Raza A (2002) Identification of a conserved *Plasmodium falciparum var* gene implicated in malaria in pregnancy. J Infect Dis 185:1207–1211

164. Salanti A, Jensen AT, Zornig HD, Staalsoe T, Joergensen L, Nielsen MA, Khattab A, Arnot DE, Klinkert MQ, Hviid L, Theander TG (2002) A sub-family of common and highly conserved *Plasmodium falciparum* var genes. Mol Biochem Parasitol 122:111–5

165. Salanti A, Staalsoe T, Lavstsen T, Jensen AT, Sowa MP, Arnot DE, Hviid L, Theander TG (2003) Selective upregulation of a single distinctly structured var gene in chondroitin sulphate A-adhering *Plasmodium falciparum* involved in pregnancy-associated malaria. Mol Microbiol 49:179–91

166. Sholapurkar SL, Mahajan RC, Gupta AN, Prasad RN (1988) Malarial parasite density in infected pregnant women from northern India. Indian J Med Res 88:228–30

167. Shulman CE, Marshall T, Dorman EK, Bulmer JN, Cutts F, Peshu N, Marsh K (2001) Malaria in pregnancy: adverse effects on haemoglobin levels and birthweight in primigravidae and multigravidae. Trop Med Int Hlth 6:770–778

168. Silamut K, Phu NH, Whitty C, Turner GDH, Louwrier K, Mai NTH, Simpson JA, Hien TT, White NJ (1999) A quantitative analysis of the microvascular sequestration of malaria parasites in the human brain. Am J Pathol 155:395–410

169. Singh N, Saxena A, Chand SK, Valecha N, Sharma VP (1998) Studies on malaria during pregnancy in a tribal area of central India (Madhya Pradesh). Southeast Asian J Trop Med Public Health 29:10–7

170. Singh N, Shukla MM, Sharma VP (1999) Epidemiology of malaria in pregnancy in central India. Bull World Health Organ 77:567–72

171. Smith JD, Chitnis CE, Craig AG, Roberts DJ, Hudson-Taylor DE, Peterson DS, Pinches R, Newbold CI, Miller LH (1995) Switches in expression of *Plasmodium falciparum var* genes correlate with changes in antigenic and cytoadherent phenotypes of infected erythrocytes. Cell 82:101–110

172. Smith JD, Miller LH (2004) Infected erythrocyte binding to hyaluronic acid and malaria in pregnant women. J Infect Dis 189:165–8

173. Smith JD, Subramanian G, Gamain B, Baruch DI, Miller LH (2000) Classification of adhesive domains in the *Plasmodium falciparum* erythrocyte membrane protein 1 family. Mol Biochem Parasitol 110:293–310

174. Staalsoe T, Giha HA, Dodoo D, Theander TG, Hviid L (1999) Detection of antibodies to variant antigens on *Plasmodium falciparum* infected erythrocytes by flow cytometry. Cytometry 35:329–336

175. Staalsoe T, Megnekou R, Fievet N, Ricke CH, Zornig HD, Leke R, Taylor DW, Deloron P, Hviid L (2001) Acquisition and decay of antibodies to pregnancy-associated variant antigens on the surface of *Plasmodium falciparum*-infected erythrocytes that protect against placental parasitemia. J Infect Dis 184:618–26

176. Staalsoe T, Shulman CE, Bulmer JN, Kawuondo K, Marsh K, Hviid L (2004) Variant surface antigen-specific IgG and protection against clinical consequences of pregnancy-associated *Plasmodium falciparum* malaria. Lancet 263:283–289

177. Steketee RW, Nahlen BL, Parise ME, Menendez C (2001) The burden of malaria in pregnancy in malaria-endemic areas. Am J Trop Med Hyg 64 (Suppl):28–35

178. Steketee RW, Wirima JJ, Bloland PB, Chilima B, Mermin JH, Chitsulo L, Breman JG (1996) Impairment of a pregnant woman's acquired ability to limit *Plasmodium falciparum* by infection with human immunodeficiency virus type-1. Am J Trop Med Hyg 55:42–49

179. Suguitan AL, Jr., Cadigan TJ, Nguyen TA, Zhou A, Leke RJ, Metenou S, Thuita L, Megnekou R, Fogako J, Leke RG, Taylor DW (2003) Malaria-associated cytokine changes in the placenta of women with pre-term deliveries in Yaounde, Cameroon. Am J Trop Med Hyg 69:574–81

180. Suguitan AL, Jr., Gowda DC, Fouda G, Thuita L, Zhou A, Djokam R, Metenou S, Leke RG, Taylor DW (2004) Lack of an association between antibodies to *Plasmodium falciparum* glycosylphosphatidylinositols and malaria-associated placental changes in Cameroonian women with preterm and full-term deliveries. Infect Immun 72:5267–73

181. Suguitan AL, Jr., Leke RG, Fouda G, Zhou A, Thuita L, Metenou S, Fogako J, Megnekou R, Taylor DW (2003) Changes in the levels of chemokines and cytokines in the placentas of women with *Plasmodium falciparum* malaria. J Infect Dis 188:1074–82

182. Sullivan AD, Nyirenda T, Cullinan T, Taylor T, Lau A, Meshnick SR (2000) Placental haemozoin and malaria in pregnancy. Placenta 21:417–421

183. Sunderland CA, Bulmer JN, Luscombe M, Redman CWG, Stirrat GM (1985) Immunohistological and biochemical evidence for a role for hyaluronic acid in the growth and development of the placenta. J Reproduct Immunol 8:197–212

184. Taylor DW, Zhou A, Marsillio LE, Thuita LW, Leke EB, Branch O, Gowda DC, Long C, Leke RF (2004) Antibodies that inhibit binding of *Plasmodium falciparum*-infected erythrocytes to chondroitin sulfate A and to the C terminus of merozoite surface protein 1 correlate with reduced placental malaria in Cameroonian women. Infect Immun 72:1603–7

185. Tegoshi T, Desowitz RS, Pirl KG, Maeno Y, Aikawa M (1992) Placental pathology in Plasmodium berghei-infected rats. Am J Trop Med Hyg 47:643–51

186. Tkachuk AN, Moormann AM, Poore JA, Rochford RA, Chensue SW, Mwapasa V, Meshnick SR (2001) Malaria enhances expression of CC chemokine receptor 5 on placental macrophages. J Infect Dis 183:967–72

187. Udeinya IJ, Miller LH, McGregor IA, Jensen JB (1983) *Plasmodium falciparum* strain-specific antibody blocks binding of infected erythrocytes to amelanotic melanoma cells. Nature 303:429–431

188. Udeinya IJ, Schmidt JA, Aikawa M, Miller LH, Green I (1981) *Falciparum* malaria-infected erythrocytes specifically bind to cultured human endothelial cells. Science 213:555–557

189. Valiyaveettil M, Achur RN, Alkhalil A, Ockenhouse CF, Gowda DC (2001) *Plasmodium falciparum* cytoadherence to human placenta: evaluation of hyaluronic acid and chondroitin 4-sulfate for binding of infected erythrocytes. Exp Parasitol 99:57–65

190. Van Eijk AM, Ayisi JG, Ter Kuile FO, Misore A, Otieno JA, Kolczak MS, Kager PA, Steketee RW, Nahlen BL (2001) Human immunodeficiency virus seropositivity and malaria as risk factors for third-trimester anemia in asymptomatic pregnant women in Western Kenya. Am J Trop Med Hyg 65:623–630

191. van Zon A, Eling W, Hermsen C, Koekkoek A (1982) Corticosterone regulation of the effector function of malarial immunity during pregnancy. Infect Immun 36:484–91

192. Verhoeff F, Brabin B, Chimsuku L, Kazembe P, Broadhead R (1999) Malaria in pregnancy and its consequences for the infant in rural Malawi. Ann Trop Med Parasitol 93 Suppl 1:S25–33

193. Verhoeff FH, Brabin BJ, Hart CA, Chimsuku L, Kazembe P, Broadhead R (1999) Increased prevalence of malaria in HIV infected pregnant women and its implications for malaria control. Trop Med Inter Hlth 4:5–12

194. Vleugels MPH, Brabin B, Eling WMC, de Graaf R (1989) Cortisol and *Plasmodium falciparum* infection in pregnant women in Kenya. Trans R Soc Trop Med Hyg 83:173–177

195. Walter PR, Garin Y, Blot P (1982) Placental pathologic changes in malaria. A histologic and ultrastructural study. Am J Pathol 109:330–342

196. Watkinson M, Rushton DI (1983) Plasmodial pigmentation of placentae and outcome of pregnancy in West African mothers. B Med J 287:251–254

197. Wickramasuriya GAW (1935) Some observations on malaria occurring in association with pregnancy. J Obstet Gynaecol Br Empire 42:816–834

198. Winter G, Chen Q, Flick K, Kremsner P, Fernandez V, Wahlgren M (2003) The 3D7var5.2 (var COMMON) type var gene family is commonly expressed in non-placental *Plasmodium falciparum* malaria. Mol Biochem Parasitol 127:179–91

199. World Health Organisation (1997) World malaria situation. Weekly Epidemiol Rec 36:269–74

200. Yamada M, Steketee R, Abramowsky C, Kida M, Wirima J, Heymann D, Rabbege J, Breman J, Aikawa M (1989) *Plasmodium falciparum* associated placental pathology: a light and electron microscopic and immunohistologic study. Am J Trop Med Hyg 41:161–168

Subject Index

Current Topics in Microbiology and Immunology

Volumes published since 1989 (and still available)

Vol. 252: **Potter, Michael; Melchers, Fritz (Eds.):** B1 Lymphocytes in B Cell Neoplasia. 2000. XIII, 326 pp. ISBN 3-540-67567-1

Vol. 253: **Gosztonyi, Georg (Ed.):** The Mechanisms of Neuronal Damage in Virus Infections of the Nervous System. 2001. approx. XVI, 270 pp. ISBN 3-540-67617-1

Vol. 254: **Privalsky, Martin L. (Ed.):** Transcriptional Corepressors. 2001. 25 figs. XIV, 190 pp. ISBN 3-540-67569-8

Vol. 255: **Hirai, Kanji (Ed.):** Marek's Disease. 2001. 22 figs. XII, 294 pp. ISBN 3-540-67798-4

Vol. 256: **Schmaljohn, Connie S.; Nichol, Stuart T. (Eds.):** Hantaviruses. 2001. 24 figs. XI, 196 pp. ISBN 3-540-41045-7

Vol. 257: **van der Goot, Gisou (Ed.):** PoreForming Toxins, 2001. 19 figs. IX, 166 pp. ISBN 3-540-41386-3

Vol. 258: **Takada, Kenzo (Ed.):** Epstein-Barr Virus and Human Cancer. 2001. 38 figs. IX, 233 pp. ISBN 3-540-41506-8

Vol. 259: **Hauber, Joachim, Vogt, Peter K. (Eds.):** Nuclear Export of Viral RNAs. 2001. 19 figs. IX, 131 pp. ISBN 3-540-41278-6

Vol. 260: **Burton, Didier R. (Ed.):** Antibodies in Viral Infection. 2001. 51 figs. IX, 309 pp. ISBN 3-540-41611-0

Vol. 261: **Trono, Didier (Ed.):** Lentiviral Vectors. 2002. 32 figs. X, 258 pp. ISBN 3-540-42190-4

Vol. 262: **Oldstone, Michael B.A. (Ed.):** Arenaviruses I. 2002. 30 figs. XVIII, 197 pp. ISBN 3-540-42244-7

Vol. 263: **Oldstone, Michael B. A. (Ed.):** Arenaviruses II. 2002. 49 figs. XVIII, 268 pp. ISBN 3-540-42705-8

Vol. 264/I: **Hacker, Jörg; Kaper, James B. (Eds.):** Pathogenicity Islands and the Evolution of Microbes. 2002. 34 figs. XVIII, 232 pp. ISBN 3-540-42681-7

Vol. 264/II: **Hacker, Jörg; Kaper, James B. (Eds.):** Pathogenicity Islands and the Evolution of Microbes. 2002. 24 figs. XVIII, 228 pp. ISBN 3-540-42682-5

Vol. 265: **Dietzschold, Bernhard; Richt, Jürgen A. (Eds.):** Protective and Pathological Immune Responses in the CNS. 2002. 21 figs. X, 278 pp. ISBN 3-540-42668X

Vol. 266: **Cooper, Koproski (Eds.):** The Interface Between Innate and Acquired Immunity, 2002. 15 figs. XIV, 116 pp. ISBN 3-540-42894-X

Vol. 267: **Mackenzie, John S.; Barrett, Alan D. T.; Deubel, Vincent (Eds.):** Japanese Encephalitis and West Nile Viruses. 2002. 66 figs. X, 418 pp. ISBN 3-540-42783X

Vol. 268: **Zwickl, Peter; Baumeister, Wolfgang (Eds.):** The Proteasome-Ubiquitin Protein Degradation Pathway. 2002. 17 figs. X, 213 pp. ISBN 3-540-43096-2

Vol. 269: **Koszinowski, Ulrich H.; Hengel, Hartmut (Eds.):** Viral Proteins Counteracting Host Defenses. 2002. 47 figs. XII, 325 pp. ISBN 3-540-43261-2

Vol. 270: **Beutler, Bruce; Wagner, Hermann (Eds.):** Toll-Like Receptor Family Members and Their Ligands. 2002. 31 figs. X, 192 pp. ISBN 3-540-43560-3

Vol. 271: **Koehler, Theresa M. (Ed.):** Anthrax. 2002. 14 figs. X, 169 pp. ISBN 3-540-43497-6

Vol. 272: **Doerfler, Walter; Böhm, Petra (Eds.):** Adenoviruses: Model and Vectors in Virus-Host Interactions. Virion and Structure, Viral Replication, Host Cell Interactions. 2003. 63 figs., approx. 280 pp. ISBN 3-540-00154-9

..: **Doerfler, Walter; Böhm, ..a (Eds.):** Adenoviruses: Model and Vectors in VirusHost Interactions. Immune System, Oncogenesis, Gene Therapy. 2004. 35 figs., approx. 280 pp. ISBN 3-540-06851-1

Vol. 274: **Workman, Jerry L. (Ed.):** Protein Complexes that Modify Chromatin. 2003. 38 figs., XII, 296 pp. ISBN 3-540-44208-1

Vol. 275: **Fan, Hung (Ed.):** Jaagsiekte Sheep Retrovirus and Lung Cancer. 2003. 63 figs., XII, 252 pp. ISBN 3-540-44096-3

Vol. 276: **Steinkasserer, Alexander (Ed.):** Dendritic Cells and Virus Infection. 2003. 24 figs., X, 296 pp. ISBN 3-540-44290-1

Vol. 277: **Rethwilm, Axel (Ed.):** Foamy Viruses. 2003. 40 figs., X, 214 pp. ISBN 3-540-44388-6

Vol. 278: **Salomon, Daniel R.; Wilson, Carolyn (Eds.):** Xenotransplantation. 2003. 22 figs., IX, 254 pp. ISBN 3-540-00210-3

Vol. 279: **Thomas, George; Sabatini, David; Hall, Michael N. (Eds.):** TOR. 2004. 49 figs., X, 364 pp. ISBN 3-540-00534X

Vol. 280: **Heber-Katz, Ellen (Ed.):** Regeneration: Stem Cells and Beyond. 2004. 42 figs., XII, 194 pp. ISBN 3-540-02238-4

Vol. 281: **Young, John A. T. (Ed.):** Cellular Factors Involved in Early Steps of Retroviral Replication. 2003. 21 figs., IX, 240 pp. ISBN 3-540-00844-6

Vol. 282: **Stenmark, Harald (Ed.):** Phosphoinositides in Subcellular Targeting and Enzyme Activation. 2003. 20 figs., X, 210 pp. ISBN 3-540-00950-7

Vol. 283: **Kawaoka, Yoshihiro (Ed.):** Biology of Negative Strand RNA Viruses: The Power of Reverse Genetics. 2004. 24 figs., IX, 350 pp. ISBN 3-540-40661-1

Vol. 284: **Harris, David (Ed.):** Mad Cow Disease and Related Spongiform Encephalopathies. 2004. 34 figs., IX, 219 pp. ISBN 3-540-20107-6

Vol. 285: **Marsh, Mark (Ed.):** Membrane Trafficking in Viral Replication. 2004. 19 figs., IX, 259 pp. ISBN 3-540-21430-5

Vol. 286: **Madshus, Inger H. (Ed.):** Signalling from Internalized Growth Factor Receptors. 2004. 19 figs., IX, 187 pp. ISBN 3-540-21038-5

Vol. 287: **Enjuanes, Luis (Ed.):** Coronavirus Replication and Reverse Genetics. 2005. 49 figs., XI, 257 pp. ISBN 3-540-21494-1

Vol. 288: **Mahy, Brain W. J. (Ed.):** Foot-and-Mouth-Disease Virus. 2005. 16 figs., IX, 178 pp. ISBN 3-540-22419X

Vol. 289: **Griffin, Diane E. (Ed.):** Role of Apoptosis in Infection. 2005. 40 figs., IX, 294 pp. ISBN 3-540-23006-8

Vol. 290: **Singh, Harinder; Grosschedl, Rudolf (Eds.):** Molecular Analysis of B Lymphocyte Development and Activation. 2005. 28 figs., XI, 255 pp. ISBN 3-540-23090-4

Vol. 291: **Boquet, Patrice; Lemichez Emmanuel (Eds.)** Bacterial Virulence Factors and Rho GTPases. 2005. 28 figs., IX, 196 pp. ISBN 3-540-23865-4

Vol. 292: **Fu, Zhen F (Ed.):** The World of Rhabdoviruses. 2005. 27 figs., X, 210 pp. ISBN 3-540-24011-X

Vol. 293: **Kyewski, Bruno; Suri-Payer, Elisabeth (Eds.):** CD4+CD25+ Regulatory T Cells: Origin, Function and Therapeutic Potential. 2005. 22 figs., XII, 332 pp. ISBN 3-540-24444-1

Vol. 294: **Caligaris-Cappio, Federico, Dalla Favera, Ricardo (Eds.):** Chronic Lymphocytic Leukemia. 2005. 25 figs., VIII, 187 pp. ISBN 3-540-25279-7

Vol. 295: **Sullivan, David J.; Krishna Sanjeew (Eds.):** Malaria: Drugs, Disease and Post-genomic Biology. 2005. 40 figs., XI, 446 pp. ISBN 3-540-25363-7

Vol. 296: **Oldstone, Michael B. A. (Ed.):** Molecular Mimicry: Infection Induced Autoimmune Disease. 2005. 28 figs., VIII, 167 pp. ISBN 3-540-25597-4

Printing: Krips bv, Meppel
Binding: Stürtz, Würzburg